Surgery

PreTest™ Self-Assessment and Review

Notice

Medicine is an ever-changing science. As new research and clinical experience broaden our knowledge, changes in treatment and drug therapy are required. The authors and the publisher of this work have checked with sources believed to be reliable in their efforts to provide information that is complete and generally in accord with the standards accepted at the time of publication. However, in view of the possibility of human error or changes in medical sciences, neither the authors nor the publisher nor any other party who has been involved in the preparation or publication of this work warrants that the information contained herein is in every respect accurate or complete, and they disclaim all responsibility for any errors or omissions or for the results obtained from use of the information contained in this work. Readers are encouraged to confirm the information contained herein with other sources. For example and in particular, readers are advised to check the product information sheet included in the package of each drug they plan to administer to be certain that the information contained in this work is accurate and that changes have not been made in the recommended dose or in the contraindications for administration. This recommendation is of particular importance in connection with new or infrequently used drugs.

Surgery
PreTest™ Self-Assessment and Review
13th Edition

Lillian S. Kao, MD, MS
Associate Professor
Department of Surgery
University of Texas Health Science Center at Houston
Houston, Texas

Tammy Lee, MD
Active Staff Surgeon
Private Practice
Houston, Texas

 Medical

New York   Chicago   San Francisco   Lisbon   London   Madrid   Mexico City
Milan   New Delhi   San Juan   Seoul   Singapore   Sydney   Toronto

Surgery: PreTest™ Self-Assessment and Review, 13th Edition

Copyright © 2012, 2009, 2006, 2003, 2001, 1998, 1995, 1992, 1989, 1987, 1985, 1982, 1978 by The McGraw-Hill Companies, Inc. All rights reserved. Printed in the United States of America. Except as permitted under the United States Copyright Act of 1976, no part of this publication may be reproduced or distributed in any form or by any means, or stored in a data base or retrieval system, without the prior written permission of the publisher.

PreTest™ is a trademark of The McGraw-Hill Companies, Inc.

1 2 3 4 5 6 7 8 9 0   DOC/DOC   17 16 15 14 13 12

ISBN 978-0-07-176121-5
MHID 0-07-176121-7

The book was set in Berkeley by Cenveo Publisher Services.
The editors were Kirsten Funk and Cindy Yoo.
The production supervisor was Sherri Souffrance.
Project management was provided by Ridhi Mathur, Cenveo Publisher Services.
The cover designer was Margaret Webster-Shapiro.
RR Donnelley was printer and binder.

This book is printed on acid-free paper.

Cataloging-in-Publication Data for this book is on file at the Library of Congress.

McGraw-Hill books are available at special quantity discounts to use as premiums and sales promotions, or for use in corporate training programs. To contact a representative please e-mail us at bulksales@mcgraw-hill.com

Student Reviewers

Jeffrey T. Bruckel
Fourth Year Medical Student
SUNY Downstate Medical Center
Class of 2010

Sabrina Islam, MD
Fourth Year Medical Student
SUNY Downstate Medical Center
Class of 2010

Jonathan P. Meizoso
Fourth Year Medical Student
University of Miami Miller School of Medicine
Class of 2012

Godwin Ofikwu, MD
PGY2 Surgical Resident
Columbia University

Elizabeth C. Pearce, MD
PGY2 Surgical Resident
Vanderbilt University Medical Center

Rory Snepar, MD
PGY1 Resident
UMDNJ
Class of 2011

Contents

Introduction

Surgery: PreTest Self-Assessment and Review, 13th Edition, is intended to provide medical students, as well as house officers and physicians, with a convenient tool for assessing and improving their knowledge of medicine. The 500+ questions in this book are similar in format and complexity to those included in Step 2 of the United States Medical Licensing Examination (USMLE). They may also be a useful study tool for Step 3.

For multiple-choice questions, the **one best** response to each question should be selected. For matching sets, a group of questions will be preceded by a list of lettered options. For each question in the matching set, select **one** lettered option that is **most** closely associated with the question. Each question in this book has a corresponding answer, a reference to a text that provides background to the answer, and a short discussion of various issues raised by the question and its answer. A listing of references for the entire book follows the last chapter.

To simulate the time constraints imposed by the qualifying examinations for which this book is intended as a practice guide, the student or physician should allot about 1 minute for each question. After answering all questions in a chapter, as much time as necessary should be spent in reviewing the explanations for each question at the end of the chapter. Attention should be given to all explanations, even if the examinee answered the question correctly. Those seeking more information on a subject should refer to the reference materials listed or to other standard texts in medicine.

Pre- and Postoperative Care

Questions

1. A 48-year-old woman develops constipation postoperatively and self-medicates with milk of magnesia. She presents to clinic, at which time her serum electrolytes are checked, and she is noted to have an elevated serum magnesium level. Which of the following represents the earliest clinical indication of hypermagnesemia?

a. Loss of deep tendon reflexes
b. Flaccid paralysis
c. Respiratory arrest
d. Hypotension
e. Stupor

2. Five days after an uneventful cholecystectomy, an asymptomatic middle-aged woman is found to have a serum sodium level of 125 mEq/L. Which of the following is the most appropriate management strategy for this patient?

a. Administration of hypertonic saline solution
b. Restriction of free water
c. Plasma ultrafiltration
d. Hemodialysis
e. Aggressive diuresis with furosemide

3. A 50-year-old patient presents with symptomatic nephrolithiasis. He reports that he underwent a jejunoileal bypass for morbid obesity when he was 39. Which of the following is a complication of jejunoileal bypass?

a. Pseudohyperparathyroidism
b. Hyperuric aciduria
c. Hungry bone syndrome
d. Hyperoxaluria
e. Sporadic unicameral bone cysts

4. Following surgery a patient develops oliguria. You believe the oliguria is due to hypovolemia, but you seek corroborative data before increasing intravenous fluids. Which of the following values supports the diagnosis of hypovolemia?

a. Urine sodium of 28 mEq/L
b. Urine chloride of 15 mEq/L
c. Fractional excretion of sodium less than 1
d. Urine/serum creatinine ratio of 20
e. Urine osmolality of 350 mOsm/kg

5. A 45-year-old woman with Crohn disease and a small intestinal fistula develops tetany during the second week of parenteral nutrition. The laboratory findings include

Na: 135 mEq/L
K: 3.2 mEq/L
Cl: 103 mEq/L
HCO_3: 25 mEq/L
Ca: 8.2 mEq/L
Mg: 1.2 mEq/L
PO_4: 2.4 mEq/L
Albumin: 2.4

An arterial blood gas sample reveals a pH of 7.42, PCO_2 of 38 mm Hg, and PO_2 of 84 mm Hg. Which of the following is the most likely cause of the patient's tetany?

a. Hyperventilation
b. Hypocalcemia
c. Hypomagnesemia
d. Essential fatty acid deficiency
e. Focal seizure

6. A patient with a nonobstructing carcinoma of the sigmoid colon is being prepared for elective resection. Which of the following reduces the risk of postoperative infectious complications?

a. A single preoperative parenteral dose of antibiotic effective against aerobes and anaerobes
b. Avoidance of oral antibiotics to prevent emergence of *Clostridium difficile*
c. Postoperative administration for 48 hours of parenteral antibiotics effective against aerobes and anaerobes
d. Postoperative administration of parenteral antibiotics effective against aerobes and anaerobes until the patient's intravenous lines and all other drains are removed
e. Redosing of antibiotics in the operating room if the case lasts for more than 2 hours

7. A 75-year-old man with a history of myocardial infarction 2 years ago, peripheral vascular disease with symptoms of claudication after walking half a block, hypertension, and diabetes presents with a large ventral hernia. He wishes to have the hernia repaired. Which of the following is the most appropriate next step in his preoperative workup?

a. He should undergo an electrocardiogram (ECG).
b. He should undergo an exercise stress test.
c. He should undergo coronary artery bypass prior to operative repair of his ventral hernia.
d. He should undergo a persantine thallium stress test and echocardiography.
e. His history of a myocardial infarction within 3 years is prohibitive for elective surgery. No further testing is necessary.

8. A previously healthy 55-year-old man undergoes elective right hemicolectomy for a stage I (T2N0M0) cancer of the cecum. His postoperative ileus is somewhat prolonged, and on the fifth postoperative day his nasogastric tube is still in place. Physical examination reveals diminished skin turgor, dry mucous membranes, and orthostatic hypotension. Pertinent laboratory values are as follows:

Arterial blood gases: pH 7.56, P_{CO_2} 50 mm Hg, P_{O_2} 85 mm Hg.
Serum electrolytes (mEq/L): Na^+ 132, K^+ 3.1, Cl^- 80; HCO_3^- 42.
Urine electrolytes (mEq/L): Na^+ 2, K^+ 5, Cl^- 6.

What is the patient's acid–base abnormality?

a. Uncompensated metabolic alkalosis
b. Respiratory acidosis with metabolic compensation
c. Combined metabolic and respiratory alkalosis
d. Metabolic alkalosis with respiratory compensation
e. Mixed respiratory acidosis and respiratory alkalosis

9. A 52-year-old man with gastric outlet obstruction secondary to a duodenal ulcer presents with hypochloremic, hypokalemic metabolic alkalosis. Which of the following is the most appropriate therapy for this patient?

a. Infusion of 0.9% NaCl with supplemental KCl until clinical signs of volume depletion are eliminated
b. Infusion of isotonic (0.15 N) HCl via a central venous catheter
c. Clamping the nasogastric tube to prevent further acid losses
d. Administration of acetazolamide to promote renal excretion of bicarbonate
e. Intubation and controlled hypoventilation on a volume-cycled ventilator to further increase P_{CO_2}

10. A 23-year-old woman is brought to the emergency room from a halfway house, where she apparently swallowed a handful of pills. The patient complains of shortness of breath and tinnitus, but refuses to identify the pills she ingested. Pertinent laboratory values are as follows:

Arterial blood gases: pH 7.45, P_{CO_2} 12 mm Hg, P_{O_2} 126 mm Hg.
Serum electrolytes (mEq/L): Na^+ 138, K^+ 4.8, Cl^- 102, HCO_3^- 8.

An overdose of which of the following drugs would be most likely to cause the acid–base disturbance in this patient?

a. Phenformin
b. Aspirin
c. Barbiturates
d. Methanol
e. Diazepam (Valium)

11. An 18-year-old previously healthy man is placed on intravenous heparin after having a pulmonary embolism (PE) after exploratory laparotomy for a small-bowel injury following a motor vehicle collision. Five days later, his platelet count is 90,000/μL and continues to fall over the next several days. The patient's serum is positive for antibodies to the heparin-platelet factor complexes. Which of the following is the most appropriate next management step?

a. Cessation of all anticoagulation therapy
b. Cessation of heparin and immediate institution of high-dose warfarin therapy
c. Cessation of heparin and institution of low-molecular-weight heparin
d. Cessation of heparin and institution of lepirudin
e. Cessation of heparin and transfusion with platelets

12. A 65-year-old man undergoes a technically difficult abdominal–perineal resection for a rectal cancer during which he receives 3 units of packed red blood cells. Four hours later, in the intensive care unit (ICU), he is bleeding heavily from his perineal wound. Emergency coagulation studies reveal normal prothrombin, partial thromboplastin, and bleeding times. The fibrin degradation products are not elevated, but the serum fibrinogen content is depressed and the platelet count is 70,000/μL. Which of the following is the most likely cause of his bleeding?

a. Delayed blood transfusion reaction
b. Autoimmune fibrinolysis
c. A bleeding blood vessel in the surgical field
d. Factor VIII deficiency
e. Hypothermic coagulopathy

13. A 78-year-old man with a history of coronary artery disease and an asymptomatic reducible inguinal hernia requests an elective hernia repair. Which of the following would be a valid reason for delaying the proposed surgery?

a. Coronary artery bypass surgery 3 months earlier
b. A history of cigarette smoking
c. Jugular venous distension
d. Hypertension
e. Hyperlipidemia

14. A 68-year-old man is admitted to the coronary care unit with an acute myocardial infarction. His postinfarction course is marked by congestive heart failure and intermittent hypotension. On the fourth day in hospital, he develops severe midabdominal pain. On physical examination, blood pressure is 90/60 mm Hg and pulse is 110 beats per minute and regular; the abdomen is soft with mild generalized tenderness and distention. Bowel sounds are hypoactive; stool Hematest is positive. Which of the following is the most appropriate next step in this patient's management?

a. Barium enema
b. Upper gastrointestinal series
c. Angiography
d. Ultrasonography
e. Celiotomy

15. A 30-year-old woman in her last trimester of pregnancy suddenly develops massive swelling of the left lower extremity. Which of the following would be the most appropriate workup and treatment at this time?

a. Venography and heparin
b. Duplex ultrasonography and heparin
c. Duplex ultrasonography, heparin, and vena caval filter
d. Duplex ultrasonography, heparin, warfarin (Coumadin)
e. Impedance plethysmography, warfarin

16. A 20-year-old woman with a family history of von Willebrand disease is found to have an activated partial thromboplastin time (aPTT) of 78 (normal = 32) on routine testing prior to cholecystectomy. Further investigation reveals a prothrombin time (PT) of 13 (normal = 12), a platelet count of 350,000/mm^3, and an abnormal bleeding time. Which of the following should be administered in the perioperative period?

a. Factor VIII
b. Platelets
c. Vitamin K
d. Aminocaproic acid
e. Desmopressin (DDAVP)

17. A 65-year-old man undergoes a low anterior resection for rectal cancer. On the fifth day in hospital, his physical examination shows a temperature of 39°C (102°F), blood pressure of 150/90 mm Hg, pulse of 110 beats per minute and regular, and respiratory rate of 28 breaths per minute. A computed tomography (CT) scan of the abdomen reveals an abscess in the pelvis. Which of the following most accurately describes his present condition?

a. Systemic inflammatory response syndrome (SIRS)
b. Sepsis
c. Severe sepsis
d. Septic shock
e. Severe septic shock

18. A victim of blunt abdominal trauma has splenic and liver lacerations as well as an unstable pelvic fracture. He is hypotensive and tachycardic with a heart rate of 150 despite receiving 2 L of crystalloid en route to the hospital. He was intubated prior to arrival due to declining mental status. He is taken emergently to the operating room for exploratory laparotomy and external fixation of his pelvic fracture. Which of the following is the best resuscitative strategy?

a. Infusion of another liter of crystalloid
b. Infusion of 500 mL of 5% albumin
c. Infusion of packed red blood cells followed by fresh-frozen plasma and platelets as indicated by the PT and platelet counts on laboratory values
d. Infusion of packed red blood cells and early administration of fresh-frozen plasma and platelets prior to return of laboratory values
e. Infusion of packed red blood cells and vitamin K

19. A 62-year-old woman undergoes a pancreaticoduodenectomy for a pancreatic head cancer. A jejunostomy is placed to facilitate nutritional repletion as she is expected to have a prolonged recovery. What is the best method for delivering postoperative nutrition?

a. Institution of enteral feeding via the jejunostomy tube after return of bowel function as evidenced by passage of flatus or a bowel movement
b. Institution of enteral feeding via the jejunostomy tube within 24 hours postoperatively
c. Institution of supplemental enteral feeding via the jejunostomy tube only if oral intake is inadequate after return of bowel function
d. Institution of a combination of immediate trophic (15 mL/h) enteral feeds via the jejunostomy tube and parenteral nutrition to provide total nutritional support
e. Complete nutritional support with total parenteral nutrition

20. A 65-year-old woman has a life-threatening pulmonary embolus 5 days following removal of a uterine malignancy. She is immediately heparinized and maintained in good therapeutic range for the next 3 days, then passes gross blood from her vagina and develops tachycardia, hypotension, and oliguria. Following resuscitation, an abdominal CT scan reveals a major retroperitoneal hematoma. Which of the following is the best next step in management?

a. Immediately reverse heparin by a calculated dose of protamine and place a vena caval filter (eg, a Greenfield filter).
b. Reverse heparin with protamine, explore and evacuate the hematoma, and ligate the vena cava below the renal veins.
c. Switch to low-dose heparin.
d. Stop heparin and observe closely.
e. Stop heparin, give fresh-frozen plasma (FFP), and begin warfarin therapy.

21. A 71-year-old man develops dysphagia for both solids and liquids and weight loss of 60 lb over the past 6 months. He undergoes endoscopy, demonstrating a distal esophageal lesion, and biopsies are consistent with squamous cell carcinoma. He is scheduled for neoadjuvant chemoradiation followed by an esophagectomy. Preoperatively he is started on total parenteral nutrition, given his severe malnutrition reflected by an albumin of less than 1. Which of the following is most likely to be a concern initially in starting total parenteral nutrition in this patient?

a. Hyperkalemia
b. Hypermagnesemia
c. Hypoglycemia
d. Hypophosphatemia
e. Hypochloremia

22. An elderly diabetic woman with chronic steroid-dependent bronchospasm has an ileocolectomy for a perforated cecum. She is taken to the ICU intubated and is maintained on broad-spectrum antibiotics, renal dose dopamine, and a rapid steroid taper. On postoperative day 2, she develops a fever of 39.2°C (102.5°F), hypotension, lethargy, and laboratory values remarkable for hypoglycemia and hyperkalemia. Which of the following is the most likely explanation for her deterioration?

a. Sepsis
b. Hypovolemia
c. Adrenal insufficiency
d. Acute tubular necrosis
e. Diabetic ketoacidosis

23. A cirrhotic patient with abnormal coagulation studies due to hepatic synthetic dysfunction requires an urgent cholecystectomy. A transfusion of FFP is planned to minimize the risk of bleeding due to surgery. What is the optimal timing of this transfusion?

a. The day before surgery
b. The night before surgery
c. On call to surgery
d. Intraoperatively
e. In the recovery room

24. On postoperative day 5, an otherwise healthy 55-year-old man recovering from a partial hepatectomy is noted to have a fever of 38.6°C (101.5°F). Which of the following is the most common nosocomial infection postoperatively?

a. Wound infection
b. Pneumonia
c. Urinary tract infection
d. Intra-abdominal abscess
e. Intravenous catheter-related infection

25. Ten days after an exploratory laparotomy and lysis of adhesions, a patient, who previously underwent a low anterior resection for rectal cancer followed by postoperative chemoradiation, is noted to have succus draining from the wound. She appears to have adequate source control—she is afebrile with a normal white blood count. The output from the fistula is approximately 150 cc per day. Which of the following factors is most likely to prevent closure of the enterocutaneous fistula?

a. Previous radiation
b. Previous chemotherapy
c. Recent surgery
d. History of malignancy
e. More than 100-cc output per day

26. A 26-year-old man is resuscitated with packed red blood cells following a motor vehicle collision complicated by a fractured pelvis and resultant hemorrhage. A few hours later the patient becomes hypotensive with a normal central venous pressure (CVP), oliguric, and febrile. Upon examination, the patient is noted to have profuse oozing of blood from his intravenous (IV) sites. Which of the following is the most likely diagnosis?

a. Hypovolemic shock
b. Acute adrenal insufficiency
c. Gram-negative bacteremia
d. Transfusion reaction
e. Ureteral obstruction

27. A 16-year-old adolescent boy with a history of severe hemophilia A is undergoing an elective inguinal hernia repair. Which of the following is the best option for preventing or treating a bleeding complication in the setting of this disease?

a. Fresh-frozen plasma
b. Combination of desmopressin and fresh-frozen plasma
c. DDAVP
d. Combination of ε-aminocaproic acid and desmopressin
e. Factor IX concentrate

28. A 59-year-old man is planning to undergo a coronary artery bypass. He has osteoarthritis and consumes nonsteroidal anti-inflammatory drugs (NSAIDs) for the pain. Which of the following is the most appropriate treatment prior to surgery to minimize his risk of bleeding from his NSAID use?

a. Begin vitamin K 1 week prior to surgery.
b. Give FFP few hours before surgery.
c. Stop the NSAIDs 1 week prior to surgery.
d. Stop the NSAIDs 3 to 4 days prior to surgery.
e. Stop the NSAIDs the day before surgery.

29. A 63-year-old man undergoes a partial gastrectomy with Billroth II reconstruction for intractable peptic ulcer disease. He presents several months postoperatively with a megaloblastic anemia. Which of the following is the best treatment for this surgical complication?

a. Transfusion with 1 unit of packed red blood cells
b. Oral iron supplementation
c. Oral vitamin B_{12} supplementation
d. Intravenous vitamin B_{12} (cyanocobalamin) supplementation
e. Oral folate supplementation

30. A 52-year-old woman undergoes a sigmoid resection with primary anastomosis for recurrent diverticulitis. She returns to the emergency room 10 days later with left flank pain and decreased urine output; laboratory examination is significant for a white blood cell (WBC) count of 20,000/mm³. She undergoes a CT scan that demonstrates new left hydronephrosis, but no evidence of an intra-abdominal abscess. Which of the following is the most appropriate next step in management?

a. Intravenous pyelogram
b. Intravenous antibiotics and repeat CT in 1 week
c. Administration of intravenous methylene blue
d. No further management if urinalysis is negative for hematuria
e. Immediate reexploration

31. A 23-year-old woman undergoes total thyroidectomy for carcinoma of the thyroid gland. On the second postoperative day, she begins to complain of a tingling sensation in her hands. She appears quite anxious and later complains of muscle cramps. Which of the following is the most appropriate initial management strategy?

a. 10 mL of 10% magnesium sulfate intravenously
b. Oral vitamin D
c. 100 µg oral Synthroid
d. Continuous infusion of calcium gluconate
e. Oral calcium gluconate

32. A 65-year-old man has an enterocutaneous fistula originating in the jejunum secondary to inflammatory bowel disease. Which of the following would be the most appropriate fluid for replacement of his enteric losses?

a. D_5W
b. 3% normal saline
c. Ringer lactate solution
d. 0.9% sodium chloride
e. 6% sodium bicarbonate solution

33. A 62-year-old man is suffering from arrhythmias on the night of his triple coronary bypass. Potassium has been administered. His urine output is 20 to 30 mL/h. Serum potassium level is 6.2. Which of the following medications counteracts the effects of potassium without reducing the serum potassium level?

a. Sodium polystyrene sulfonate (Kayexalate)
b. Sodium bicarbonate
c. 50% dextrose
d. Calcium gluconate
e. Insulin

34. An in-hospital workup of a 78-year-old hypertensive, mildly asthmatic man who is receiving chemotherapy for colon cancer reveals symptomatic gallstones. Preoperative laboratory results are notable for a hematocrit of 24% and urinalysis with 18 to 25 WBCs and gram-negative bacteria. On call to the operating room, the patient receives intravenous penicillin. His abdomen is shaved in the operating room. An open cholecystectomy is performed and, despite a lack of indications, the common bile duct is explored. The wound is closed primarily with a Penrose drain exiting a separate stab wound. On postoperative day 3, the patient develops a wound infection. Which of the following changes in the care of this patient could have decreased the chance of a postoperative wound infection?

a. Increasing the length of the preoperative hospital stay to prophylactically treat the asthma with steroids
b. Treating the urinary infection prior to surgery
c. Shaving the abdomen the night prior to surgery
d. Continuing the prophylactic antibiotics for 3 postoperative days
e. Using a closed drainage system brought out through the operative incision

35. A 72-year-old man undergoes a subtotal colectomy for a cecal perfora-tion due to a sigmoid colon obstruction. He has had a prolonged recovery and has been on total parenteral nutrition (TPN) for 2 weeks postopera-tively. After regaining bowel function, he experienced significant diarrhea. Examination of his abdominal wound demonstrates minimal granulation tissue. He complains that he has lost his taste for food. He also has increased hair loss and a new perioral pustular rash. Which of the following deficien-cies does he most likely have?

a. Zinc
b. Selenium
c. Molybdenum
d. Chromium
e. Thiamine

36. A 12-year-old boy with a femur fracture after a motor vehicle collision undergoes operative repair. After induction of anesthesia, he develops a fever of 40°C (104°F), shaking rigors, and blood-tinged urine. Which of the following is the best treatment option?

a. Alkalinization of the urine, administration of mannitol, and continuation with the procedure
b. Administration of dantrolene sodium and continuation with the procedure
c. Administration of dantrolene sodium and termination of the procedure
d. Administration of intravenous steroids and an antihistamine agent with con-tinuation of the procedure
e. Administration of intravenous steroids and an antihistamine agent with termina-tion of the procedure

37. A 24-year-old Jehovah's Witness who was in a high-speed motorcycle collision undergoes emergent splenectomy. His estimated blood loss was 1500 mL. Which of the following strategy should be employed for his resuscitation?

a. Vasopressors should be primarily utilized for maintenance of his blood pressure.
b. Synthetic colloids should be administered as the primary resuscitation fluid in a 3:1 ratio to replace the volume of blood lost.
c. 0.9% normal saline should be administered in a 1:1 ratio to replace the volume of blood lost.
d. 0.45% normal saline should be administered in a 3:1 ratio to replace the volume of blood lost.
e. Lactated Ringer solution should be administered in a ratio of 3:1 to replace the blood lost.

38. A 60-kg, 53-year-old man with no significant medical problems undergoes lysis of adhesions for a small-bowel obstruction. Postoperatively, he has high nasogastric output and low urine output. What is the most appropriate management of his fluids?

a. Infusion of D5 0.45% normal saline at 100 mL/h
b. Infusion of D5 0.9% normal saline at 100 mL/h
c. Infusion of D5 lactated Ringer at 100 mL/h
d. Replacement of nasogastric tube losses with lactated Ringer in addition to maintenance fluids
e. Replacement of nasogastric tube losses with 0.45% normal saline with 20 mEq/L of potassium chloride in addition to maintenance fluids

39. Four days after surgical evacuation of an acute subdural hematoma, a 44-year-old man becomes mildly lethargic and develops asterixis. He has received 2400 mL of 5% dextrose in water intravenously each day since surgery, and he appears well hydrated. Pertinent laboratory values are as follows:

Serum electrolytes (mEq/L): Na$^+$ 118, K$^+$ 3.4, Cl$^-$ 82, HCO$_3^-$ 24
Serum osmolality: 242 mOsm/L
Urine sodium: 47 mEq/L
Urine osmolality: 486 mOsm/L

Which of the following is the best treatment of his hyponatremia?

a. Insulin infusion to keep his glucose level less than 110 mg/dL
b. Slow infusion of 3% normal saline until neurologic symptoms are improved
c. Rapid infusion of 3% normal saline to correct the sodium to normal
d. Desmopressin (DDAVP) administration
e. Administration of a loop diuretic

40. A 43-year-old woman develops acute renal failure following an emergency resection of a leaking abdominal aortic aneurysm. One week after surgery, the following laboratory values are obtained:

Serum electrolytes (mEq/L): Na^+ 127, K^+ 5.9, Cl^- 92, HCO_3^- 15
Blood urea nitrogen: 82 mg/dL
Serum creatinine: 6.7 mg/dL

The patient has gained 4 kg since surgery and is mildly dyspneic at rest. Eight hours after these values are reported, the following electrocardiogram is obtained. Which of the following is the most appropriate initial treatment in the management of this patient?

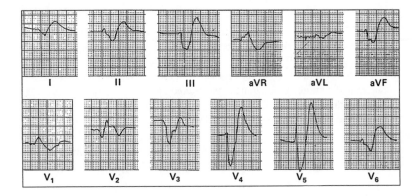

a. 10 mL of 10% calcium gluconate
b. 0.25 mg digoxin every 3 hours for 3 doses
c. Oral Kayexalate
d. 100 mg lidocaine
e. Emergent hemodialysis

41. A 63-year-old man with a 40-pack per year smoking history undergoes a low anterior resection for rectal cancer and on postoperative day 5 develops a fever, new infiltrate on chest x-ray, and leukocytosis. He is transferred to the ICU for treatment of his pneumonia because of clinical deterioration. Which of the following is a sign of early sepsis?

a. Respiratory acidosis
b. Decreased cardiac output
c. Hypoglycemia
d. Increased arteriovenous oxygen difference
e. Peripheral vasodilation

42. A 60-year-old woman with no previous medical problems undergoes a total colectomy with diverting ileostomy for a cecal perforation secondary to a sigmoid stricture. Postoperatively, she has 2 L of ileostomy output per day. Her heart rate is 110 beats per minute, her respiratory rate is 24 breaths per minute, and her oxygen saturation is 98% on 2-L nasal cannula (NC). Her hemoglobin levels have been stable postoperatively at 9.0 mg/dL. Her other laboratory values on postoperative day 6 are as follows:

Na$^+$: 128
K$^+$: 3.0
Cl$^-$: 102
HCO$_3^-$: 20

Which of the following statements is the best strategy for correcting her acid–base disorder?

a. Her maintenance fluids should be changed to 0.9% normal saline with 20 mEq/L of potassium chloride.
b. She should be intubated to correct her tachypnea and prevent respiratory alkalosis.
c. She should be transfused 2 units of packed red blood cells.
d. She should be treated with fluid replacement and stool-bulking agents.
e. She should undergo immediate dialysis.

43. A 39-year-old man is undergoing resuscitation with blood products for an upper GI bleed. He is suspected of having a hemolytic transfusion reaction. Which of the following is appropriate in the management of this patient?

a. Removal of nonessential foreign body irritants, for example, Foley catheter
b. Fluid restriction
c. 0.1 M HCl infusion
d. Steroids
e. Fluids and mannitol

44. A 45-year-old woman undergoes an uneventful laparoscopic cholecystectomy for which she receives 1 dose of cephalosporin. One week later, she returns to the emergency room with fever, nausea, and copious diarrhea and is suspected of having pseudomembranous colitis. She is afebrile and has no peritoneal signs on abdominal examination. She has a mild leukocytosis with a left shift. Which of the following is the appropriate initial management strategy?

a. Administration of an antidiarrheal agent
b. Exploratory laparotomy with left hemi-colectomy and colostomy
c. Exploratory laparotomy with subtotal abdominal colectomy and ileostomy
d. Administration of intravenous vancomycin
e. Administration of oral metronidazole

45. A 42-year-old man sustains a gunshot wound to the abdomen and is in shock. Multiple units of packed red blood cells are transfused in an effort to resuscitate him. He complains of numbness around his mouth and displays carpopedal spasm. An electrocardiogram demonstrates a prolonged QT interval. Which of the following is the most appropriate treatment?

a. Intravenous bicarbonate
b. Intravenous potassium
c. Intravenous calcium
d. Intravenous digoxin
e. Intravenous parathyroid hormone

Questions 46 to 49

A patient has a calculated basal energy expenditure of 2000 kcal/day. Match the following clinical situations with the appropriate daily energy requirement. Each lettered option may be used once, more than once, or not at all.

a. 1800 kcal/day
b. 2000 kcal/day
c. 2200 kcal/day
d. 3000 kcal/day
e. 4000 kcal/day

46. Starvation

47. Multiple organ failure

48. Third-degree burns involving 60% of body surface area

49. After surgery

Pre- and Postoperative Care

Answers

1. The answer is a. *(Brunicardi, p 63.)* The earliest clinical indication of hypermagnesemia is loss of deep tendon reflexes. States of magnesium excess are characterized by generalized neuromuscular depression. Clinically, severe hypermagnesemia is rarely seen except in those patients with advanced renal failure treated with magnesium-containing antacids. However, hypermagnesemia is produced intentionally by obstetricians who use parenteral magnesium sulfate ($MgSO_4$) to treat preeclampsia. $MgSO_4$ is administered until depression of the deep tendon reflexes is observed, a deficit that occurs with modest hypermagnesemia (over 4 mEq/L). Greater elevations of magnesium produce progressive weakness, which culminates in flaccid quadriplegia and in some cases respiratory arrest due to paralysis of the chest bellows mechanism. Hypotension may occur because of the direct arteriolar relaxing effect of magnesium. Changes in mental status occur in the late stages of the syndrome and are characterized by somnolence that progresses to coma.

2. The answer is b. *(Brunicardi, pp 61-62.)* The initial, and often definitive, management of hyponatremia is free-water restriction. Symptomatic hyponatremia, which occurs at serum sodium levels less than or equal to 120 mEq/L, can result in headache, seizures, coma, and signs of increased intracranial pressure and may require infusion of hypertonic saline. Rapid correction should be avoided so as not to cause central pontine myelinolysis, manifested by neurologic symptoms ranging from seizures to brain damage and death. Additionally, a search for the underlying etiology of the hyponatremia should be undertaken. Acute severe hyponatremia sometimes occurs following elective surgical procedures due to a combination of appropriate stimulation of antidiuretic hormone and injudicious administration of excess free water in the first few postoperative days. Other potential etiologies include hyperosmolarity with free-water shifts from the intra- to the extracellular compartment (eg, hyperglycemia), sodium depletion (eg, gastrointestinal or renal losses, insufficient intake), dilution (eg, drug-induced), and the syndrome of inappropriate secretion of antidiuretic hormone (SIADH).

3. The answer is d. (*Mulholland, pp 716-717.*) Any patient who has lost much of the ileum (whether from injury, disease, or elective surgery) is at high risk of developing enteric hyperoxaluria if the colon remains intact. Calcium oxalate stones can subsequently develop due to excessive absorption of oxalate from the colon. Normally, fatty acids are absorbed by the terminal ileum, and calcium and oxalate combine to form an insoluble compound that is not absorbed. In the absence of the terminal ileum, unabsorbed fatty acids reach the colon, where they combine with calcium, leaving free oxalate to be absorbed. Unabsorbed fatty acids and bile acids in the colon also promote oxalate uptake by the colon. Subsequently, the excess oxalate is excreted by the kidneys, promoting calcium oxalate stone formation.

Hungry bone syndrome refers to rapid remineralization of bones leading to hypocalcemia and can be seen postoperatively in patients with secondary or tertiary hyperparathyroidism. Pseudohyperparathyroidism refers to hypercalcemia associated with the production of parathyroid-related peptide. A unicameral bone cyst is a benign lesion found in children.

4. The answer is c. (*Townsend, pp 621-622.*) A fractional excretion of sodium (FENa) is calculated as (urine sodium × serum creatinine) ÷ (serum sodium × urinary creatinine) × 100. A FENa less than 1% supports a prerenal etiology for the patient's oliguria. When oliguria occurs postoperatively, it is important to differentiate between low output caused by the physiologic response to intravascular hypovolemia and that caused by acute tubular necrosis. A FENa of less than 1% in an oliguric setting indicates aggressive sodium reclamation in the tubules. Values above this suggest a tubular injury such that Na cannot be appropriately reclaimed. In the setting of postoperative hypovolemia, all findings would reflect the kidney's efforts to retain volume: the urine sodium would be below 20 mEq/L, the urine chloride would not be helpful except in the metabolically alkalotic patient, the urine osmolality would be over 500 mOsm/kg, the urine/serum creatinine ratio would be above 20, and the blood urea nitrogen (BUN)/creatinine ratio would be above 20.

5. The answer is c. *(Brunicardi, p 63.)* Magnesium deficiency is common in malnourished patients and patients with large gastrointestinal fluid losses. The neuromuscular effects resemble those of calcium deficiency—namely, paresthesia, hyperreflexia, muscle spasm, and, ultimately, tetany. The cardiac effects are more like those of hypercalcemia. An electrocardiogram therefore provides a rapid means of differentiating between hypocalcemia (prolonged QT interval, T-wave inversion, heart blocks) and hypomagnesemia (prolonged QT and PR intervals, ST segment depression, flattening or inversion of p waves, torsade de pointes). Hypomagnesemia also causes potassium wasting by the kidney. Many hospital patients with refractory hypocalcemia will be found to be magnesium deficient. Often this deficiency becomes manifest during the response to parenteral nutrition when normal cellular ionic gradients are restored. A normal blood pH and arterial Pco_2 rule out hyperventilation. The serum calcium in this patient is normal when adjusted for the low albumin (add 0.8 mg/dL per 1 g/dL decrease in albumin). Hypomagnesemia causes functional hypoparathyroidism, which can lower serum calcium and thus result in a combined defect.

6. The answer is a. *(Townsend, pp 265-266.)* The appropriate dosing and timing of antibiotic prophylaxis to prevent surgical site infections in an elective procedure is a single dose, no greater than 1 hour prior to the incision. Additionally, most textbooks recommend use of an oral, nonabsorbable antibiotic regimen effective against aerobes and anaerobes in combination with a mechanical bowel preparation before elective colon resections. There is no evidence to support the continuation of antibiotics for more than 24 hours after an elective operation has been completed, and this practice should be avoided to prevent increasing microbial drug resistance. For complex, prolonged procedures, redosing of antibiotics may be appropriate during the procedure based on the drug's half-life. Broad-spectrum antibiotic coverage, including against anaerobic organisms, is required only in cases where such flora are anticipated, such as during colon resections.

7. The answer is d. *(Townsend, pp 252-256.)* The patient should undergo persantine thallium stress testing followed by echocardiography to assess his need for coronary angiogram with possible need for angioplasty, stenting, or surgical revascularization prior to repair of his hernia. Although exercise stress testing is an appropriate method for evaluating a patient's cardiac function preoperatively, this patient's functional status is limited by his peripheral vascular disease and therefore a pharmacologic stress test would be the preferred method of cardiac evaluation. An ECG should be performed in this patient with a history of cardiovascular disease, hypertension, and diabetes, but a normal ECG would not preclude further workup. While myocardial infarction (MI) within 6 months of surgery is considered to increase a patient's risk for a cardiac complication after surgery using Goldman's criteria, a remote history of MI is not prohibitive for surgery in and of itself.

8. The answer is d. *(Townsend, pp 81-85.)* The patient has a metabolic alkalosis secondary to gastric losses of HCl, with compensatory hypoventilation as reflected by the elevated arterial pH and PCO_2 and supported by the absence of clinical lung disease. The PCO_2 would be normal if the metabolic alkalosis was uncompensated. A respiratory acidosis with metabolic compensation would be characterized by decreased pH, increased PCO_2 levels, and increased bicarbonate levels. Mixed acid–base abnormalities should be suspected when the pH is normal, but the PCO_2 and bicarbonate levels are abnormal or if the compensatory responses appear to be excessive or inadequate. The combination of respiratory acidosis and respiratory alkalosis is impossible.

9. The answer is a. *(Townsend, pp 88-89.)* Infusion of 0.9% normal saline (sodium chloride) will correct his hypovolemia and his metabolic alkalosis. The development of a clinically significant metabolic alkalosis is secondary not only to the loss of acid or addition of alkali but also to renal responses that maintain the alkalosis (paradoxical aciduria). The normal kidney can tremendously augment its excretion of acid or alkali in response to changes in ingested load. However, in the presence of significant volume depletion and consequent excessive salt and water retention, the tubular maximum for bicarbonate reabsorption is increased. Correction of volume depletion alone is usually sufficient to correct the alkalosis, since the kidney will then excrete the excess bicarbonate. HCl infusion is usually unnecessary. Acetazolamide can be utilized to increase renal excretion of bicarbonate but should be avoided in volume-depleted individuals. Moreover, to the extent that acetazolamide causes natriuresis, it will exacerbate the volume depletion.

10. The answer is b. *(Brunicardi, pp 59-60.)* This patient's history of tinnitus in conjunction with her mixed metabolic acidosis-respiratory alkalosis is consistent with salicylate intoxication. Salicylates directly stimulate the respiratory center and produce respiratory alkalosis. By building up an accumulation of organic acids, salicylates also produce a concomitant metabolic acidosis. The patient is in a state of metabolic acidosis as shown by a markedly increased anion gap of 28 mEq unmeasured anions per liter of plasma. However, the respiratory response is greater than can be explained by a compensatory response; respiratory compensation alone would not result in an alkalemic pH. The disturbance cannot be pure respiratory alkalosis, since the serum bicarbonate does not drop below 15 mEq/L as a result of renal compensation and the anion gap does not vary by more than 1 to 2 mEq/L from its normal value of 12 in response to a respiratory disturbance. The renal response to hyperventilation involves wasting of bicarbonate and compensatory retention of chloride; it does not involve a change in the concentration of unmeasured anions, such as albumin and organic acids.

Phenformin and methanol overdoses also produce high-anion-gap metabolic acidosis, but without the simultaneous respiratory disturbance. Sedatives, such as barbiturates or diazepam, would result in hypoventilation with respiratory acidosis.

11. The answer is d. (*Brunicardi, pp 784-785.*) The patient has heparin-induced thrombocytopenia (HIT), which is a complication of heparin therapy, at both prophylactic and therapeutic doses. HIT is mediated by antibodies to the complexes formed by binding of heparin to platelet factor 4. In a previously unexposed patient, HIT typically manifests after 5 days as a decrease in platelet counts by 50% of the highest preceding value or to a level less than 100,000/mm^3. Complications of HIT are related to venous and/or arterial thromboembolic phenomena. Treatment of HIT consists of cessation of heparin (including low-molecular-weight heparins), institution of a nonheparin anticoagulant such as a direct thrombin inhibitor (examples include lepirudin and argatroban), and conversion to oral warfarin when appropriate. Cessation of heparin alone is inadequate to prevent thromboembolic complications, and warfarin should not be started until the platelet count is above 100,000/mm^3. Platelet transfusion is not indicated, as HIT results in thrombotic rather than hemorrhagic complications.

12. The answer is c. (*Townsend, pp 116-119, 131, 329-330.*) Whenever significant bleeding is noted in the early postoperative period, the presumption should always be that it is due to an error in surgical control of blood vessels in the operative field. Hematologic disorders that are not apparent during the long operation are most unlikely to surface as problems postoperatively. Blood transfusion reactions can cause diffuse loss of clot integrity; the sudden appearance of diffuse bleeding during an operation may be the only evidence of an intraoperative transfusion reaction. In the postoperative period, transfusion reactions usually present as unexplained fever, apprehension, and headache—all symptoms difficult to interpret in the early postoperative period. Factor VIII deficiency (hemophilia) would almost certainly be known by history in a 65-year-old man, but, if not, intraoperative bleeding would have been a problem earlier in this long operation. Moreover, factor VIII deficiency causes prolongation of the partial thromboplastin time (PTT), which is normal in this patient. Severely hypothermic patients will not be able to form clots effectively, but clot dissolution does not occur. Care should be taken to prevent the development of hypothermia during long operations through the use of warmed intravenous fluid, gas humidifiers, and insulated skin barriers.

13. The answer is c. *(Townsend, pp 252-256.)* The work of Goldman and others has served to identify risk factors for perioperative myocardial infarction. The highest likelihood is associated with recent myocardial infarction: the more recent the event, the higher the risk up to 6 months. It should be noted, however, that the risk never returns to normal. A non-Q-wave infarction may not have destroyed much myocardium, but it leaves the surrounding area with borderline perfusion, thus the particularly high risk of subsequent perioperative infarction. Evidence of congestive heart failure, such as jugular venous distention, or S3 gallop also carries a high risk, as does the frequent occurrence of ectopic beats. Old age (>70 years) and emergency surgery are risk factors independent of these others. Coronary revascularization by coronary artery bypass graft (CABG) tends to protect against myocardial infarction. Smoking, diabetes, hypertension, and hyperlipidemia (all of which predispose to coronary artery disease) are surprisingly not independent risk factors, although they may increase the death rate should an infarct occur. The value of this information and data derived from further testing is that it identifies the patient who needs to be monitored invasively with a systemic arterial catheter and pulmonary arterial catheter. Most perioperative infarcts occur postoperatively when the third-space fluids return to the circulation, which increases the preload and the myocardial oxygen consumption. This generally occurs around the third postoperative day.

14. The answer is c. *(Brunicardi, pp 730-736.)* In the absence of perito-neal signs, angiography is the diagnostic test of choice for acute mesenteric ischemia. Patients with peritoneal signs should undergo emergent laparo-tomy. Acute mesenteric ischemia may be difficult to diagnose. The condi-tion should be suspected in patients with either systemic manifestations of arteriosclerotic vascular disease or low cardiac-output states associated with a sudden development of abdominal pain that is out of proportion to the physical findings. Because of the risk of progression to small-bowel infarc-tion, acute mesenteric ischemia is an emergency and timely diagnosis is essential. Although patients may have lactic acidosis or leukocytosis, these are late findings. Abdominal films are generally unhelpful and may show a nonspecific ileus pattern. Since the pathology involves the small bowel, a barium enema is not indicated. Upper gastrointestinal series and ultrasonog-raphy are also of limited value. CT scanning is a good initial test, but should still be followed by angiography in a patient with clinically suspected acute mesenteric ischemia, even in the absence of findings on the CT scan. In addi-tion to establishing the diagnosis in this stable patient, angiography may also assist with operative planning and elucidation of the etiology of the acute mesenteric ischemia. The cause may be embolic occlusion or thrombosis of the superior mesenteric artery, primary mesenteric venous occlusion, or nonocclusive mesenteric ischemia secondary to low-cardiac output states. A mortality of 50% to 75% is reported. The majority of affected patients are at high operative risk, but early diagnosis followed by revascularization or resectional surgery or both are the only hope for survival. Celiotomy must be performed once the diagnosis of arterial occlusion or bowel infarction has been made. Initial treatment of nonocclusive mesenteric ischemia includes measures to increase cardiac output and blood pressure. Laparotomy should be performed if peritoneal signs develop.

15. The answer is b. *(Brunicardi, pp 781-789.)* Duplex ultrasound is the diagnostic modality of choice for detection of infrainguinal deep venous thrombosis (DVT). Although venography is the gold standard, it is no longer routinely used, given the risks of local (thrombosis, pain) and contrast-related (allergic reaction, renal failure) complications. Impedance plethysmography, which measures changes in volume in the lower extrem-ity as related to blood flow, is also used infrequently due to the superiority of duplex scanning in detecting DVTs. In pregnant women, anticoagula-tion for treatment of DVT is achieved with heparin, which does not cross the placenta, rather than warfarin, which is associated with the risk of spontaneous abortion and birth defects. The vena caval filter is not indicated because there is no contraindication to heparin therapy and no evidence of failure of anticoagulation therapy (pulmonary embolus in the face of adequate anticoagulation).

16. The answer is e. (*Townsend, p 119.*) The patient's elevated aPTT, normal PT, and abnormal bleeding time are consistent with her von Willebrand disease (vWD). von Willebrand factor (vWF) is an important stimulus for platelet aggregation at the site of tissue injury and a major carrier protein for circulating factor VIII. There are three major groups of vWD. Type I, inherited as an autosomal dominant trait, has decreased levels of vWF. Type II is variably inherited and has qualitative defects in vWF. Type III is an autosomal recessive severe bleeding disorder with absent levels of vWF. Patients with vWD present with mucosal bleeding, petechiae, epistaxis, and menorrhagia. vWD produces a depressed ristocetin cofactor assay (which measures the effectiveness of vWF in agglutinating platelets when stimulated with the antibiotic ristocetin). These patients do not generally require treatment unless they need surgery or are severely injured. DDAVP, a synthetic analogue of vasopressin, activates receptors that result in release of vWF from storage sites and causes shortening in the bleeding time in patients with type I vWD and some patients with type II vWD. vWF prevents inactivation of factor VIII; administration of DDAVP results in normalization of factor VIII activities. Transfusion of cryoprecipitate provides vWF, whereas infusions of high-purity concentrates of factor VIII:C are not effective because of the lack of vWF. Vitamin K is used perioperatively to reverse coagulopathy due to warfarin or liver disease and is not indicated in this scenario. Aminocaproic acid inhibits fibrinolysis and is not indicated for treating vWD.

17. The answer is b. (*Townsend, p 156.*) The correct diagnosis is sepsis. Systemic inflammatory response syndrome (SIRS) involves 2 or more of the following: temperature >38°C (100°F) or <36°C (97°F), heart rate >90 beats per minute, respiratory rate >20 or $PaCO_2$ <32 mm Hg, WBC count >12,000 or <4000/mm^3 or >10% immature neutrophils. Sepsis = SIRS + documented infection. Severe sepsis = sepsis + organ dysfunction or hypoperfusion (lactic acidosis, oliguria, or altered mental status). Septic shock = sepsis + organ dysfunction + hypotension (systolic blood pressure <90 mm Hg or >90 mm Hg with vasopressors).

18. The answer is d. *(Brunicardi, pp 78-83.)* The patient is in class IV hemorrhagic shock, which represents a loss of more than 40% of circulating blood volume. He requires massive blood transfusion. The term massive blood transfusion is defined as a single transfusion greater than 10 units of packed red blood cells (PRBCs) transfused over a period of 24 hours. There is evidence to suggest that severely injured trauma patients arrive at the hospital coagulopathic. Furthermore, when large amounts of banked blood are transfused, the recipient develops dilutional thrombocytopenia and deficiencies in factors V and VIII. Recent studies have suggested that early administration of fresh-frozen plasma (FFP) and platelets decreases mortality and that a 1:1 ratio of PRBC:FFP should be initiated upon recognition of the need for massive transfusion. Waiting to administer FFP and platelets until laboratory values confirm coagulopathy is no longer recommended. Moreover, excessive crystalloid infusion should be avoided. Albumin has no role in damage control resuscitation. Vitamin K will take days to replace the clotting factors. This patient needs to have his coagulopathy corrected immediately to prevent death from hemorrhagic shock.

19. The answer is b. *(Brunicardi, pp 41-44.)* Early enteral nutrition is recommended in patients predicted to have a prolonged recovery after surgery. The misconception that the entire bowel does not function in the early postoperative period is still widely held. Intestinal motility and absorption studies have clarified the patterns by which bowel activity resumes. The stomach remains uncoordinated in its muscular activity and does not empty efficiently for about 24 hours after abdominal procedures. The small bowel functions normally within hours of surgery and is able to accept nutrients promptly, either by nasoduodenal or percutaneous jejunal feeding catheters or, after 24 hours, by gastric emptying. The colon is stimulated in large measure by the gastrocolic reflex but ordinarily is relatively inactive for 3 to 4 days. Well-nourished patients who undergo uncomplicated surgical procedures can tolerate up to 10 days without full nutritional support before significant problems with protein breakdown begin to occur. Enteral nutrition is preferred over parenteral nutrition because of decreased risks of nosocomial infections and catheter-related complications and increased benefit in preventing mucosal atrophy.

20. The answer is a. *(Brunicardi, pp 784-789.)* Immediate reversal of heparin anticoagulation is indicated in a heparinized patient with significant life-threatening hemorrhage. Protamine sulfate is a specific antidote to heparin and is given at 1 mg for each 100 units heparin. It is given in cases when hemorrhage begins shortly after a bolus of heparin. For a patient who is undergoing heparin therapy, the dose should be based on the half-life of heparin (90 minutes). Since protamine is also an anticoagulant, only half the calculated circulating heparin should be reversed. The indications for inferior vena cava (IVC) filter placement fall into three categories: a failure or complication of anticoagulation, a known free-floating venous clot, and a prior history of PE. In this critically ill patient, exploration of the retroperitoneal space would be surgically challenging and unnecessary.

21. The answer is d. *(Townsend, pp 168-175.)* Hypophosphatemia is a complication of refeeding syndrome, which occurs in malnourished patients who are administered with intravenous glucose. During periods of starvation, electrolytes are shifted to the extracellular space to maintain adequate serum concentrations. With refeeding, insulin levels rise and electrolytes are shifted back intracellularly, resulting in potential hypokalemia, hypomagnesemia, and hypophosphatemia. Additionally, refeeding results in an increased cellular need for phosphorus for energy production (ATP) and glucose metabolism. Early complications of TPN also include hyperglycemia, hyperchloremic acidosis, and volume overload with resultant heart failure. TPN, particularly in the extremely malnourished patient, should be started slowly; magnesium, potassium, and phosphate levels should be repleted; and dextrose infusions should be limited to prevent complications of refeeding.

22. The answer is c. *(Brunicardi, pp 338, 1402-1403.)* Acute adrenal insufficiency can occur in patients with severe stress, infection, or trauma or as a result of abrupt cessation or too rapid tapering of chronic glucocorticoid therapy, and is classically manifested as changing mental status, increased temperature, cardiovascular collapse, hypoglycemia, and hyperkalemia. The diagnosis can be difficult to make and requires a high index of suspicion. Its clinical presentation is similar to that of sepsis; however, sepsis is generally associated with hyperglycemia and no significant change in potassium. The treatment for adrenal crisis is intravenous steroids, volume resuscitation, and other supportive measures to treat any new or ongoing stress. Dexamethasone should be used as steroid replacement when additional testing with an adrenocorticotropic hormone (ACTH) stimulation test is planned, since hydrocortisone can interfere with measurement of cortisol levels. Steroid treatment can be subsequently converted to oral medication and tapered after treatment of the adrenal crisis.

23. The answer is c. *(Brunicardi, p 75.)* Transfusions with FFP to replenish vitamin K–dependent clotting factors should be administered on call to the operating room. The timing of transfusion is dependent on the quantity of each factor delivered and its half-life. The half-life of the most stable clotting factor, factor VII, is 4 to 6 hours. Thus, transfusion of FFP on call to the operating room ensures that the transfusion is complete prior to the incision, with circulating factors to cover the operative and immediate postoperative period.

24. The answer is c. *(Brunicardi, pp 336-337.)* The most common nosocomial infection is a urinary tract infection. Treatment consists of removal of an indwelling catheter as soon as possible and antibiotic therapy for cultures with greater than 100,000 CFU/mL. Pneumonias, wound infections, intra-abdominal abscesses, and catheter-related bloodstream infections are also all causes of nosocomial infections, and a workup of a postoperative fever should also include careful examination of the patient and other diagnostic tests as appropriate (chest x-ray, blood cultures, abdominal/pelvic CT scan).

25. The answer is a. *(Brunicardi, p 998.)* Factors that predispose to fistula formation and may prevent closure include *f*oreign body, *r*adiation, *i*nflammation, *e*pithelialization of the tract, *n*eoplasm, *d*istal obstruction, and steroids. (Recall the list of aforementioned factors with "FRIENDS.") Factors that result in unhealthy or abnormal tissue surrounding the enterocutaneous fistula decrease the likelihood of spontaneous resolution. For example, radiation therapy, such as used for treatment of pelvic gynecologic and rectal malignancies, can result in chronic injury to the small intestine characterized by fibrosis and poor wound healing. High-output fistulas, defined as those with more than 500 cc per day output, are usually proximal and unlikely to close. Treatment consists of source control, nutritional supplementation, wound care, and delayed surgical intervention if the fistula fails to close.

26. The answer is d. *(Townsend, p 131.)* Transfusion reactions can be categorized into hemolytic versus allergic nonhemolytic reactions. Hemolytic transfusion reactions are caused by complement-mediated destruction of transfused red blood cells by the recipient's preexisting antibodies. Severe hemolytic transfusion reactions usually involve the transfusion of ABO-incompatible blood, with fatalities occurring in 1 in 600,000 units.

Peptides from the complement, released into the blood as the red blood cells are rapidly destroyed, cause hypotension, activate coagulation, and lead to disseminated intravascular coagulation (DIC). Symptoms of a hemolytic transfusion reaction include fever, chills, pain and redness along the infused vein, oozing from IV sites, respiratory distress, anxiety, hypotension, and oliguria. The patient would have a low CVP with hypovolemic shock. Acute adrenal insufficiency, gram-negative bacteremia, and ureteral obstruction would not cause oozing from the IV sites.

27. The answer is d. *(Townsend, pp 118-119.)* Hemophilia A is a coagulation disorder resulting from a deficiency or abnormality of factor VIII. Desmopressin (DDAVP) is a synthetic analogue of antidiuretic hormone that increases levels of factor VIII and von Willebrand factor. DDAVP can be used alone for mild hemophilia A, but is ineffective in severe forms of the disease. For severe hemophilia A, DDAVP is given in combination with an inhibitor of fibrinolysis such as ε-aminocaproic acid (AMICAR). Although FFP contains factor VIII, the levels are too low to prevent or control bleeding in hemophiliacs. Other agents used in treatment of hemophilia A include cryoprecipitate and specific factor VIII concentrates.

28. The answer is d. *(Townsend, p 122.)* NSAIDs such as aspirin block platelet function by causing a reversible defect in the enzyme cyclooxygenase. Unlike aspirin which permanently acetylates cyclooxygenase and leaves affected platelets dysfunctional throughout their 7-day life span, NSAIDs cause a reversible defect that lasts 3 to 4 days. Therefore, the patient's platelets will be functional for surgery if he stops taking the NSAIDs 3 to 4 days prior to the date of surgery. The patient would not benefit from FFP or vitamin K since he does not have problems with his clotting factors.

29. The answer is d. *(Townsend, pp 1252-1253.)* Either megaloblastic anemia due to vitamin B_{12} deficiency (due to lack of intrinsic factor, which is necessary for B_{12} absorption and is normally produced by the parietal cells of the stomach) or microcytic anemia due to iron deficiency (due to decreased iron intake and impaired absorption in the duodenum) can result after partial gastrectomy. While folate deficiency can also cause megaloblastic anemia, it is rare after partial gastrectomy. Oral B_{12} is not a reliable method for correcting B_{12} deficiency; intravenous cyanocobalamin should be administered every 3 to 4 months for life. Other complications of partial gastrectomy includes osteoporosis secondary to impaired calcium absorption due to the Billroth II reconstruction (since calcium is normally absorbed in the proximal intestine—duodenum and jejunum). Also, fatty acids may also be malabsorbed due to inadequate mixing of bile salts and lipase with ingested fat, and therefore steatorrhea may result.

30. The answer is a. (*Townsend, pp 2263-2264.*) The patient should undergo an intravenous pyelogram for a suspected ureteral injury. After gynecologic surgeries, colorectal surgery is the most common cause of iatrogenic ureteral injuries. Intraoperatively, intravenous administration of methylene blue or indigocyanine green may facilitate identification of an injury. However, delay in diagnosis is common, and patients may present with flank pain, fevers, and signs of sepsis, ileus, or decreased urine output. CT scan may demonstrate hydronephrosis or a fluid collection (urinoma). Initial diagnosis and management should include urinalysis, although hematuria may not always be present; percutaneous nephrostomy tube or retrograde ureteral catheterization; percutaneous drainage of fluid collections; and identification of the location of ureteral injury. Surgical management should be delayed if diagnosis is late (10-14 days), and operative strategy is dependent on the location of the injury. Diagnostic imaging such as a pyelogram or nuclear medicine scan may be helpful to identify the site of the injury.

31. The answer is d. (*Townsend, pp 80-81, 951, 959-960.*) Intravenous calcium infusion is the treatment for severe, symptomatic hypocalcemia, although, typically, oral calcium supplementation (up to 1-2 g every 4 hours) is sufficient in patients with mild symptoms. Since postthyroidectomy hypocalcemia is usually due to transient ischemia of the parathyroid glands and is self-limited, in most cases the problem is resolved in several days. In cases of persistent hypocalcemia, vitamin D preparations may be necessary. There is no role for thyroid hormone replacement or magnesium sulfate in the treatment of hypocalcemia.

32. The answer is c. (*Brunicardi, p 54.*) Bile and the fluids found in the duodenum, jejunum, and ileum all have an electrolyte content similar to that of Ringer lactate. Saliva, gastric juice, and right colon fluids have high K^+ and low Na^+ content. Pancreatic secretions are high in bicarbonate. It is important to consider these variations in electrolyte patterns when calculating replacement requirements following gastrointestinal losses.

33. The answer is d. *(Brunicardi, pp 56-57.)* Calcium gluconate does not affect the serum potassium level but rather counteracts the myocardial effects of hyperkalemia. Reduction in an elevated serum potassium level, however, is important to avoid the cardiovascular complications that ultimately culminate in cardiac arrest. Kayexalate is a cation exchange resin that is instilled into the gastrointestinal tract and exchanges sodium for potassium ions. Its use is limited to semiacute and chronic potassium elevations. Sodium bicarbonate causes a rise in serum pH and shifts potassium intracellularly. Administration of glucose initiates glycogen synthesis and uptake of potassium. Insulin can be used in conjunction with this to aid in the shift of potassium intracellularly.

34. The answer is b. *(Brunicardi, pp 222-224.)* The determinants of a postoperative wound infection include factors predetermined by the status of the patient (eg, age, obesity, steroid dependence, multiple diagnoses [more than three], immunosuppression) and by the type of procedure (eg, contaminated versus clean, emergent versus elective). However, there are several factors that can be optimized by the surgeon. Decreasing the bacterial inoculum and virulence by limiting the patient's prehospital stay, clipping the operative site in the operating room, administering perioperative antibiotics (within a 24-hour period surrounding operation) with an appropriate antimicrobial spectrum, treating remote infections, avoiding breaks in technique, using closed drainage systems (if needed at all) that exit the skin away from the surgical incision, and minimizing the duration of the operation have all been shown to decrease postoperative infection. Making a wound less favorable to infection requires attention to basic Halstedian principles of hemostasis, anatomic dissection, and gentle handling of tissues as well as limiting the amount of foreign body and necrotic tissue in the wound. Although they are the most difficult factors to influence, host defense mechanisms can be improved by optimizing nutritional status, tissue perfusion, and oxygen delivery.

35. The answer is a. *(Townsend, pp 163-165.)* The patient has a zinc deficiency. Alopecia, poor wound healing, night blindness or photophobia, anosmia, neuritis, and skin rashes are all characteristic of patients with zinc deficiency, which often results in the setting of excessive diarrhea. Selenium deficiency is characterized by the development of a cardiomyopathy. Molybdenum deficiency is manifested by encephalopathy due to toxic accumulation of sulfur-containing amino acids. Chromium deficiency can occur in patients on long-term TPN and is characterized by difficult-to-control hyperglycemia and peripheral neuropathy and encephalopathy. Thiamine deficiency results in beriberi, which includes symptoms of encephalopathy and peripheral neuropathy; patients with beriberi can also develop cardiovascular symptoms and cardiac failure.

36. The answer is c. (*Brunicardi, pp 1750-1751.*) The patient is manifesting symptoms of malignant hyperthermia (fevers, rigors, and myoglobinuria), which is treated by administration of dantrolene, immediate discontinuation of offending medication (which can include succinylcholine or halothane-based inhalational anesthetics), and supportive cooling measures. While urine alkalinization, loop diuretics, and mannitol are appropriate treatment measures for rhabdomyolysis, the underlying problem in this patient is malignant hyperthermia, which, because of its associated mortality of 30% in severe cases, should be treated first and foremost. Malignant hyperthermia is not a manifestation of anaphylactic shock, and therefore steroids and antihistamines have no role in its treatment.

37. The answer is e. (*Townsend, p 98.*) Normal saline and lactated Ringer solution are examples of isotonic solutions, both of which can be used to replace the volume of blood lost in a ratio of 3:1. One caveat of administering large volumes of normal saline is that a non-anion-gap metabolic acidosis can result from increased chloride concentrations. Hypotonic saline solutions such as 0.45% normal saline should not be used for acute resuscitation in hemorrhagic shock but are appropriate for postoperative fluid maintenance in the hemodynamically stable patient. The use of colloids in resuscitation of patients in hemorrhagic shock is controversial; in general, however, colloids can be used to replace blood volume lost in a ratio of 1:1. The definitive treatment of hypovolemic shock is fluid resuscitation, not initiation of vasopressors.

38. The answer is d. (*Brunicardi, pp 54-63; Townsend, p 98.*) This postoperative patient requires replacement of nasogastric tube losses in addition to maintenance fluids. In an otherwise healthy individual, maintenance fluids are calculated based on body weight as 4 mL/kg/h for the first 10 kg, 2 mL/kg/h for the second 10 kg, and 1 mL/kg/h for every additional kg body weight. A 60-kg man requires 100 mL of fluid per hour or 2400 mL of fluid per day. Five percent dextrose in 0.45% normal saline with or without potassium chloride (depending on renal function) would be an appropriate maintenance fluid. Both lactated Ringer and normal saline, which are isotonic, can be used to replace gastrointestinal losses.

39. The answer is b. *(Brunicardi, pp 61-62.)* The patient presented has the SIADH. Although this syndrome is associated primarily with diseases of the central nervous system or of the chest (eg, oat cell carcinoma of the lung), excessive amounts of antidiuretic hormone are also present in most postoperative patients. The pathophysiology of SIADH involves an inability to dilute the urine; administered water is therefore retained, which produces dilutional hyponatremia. Body sodium stores and fluid balance are normal, as evidenced by the absence of the clinical findings suggestive of abnormalities of extracellular fluid volume. For mild asymptomatic hyponatremia, the appropriate therapy is to restrict water ingestion to a level below the patient's ability to excrete water. Hypertonic (3%) saline can be used to correct severe hyponatremia with neurologic manifestations, but should be infused slowly. Rapid correction of hyponatremia can lead to central pontine myelinolysis. Hyperglycemia cannot account for the hyponatremia seen in this patient because the serum osmolality, as well as the serum sodium, is depressed. Hyponatremia resulting from hyperglycemia would be associated with an elevated serum osmolality. Therefore, insulin infusion would not correct the hyponatremia. Desmopressin can be used to treat diabetes insipidus resulting from a traumatic brain injury, but is not indicated for SIADH. Loop diuretics are used in treating hypervolemic hyponatremia.

40. The answer is a. *(Brunicardi, pp 56-57.)* The electrocardiogram demonstrates changes that are essentially diagnostic of severe hyperkalemia. Correct treatment for the affected patient includes discontinuation of exogenous sources of potassium, administration of a source of calcium ions (which will immediately oppose the myocardial effects of potassium), and administration of sodium bicarbonate (which, by producing a mild alkalosis, will shift potassium into cells); each will temporarily reduce serum potassium concentration. Infusion of glucose and insulin would also effect a temporary transcellular shift of potassium. However, these maneuvers are only temporarily effective; definitive treatment calls for removal of potassium from the body. The sodium-potassium exchange resin sodium polystyrene sulfonate (Kayexalate) would accomplish this removal, but over a period of hours and at the price of adding a sodium ion for each potassium ion that is removed. Hemodialysis or peritoneal dialysis is probably required for this patient, since these procedures also rectify the other consequences of acute renal failure, but they would not be the first line of therapy, given the acute need to reduce the potassium level. Both lidocaine and digoxin would be not only ineffective but contraindicated, since they would further depress the myocardial conduction system.

41. The answer is e. (*Brunicardi, pp 128-129.*) It is important to identify and treat occult or early sepsis before it progresses to septic shock and the associated complications of multiple organ failure. An immunocompromised host may not manifest some of the more typical signs and symptoms of infection, such as elevated temperature and white cell count; this forces the clinician to focus on more subtle signs and symptoms. Early sepsis is a physiologically hyperdynamic, hypermetabolic state representing a surge of catecholamines, cortisol, and other stress-related hormones. Changing mental status, tachypnea that leads to respiratory alkalosis, and flushed skin are often the earliest manifestations of sepsis. Intermittent hypotension requiring increased fluid resuscitation to maintain adequate urine output is characteristic of occult sepsis. Hyperglycemia and insulin resistance during sepsis are typical in diabetic as well as nondiabetic patients. This relates to the gluconeogenic state of the stress response. The cardiovascular response to early sepsis is characterized by an increased cardiac output, decreased systemic vascular resistance, and decreased peripheral utilization of oxygen, which yields a decreased arteriovenous oxygen difference.

42. The answer is d. (*Brunicardi, pp 58-61.*) The patient has a non-anion-gap metabolic acidosis, ($[Na^+] - [Cl^- + HCO_3^-] = [128] - [102 + 20] = 6$), secondary to high output from her ileostomy with gastrointestinal losses of bicarbonate. This should be managed with fluid replacement and stool-bulking agents. The ionic composition of small-bowel fluid is Na^+ 140, K^+ 5, Cl^- 104, and HCO_3^- 30. Patients with large ileostomy outputs are at risk for dehydration with accompaning hyponatremia, hypokalemia, and non-anion-gap metabolic acidosis. Infusion of additional normal saline and potassium chloride will exacerbate the non-anion-gap acidosis. The patient's tachypnea and respiratory alkalosis are compensatory mechanisms for her metabolic acidosis. Treatment should be targeted at the primary metabolic abnormality. Given that her oxygenation is adequate, there is no indication for intubation. Transfusion is not indicated as the etiology of the patient's hypovolemia is not hemorrhage. Renal failure can result in an anion-gap, uremic acidosis and hyperkalemia, both of which may be indications for dialysis. However, this patient is volume depleted.

43. The answer is e. *(Townsend, p 131.)* Hemolytic transfusion reactions lead to hypotension and oliguria. The increased hemoglobin in the plasma will be cleared via the kidneys, which leads to hemoglobinuria. Placement of an indwelling Foley catheter with subsequent demonstration of oliguria and hemoglobinuria not only confirms the diagnosis of a hemolytic transfusion reaction but is useful in monitoring corrective therapy. Treatment begins with discontinuation of the transfusion, followed by aggressive fluid resuscitation to support the hypotensive episode and increase urine output. Inducing diuresis through aggressive fluid resuscitation and osmotic diuretics is important to clear the hemolyzed red cell membranes, which can otherwise collect in glomeruli and cause renal damage. Alkalinization of the urine (pH >7) helps prevent hemoglobin clumping and renal damage. Steroids do not have a role in the treatment of hemolytic transfusion reactions.

44. The answer is e. *(Brunicardi, p 1057.)* Treatment of *C difficile* colitis is metronidazole for first-line therapy and oral vancomycin as a second-tier agent. Recurrence appears in up to 20% of patients. Indications for surgical treatment are intractable disease, failure of medical therapy, toxic megacolon, and colonic perforation; surgical therapy consists of subtotal colectomy with end ileostomy. The diagnosis can be made by either detection of the characteristic appearance of pseudomembranes on endoscopy or detection of either toxin A or toxin B in the stool. Anti-diarrheal agents are contraindicated in suspected *C difficile* colitis as they may prolong the infection.

45. The answer is c. *(Brunicardi, pp 80-81.)* Hypocalcemia is associated with physical findings including spasm of the muscles of the forearm and hand when a blood pressure cuff is inflated (Trousseau sign) and spasm of the facial muscles when the facial nerve is stimulated (Chvostek sign). Hypocalcemia is also associated with a prolonged QT interval and may be aggravated by both hypomagnesemia and alkalosis. Additionally, massive transfusion is associated with hypocalcemia secondary to chelation with citrate in banked blood. Severe, symptomatic hypocalcemia, encountered most frequently following parathyroid or thyroid surgery or in patients with acute pancreatitis, should be treated with intravenous calcium gluconate. The myocardium is very sensitive to calcium levels; therefore, calcium is considered a positive inotropic agent. Calcium increases the contractile strength of cardiac muscle as well as the velocity of shortening. In its absence, the efficiency of the myocardium decreases. Hypocalcemia often occurs with hypoproteinemia, even though the ionized serum calcium fraction remains normal.

46 to 49. The answers are 46-a, 47-d, 48-e, 49-c. (*Mulholland, pp 177-178.*) Basal metabolic rate is the energy required to maintain cell integrity in the resting state at a normal physiologic temperature. The basal energy expenditure decreases with advancing age and varies with sex and body size. The patient's clinical condition also impacts the basal energy expenditure. During starvation, the metabolic rate is decreased by 10%. Trauma, stress, sepsis, burns, and surgery all increase the metabolic rate. The basal energy expenditure can be multiplied by a stress factor to better approximate caloric requirements. The stress factor after a routine operation is 1.1, multiple organ failure or severe injury is 1.5, and more than 50% body surface area burns is 2.0.

Critical Care: Anesthesiology, Blood Gases, and Respiratory Care

Questions

50. A 75-year-old thin cachectic woman undergoes a tracheostomy for failure to wean from the ventilator. One week later, she develops significant bleeding from the tracheostomy. Which of the following would be an appropriate initial step in the management of this problem?

a. Remove the tracheostomy and place pressure over the wound.
b. Deflate the balloon cuff on the tracheostomy.
c. Attempt to reintubate the patient with an endotracheal tube.
d. Upsize the tracheostomy.
e. Perform fiberoptic evaluation immediately.

51. A 53-year-old woman has been intubated for several days after sustaining a right pulmonary contusion after a motor vehicle collision as well as multiple rib fractures. Which of the following is a reasonable indication to attempt extubation?

a. Negative inspiratory force (NIF) of −15 cm H_2O
b. Po_2 of 60 mm Hg while breathing 30% inspired Fio_2 with a positive end-expiratory pressure (PEEP) of 10 cm H_2O
c. Spontaneous respiratory rate of 35 breaths per minute
d. A rapid shallow breathing index of 80
e. Minute ventilation of 18 L/min

52. A 19-year-old man receives un-cross-matched blood during resuscitation after a gunshot wound to the abdomen. He develops fever, tachycardia, and oliguria during the transfusion and is diagnosed as having a hemolytic reaction. Which of the following is the most appropriate next step in the management of this patient?

a. Administration of a loop diuretic such as furosemide
b. Treating anuria with fluid and potassium replacement
c. Acidifying the urine to prevent hemoglobin precipitation in the renal tubules
d. Removing foreign bodies, such as Foley catheters, which may cause hemorrhagic complications
e. Stopping the transfusion immediately

53. A 74-year-old woman with a history of a previous total abdominal hysterectomy presents with abdominal pain and distention for 3 days. She is noted on plain films to have dilated small-bowel and air-fluid levels. She is taken to the operating room for a small-bowel obstruction. Which of the following inhalational anesthetics should be avoided because of accumulation in air-filled cavities during general anesthesia?

a. Diethyl ether
b. Nitrous oxide
c. Halothane
d. Methoxyflurane
e. Trichloroethylene

54. A 61-year-old alcoholic man presents with severe epigastric pain radiating to his back. His amylase and lipase are elevated, and he is diagnosed with acute pancreatitis. Over the first 48 hours, he is determined to have 6 Ranson's criteria, including a Pa_{O_2} less than 60 mm Hg. His chest x-ray reveals bilateral pulmonary infiltrates, and his wedge pressure is low. Which of the following criteria must be met to make a diagnosis of adult respiratory distress syndrome (ARDS)?

a. Hypoxemia defined as a Pa_{O_2}/Fi_{O_2} ratio of less than 200
b. Hypoxemia defined as a Pa_{O_2} of less than 60 mm Hg
c. A pulmonary capillary wedge pressure greater than 18 mm Hg
d. Lack of improvement in oxygenation with administration of a test dose of furosemide
e. Presence of a focal infiltrate on chest x-ray

55. A 50-year-old man has respiratory failure due to pneumonia and sepsis after undergoing splenectomy for a traumatic injury. Which of the following management strategies will improve tissue oxygen uptake (ie, shifting the oxygen dissociation curve, depicted here, to the right)?

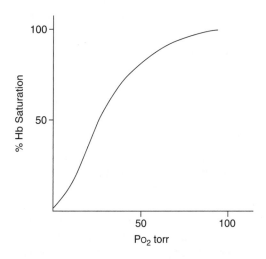

a. Transfusion of banked blood to correct acute anemia
b. Correction of acute anemia with erythropoietic stimulating agent
c. Administration of bicarbonate to promote metabolic alkalosis
d. Hypoventilation to increase the $Paco_2$
e. Administration of an antipyretic to lower the patient's temperature

56. A 64-year-old man with history of severe emphysema is admitted for hematemesis. The bleeding ceases soon after admission, but the patient becomes confused and agitated. Arterial blood gases are as follows: pH 7.23; Po_2 42 mm Hg; Pco_2 75 mm Hg. Which of the following is the best initial therapy for this patient?

a. Correct hypoxemia with high-flow nasal O_2
b. Correct acidosis with sodium bicarbonate
c. Administer 10 mg intravenous dexamethasone
d. Administer 2 mg intravenous Ativan
e. Intubate the patient

57. A 62-year-old woman with a history of coronary artery disease presents with a pancreatic head tumor and undergoes a pancreaticoduodenectomy. Postoperatively, she develops a leak from the pancreaticojejunostomy anastomosis and becomes septic. A Swan-Ganz catheter is placed, which demonstrates an increased cardiac output and decreased systemic vascular resistance. She also develops acute renal failure and oliguria. Which of the following is an indication to start dopamine?

a. To increase splanchnic flow
b. To increase coronary flow
c. To decrease heart rate
d. To lower peripheral vascular resistance
e. To inhibit catecholamine release

58. A 29-year-old woman on oral contraceptives presents with abdominal pain. A computed tomography (CT) scan of the abdomen demonstrates a large hematoma of the right liver with the suggestion of an underlying liver lesion. Her hemoglobin is 6, and she is transfused 2 units of packed red blood cells and 2 units of fresh frozen plasma. Two hours after starting the transfusion, she develops respiratory distress and requires intubation. She is not volume overloaded clinically, but her chest x-ray shows bilateral pulmonary infiltrates. Which of the following is the management strategy of choice?

a. Continue the transfusion and administer an antihistamine
b. Stop the transfusion and administer a diuretic
c. Stop the transfusion, perform bronchoscopy, and start broad-spectrum empiric antibiotics
d. Stop the transfusion and continue supportive respiratory care
e. Stop the transfusion and send a Coombs test

59. A 68-year-old hypertensive man undergoes successful repair of a ruptured abdominal aortic aneurysm. He receives 9 L Ringer lactate solution and 4 units of whole blood during the operation. Two hours after transfer to the surgical intensive care unit, the following hemodynamic parameters are obtained: systemic blood pressure (BP) 90/60 mm Hg, pulse 110 beats per minute, central venous pressure (CVP) 7 mm Hg, pulmonary artery pressure 28/10 mm Hg, pulmonary capillary wedge pressure (PCWP) 8 mm Hg, cardiac output 1.9 L/min, systemic vascular resistance 1400 (dyne·s)/cm^5 (normal is 900-1300), Pao_2 140 mm Hg (Fio_2: 0.45), urine output 15 mL/h (specific gravity: 1.029), and hematocrit 35%. Given this data, which of the following is the most appropriate next step in management?

a. Administration of a diuretic to increase urine output
b. Administration of a vasopressor agent to increase systemic blood pressure
c. Administration of a fluid challenge to increase urine output
d. Administration of a vasodilating agent to decrease elevated systemic vascular resistance
e. A period of observation to obtain more data

60. A 59-year-old man with a history of myocardial infarction 2 years ago undergoes an uneventful aortobifemoral bypass graft for aortoiliac occlusive disease. Six hours later he develops ST segment depression, and a 12-lead electrocardiogram (ECG) shows anterolateral ischemia. His hemodynamic parameters are as follows: systemic BP 70/40 mm Hg, pulse 100 beats per minute, CVP 18 mm Hg, PCWP 25 mm Hg, cardiac output 1.5 L/min, and systemic vascular resistance 1000 (dyne · s)/cm^5. Which of the following is the single best pharmacologic intervention for this patient?

a. Sublingual nitroglycerin
b. Intravenous nitroglycerin
c. A short-acting β-blocker
d. Sodium nitroprusside
e. Dobutamine

61. A 56-year-old man undergoes a left upper lobectomy. An epidural catheter is inserted for postoperative pain relief. Ninety minutes after the first dose of epidural morphine, the patient complains of itching and becomes increasingly somnolent. Blood-gas measurement reveals the following: pH 7.24, $Paco_2$ 58, Pao_2 100, and HCO_3^- 28. Which of the following is the most appropriate initial therapy for this patient?

a. Endotracheal intubation
b. Intramuscular diphenhydramine (Benadryl)
c. Epidural naloxone
d. Intravenous naloxone
e. Alternative analgesia

62. A 71-year-old man returns from the operating room (OR) after undergoing a triple coronary bypass. His initial cardiac index is 2.8 L/ (min·m²). Heart rate is then noted to be 55 beats per minute, BP is 110/80 mm Hg, wedge pressure is 15, and his cardiac index has dropped to 1.6 L/(min·m²). He has a normal left ventricle. Which of the following maneuvers will increase his cardiac output?

a. Increase his peripheral vascular resistance.
b. Increase his CVP.
c. Increase his heart rate to 90 by electrical pacing.
d. Increase his blood viscosity.
e. Increase his inspired O_2 concentration.

63. A 73-year-old woman with a long history of heavy smoking undergoes femoral artery-popliteal artery bypass for rest pain in her left leg. Because of serious underlying respiratory insufficiency, she continues to require ventilatory support for 4 days after her operation. As soon as her endotracheal tube is removed, she begins complaining of vague upper abdominal pain. She has daily fever spikes of 39°C (102.2°F) and a leukocyte count of 18,000/mL. An upper abdominal ultrasonogram reveals a dilated gallbladder, but no stones are seen. A presumptive diagnosis of acalculous cholecystitis is made. Which of the following is the next best step in her treatment?

a. Nasogastric suction and broad-spectrum antibiotics
b. Immediate cholecystectomy with operative cholangiogram
c. Percutaneous drainage of the gallbladder
d. Endoscopic retrograde cholangiopancreatography (ERCP) to visualize and drain the common bile duct
e. Provocation of cholecystokinin release by cautious feeding of the patient

64. A 32-year-old man undergoes a distal pancreatectomy, splenectomy, and partial colectomy for a gunshot wound to the left upper quadrant of the abdomen. One week later he develops a shaking chill in conjunction with a temperature spike of 39.4°C (103°F). His blood pressure is 70/40 mm Hg, pulse is 140 beats per minute, and respiratory rate is 45 breaths per minute. He is transferred to the intensive care unit (ICU), where he is intubated and a Swan-Ganz catheter is placed. Which of the following is consistent with the expected initial Swan-Ganz catheter readings?

a. An increase in cardiac output
b. An increase in peripheral vascular resistance
c. An increase in pulmonary artery pressure
d. An increase in PCWP
e. An increase in central venous pressure

65. A 43-year-old trauma patient develops acute respiratory distress syndrome (ARDS) and has difficulty oxygenating despite increased concentrations of inspired O_2. After the positive end-expiratory pressure (PEEP) is increased, the patient's oxygenation improves. What is the mechanism by which this occurs?

a. Decreasing dead-space ventilation
b. Decreasing the minute ventilation requirement
c. Increasing tidal volume
d. Increasing functional residual capacity
e. Redistribution of lung water from the interstitial to the alveolar space

66. A 27-year-old man was assaulted and stabbed on the left side of the chest between the areola and the sternum. He is hemodynamically unstable with jugular venous distention, distant heart sounds, and hypotension. Which of the following findings would be consistent with a diagnosis of hemodynamically significant cardiac tamponade?

a. More than a 10 mm Hg decrease in systolic blood pressure at the end of the expiratory phase of respiration
b. Decreased right atrial pressures on Swan-Ganz monitoring
c. Equalization of pressures across the 4 chambers on Swan-Ganz monitoring
d. Compression of the left ventricle on echocardiography
e. Overfilling of the right atrium

67. A 55-year-old woman requires an abdominoperineal operation for rectal cancer. She has a history of stable angina. Which of the following clinical markers is most likely to predict a cardiac event during her non-cardiac surgery and should prompt further cardiac workup prior to her operation?

a. Abnormal electrocardiogram
b. Prior stroke
c. Unstable angina
d. Uncontrolled hypertension
e. Her age

68. A 70-kg woman is to undergo nail removal from her right ring finger in the ambulatory surgery clinic. Which of the following is the most appropriate option for local anesthesia?

a. Digital block with 1% lidocaine without epinephrine up to 4.5 mg/kg
b. Digital block with 1% lidocaine with epinephrine up to 4.5 mg/kg
c. Digital block with 1% lidocaine with epinephrine up to 7 mg/kg
d. Local injection around the nail bed with 1% lidocaine with epinephrine up to 4.5 mg/kg
e. Local injection around the nail bed with 1% lidocaine with epinephrine up to 7 mg/kg/mL

69. A 22-year-old man sustains severe blunt trauma to the back. He notes that he cannot move his lower extremities. He is hypotensive and bradycardic. Which of the following is the best initial management of the patient?

a. Administration of phenylephrine
b. Administration of dopamine
c. Administration of epinephrine
d. Intravenous fluid bolus
e. Placement of a transcutaneous pacer

70. A 58-year-old woman with multiple comorbidities and previous cardiac surgery is in a high-speed motor vehicle collision. She is intubated for airway protection. Because of hemodynamic instability, a central venous catheter is placed in the right subclavian vein. While the surgeon is securing the catheter, the cap becomes displaced and air enters the catheter. Suddenly, the patient becomes tachycardic and hypotensive. What is the best next maneuver?

a. Decompression of the right chest with a needle in the second intercostal space
b. Placement of a right chest tube
c. Withdrawal of the central venous catheter several centimeters
d. Placement of the patient in a left lateral decubitus Trendelenburg position
e. Bilateral "clamshell" thoracotomy with aortic cross-clamping

71. A 30-year-old man is scheduled for a laparoscopic cholecystectomy for biliary colic. He reports a family history of prolonged paralysis during general anesthesia. Which of the following medications should be avoided during his procedure?

a. Succinylcholine
b. Vecuronium
c. Pancuronium
d. Halothane
e. Etomidate

72. An 18-year-old woman develops urticaria and wheezing after an injection of intravenous contrast for an abdominal CT scan. Her blood pressure is 120/60 mm Hg, heart rate is 155 beats per minute, and respiratory rate is 30 breaths per minute. Which of the following is the most appropriate immediate therapy?

a. Intubation
b. Epinephrine
c. β-Blockers
d. Iodine
e. Fluid challenge

73. A patient develops a fever and tachycardia during a blood transfusion after a redo coronary artery bypass procedure. The nurse subsequently discovers that there was a mix-up in the cross-match because of a labeling error. Which of the following is diagnostic in a patient with an immediate hemolytic reaction secondary to a blood transfusion?

a. Serum haptoglobin above 50 mg/dL
b. Indirect bilirubin greater than 5 mg/dL
c. Direct bilirubin greater than 5 mg/dL
d. Positive Coombs test
e. Myoglobinuria

74. A 72-year-old man with diabetes, renal insufficiency, and coronary artery disease presents in septic shock from emphysematous cholecystitis. His oxygen saturation is 100% on 6-L nasal cannula and his hemoglobin is 7.2 mg/dL. His mixed venous oxygen saturation is 58%. Which of the following treatment options will improve his oxygen delivery the most?

a. Increase his inspired oxygen concentration
b. Transfer him to a hyperbaric chamber
c. Administer ferrous sulfate
d. Administer an erythropoietic agent
e. Transfuse two units of packed red blood cells 7

75. An obese 50-year-old woman undergoes a laparoscopic cholecystectomy. In the recovery room, she is found to be hypotensive and tachycardic. Her arterial blood gases reveal a pH of 7.29, Pa_{O_2} of 60 mm Hg, and Pa_{CO_2} of 54 mm Hg. Which of the following is the most likely cause of this patient's problem?

a. Acute pulmonary embolism
b. Carbon dioxide (CO_2) absorption from induced pneumoperitoneum
c. Alveolar hypoventilation
d. Pulmonary edema
e. Atelectasis from a high diaphragm

76. A 65-year-old man who had a 25-lb weight loss over the previous 6 months is diagnosed with adenocarcinoma of the distal esophagus. He undergoes a transhiatal esophagectomy complicated by a cervical leak. He is receiving enteral feeds through a jejunostomy tube. After a week, his physicians wish to assess his nutritional resuscitation. Which of the following is the most accurate measure of adequacy of his nutritional support?

a. Urinary nitrogen excretion level
b. Total serum protein level
c. Serum albumin level
d. Serum transferrin level
e. Respiratory quotient

77. A 63-year-old man with multiple rib fractures and a pulmonary contusion requires prolonged intubation. He is unable to be weaned from the ventilator and is on a volume control mode. He has a tracheostomy and a percutaneous gastrotomy in place through which he is being fed. The surgeon orders a respiratory quotient (RQ), which is the ratio of the rate of carbon dioxide production over the rate of oxygen uptake. The RQ is 1. Based on this information, which of the following is the next step in his management?

a. Decrease the inspired concentration of oxygen
b. Decrease the rate on the ventilator
c. Increase the rate on the ventilator
d. Decrease the carbohydrates in his enteral feeds
e. Increase the total number of calories in his enteral feeds

78. A 22-year-old woman is involved in a major motor vehicle accident and receives a tracheostomy during her hospitalization. Five days after placement of the tracheostomy she has some minor bleeding around the tracheostomy site. Which of the following is the most appropriate immediate therapy?

a. Removal of tracheostomy at bedside.
b. Exchange the tracheostomy at bedside.
c. Exchange the tracheostomy in the operating room.
d. Bronchoscopic evaluation of the trachea at bedside.
e. Bronchoscopic evaluation of the trachea in the operating room.

79. A 72-year-old man undergoes resection of an abdominal aneurysm. He arrives in the ICU with a core temperature of 33°C (91.4°F) and shivering. Which of the following is a physiologic consequence of the shivering?

a. Rising mixed venous O_2 saturation
b. Increased production of CO_2
c. Decreased consumption of O_2
d. Rising base excess
e. Decreased minute ventilation

80. A 39-year-old woman with a known history of von Willebrand disease has a ventral hernia after a previous cesarean section and desires to undergo elective repair. Which of the following should be administered preoperatively?

a. High-purity factor VIII: C concentrates
b. Low-molecular-weight dextran
c. Fresh-frozen plasma (FFP)
d. Cryoprecipitate
e. Whole blood

81. You are the physician on call for the extracorporeal membrane oxygenation (ECMO) service. There are 5 calls today, but only one machine and one technologist available. Which of the following patients is the most appropriate recipient of this service?

a. A 1-day-old, full-term, anencephalic 4-kg boy suffering from meconium aspiration syndrome and hypoxia
b. A 75-year-old man with Alzheimer disease, severe pneumonia, and elevated pulmonary arterial pressure
c. A neonate with a diagnosis of severe pulmonary hypoplasia who is in respiratory failure
d. A 5-year-old girl with rhabdomyosarcoma metastatic to the lungs
e. A 3-day-old boy preoperative for a congenital diaphragmatic hernia

82. A 72-year-old man has multiple injuries and an altered sensorium after a high-speed motor vehicle collision. He is intubated for his decreased mental status. During intubation, a large amount of gastric contents are noted in the posterior pharynx and he aspirates. Which of the following is the appropriate initial treatment?

a. Bronchoscopy for aspiration of particulate matter
b. Steroids
c. Prophylactic antibiotics
d. Inhaled nitric oxide
e. High positive end-expiratory pressure

83. A patient with severe neurological devastation after head trauma has a prolonged course in the intensive care unit. He has been mechanically ventilated for his entire hospital stay. Which of the following clinical findings is diagnostic of a ventilator-associated pneumonia?

a. White blood cell count of greater than 12,000/mL
b. Greater than 10,000 colony-forming U/mL of an organism on bronchoalveolar lavage
c. Greater than 10,000 colony-forming U/mL of an organism on bronchoalveolar lavage
d. Purulent tracheal secretions
e. Right lower lobe infiltrate on chest x-ray

84. Shortly after the administration of an inhalational anesthetic and succinylcholine for intubation prior to an elective inguinal hernia repair in a 10-year-old boy, he becomes markedly febrile, displays a tachycardia of 160, and his urine changes color to a dark red. Which of the following is the most appropriate treatment at this time?

a. Complete the procedure but pretreat with dantrolene prior to future elective surgery.
b. Administer inhalational anesthetic agents.
c. Administer succinylcholine.
d. Hyperventilate with 100% O_2.
e. Acidify the urine to prevent myoglobin precipitation in the renal tubules.

85. A 42-year-old man has had a rocky course for the 3 days following a bowel resection for intestinal perforation due to inflammatory bowel disease. His CVP had been 12 to 14 but is now 6, in the face of diminished blood pressure and oliguria. Which of the following is the most likely etiology of his hypotension?

a. Pulmonary embolism
b. Hypervolemia
c. Positive-pressure ventilation
d. Pneumothorax
e. Gram-negative sepsis

86. Acute renal failure occurs following aortic angiography in a 72-year-old man. His weight has been rising, his lungs show rales at both bases, and he is dyspneic. His fractional excretion of sodium is greater than 1. He has eosinophilia on his peripheral smear, an elevated erythrocyte sedimentation rate, and proteinuria with microscopic hematuria. Which of the following is the most likely cause of his renal failure?

a. Hypovolemia
b. Renal artery cholesterol embolism
c. Acute tubular necrosis
d. Cardiogenic shock
e. Aortic dissection

87. A 55-year-old woman has been hospitalized because of recurrent pancreatitis, ARDS, prolonged ileus, and need for parenteral nutrition. She demonstrates weakness, lassitude, orthostatic hypotension, nausea, and fever. Which of the following abnormalities is most likely to explain these symptoms?

a. Hypothermia
b. Hypokalemia
c. Hyperglycemia
d. Hyponatremia
e. Hypervolemia

88. A 19-year-old man sustains severe lower-extremity trauma, including a femur fracture and a crush injury to his foot. He requires vascular reconstruction of the popliteal artery. On the day after surgery, he becomes dyspneic and hypoxemic and requires intubation and mechanical ventilation. Which of the following is the most likely etiology of his decompensation?

a. Aspiration
b. Atelectasis
c. Fat embolism syndrome
d. Fluid overload
e. Pneumonia

89. A 33-year-old woman is brought to the emergency room from the scene of a severe motor vehicle accident. She is combative, confused, uncooperative, and appears dusky and dyspneic. Which of the following is the most appropriate management of her airway?

a. Awake endotracheal intubation is indicated in patients with penetrating ocular injury.
b. Steroids have been shown to be of value in the treatment of aspiration of acidic gastric secretions.
c. The stomach may be assumed to be empty only if a history is obtained indicating no ingestion of food or liquid during the prior 8 hours.
d. Intubation should be performed as soon as possible (in the emergency room) if the patient is unstable.
e. Cricothyroidotomy is contraindicated in the presence of maxillofacial injuries.

90. Following a boating injury in an industrial-use river, a patient begins to display fever, tachycardia, and a rapidly expanding area of erythema, blistering, and drainage from a flank wound. An x-ray shows gas in the soft tissues. Which of the following measures is most appropriate?

a. Administration of an antifungal agent
b. Administration of antitoxin
c. Wide debridement
d. Administration of hyperbaric O_2
e. Early closure of tissue defects

91. Following pelvic gynecologic surgery, a 34-year-old woman becomes dyspneic, her peripheral arterial O_2 saturation falls from 94% to 81%, and her measured PaO_2 is 52 on a 100% non-rebreather mask. She is hemodynamically stable. A CT angiogram is consistent with a right lower lobe pulmonary embolus. Which of the following is the next step in her management?

a. Systemic anticoagulation with heparin infusion
b. Systemic anticoagulation with warfarin
c. Placement of an inferior vena cava filter
d. Thrombolytic therapy
e. Open pulmonary embolectomy

92. A 72-year-old woman who is planning to undergo ventral hernia repair is on warfarin for atrial fibrillation. She is advised to cease her warfarin several days before her surgery and is hospitalized preoperatively for heparinization. During her hospital stay, she complains of severe abdominal and flank pain. Her prothrombin time (PT) is normal, but her activated partial thromboplastin time (aPTT) is elevated. An abdominal CT scan demonstrates a large retroperitoneal hematoma. Which of the following should be administered to reverse the effects of the heparin?

a. Thrombin
b. Vitamin K
c. Protamine sulfate
d. Aprotinin
e. Platelet transfusion

93. A 42-year-old man who was in a house fire is transferred to your burn unit. He has singed nose hairs and facial burns. Direct laryngoscopy in the emergency room demonstrates pharyngeal edema and mucosal sloughing. He has 60% total body surface area burns. Which of the following is the next step in the management of this patient?

a. Hyperbaric oxygen
b. Intravenous steroids
c. Inhaled steroids
d. Bronchoscopy
e. Intubation

94. A 24-year-old man presents in septic shock from an empyema. He is febrile to 103°F, tachycardic in the 120s, and hypotensive to the 90s. His oxygen saturation is 98% on 2-L oxygen. His white blood cell count is 25,000/mL and creatinine is 0.8 mg/dL. His blood pressure does not respond to fluid administration despite a CVP of 15. Which of the following therapies is indicated in managing this patient?

a. Intubation
b. Recombinant human activated protein C
c. Epinephrine
d. Norepinephrine
e. Dobutamine

Questions 95 to 97

Match the side effects with the appropriate agent. Each lettered option may be used once, more than once, or not at all.

a. Nitrous oxide (N_2O)
b. Succinylcholine
c. Midazolam
d. Pancuronium
e. Morphine

95. A 65-year-old man with a 35% body surface area (BSA) burn develops hyperkalemia after induction.

96. An acutely injured patient becomes hypotensive shortly after induction.

97. A patient with a bowel obstruction develops increasingly distended loops of bowel after induction.

Questions 98 to 100

For each clinical problem, select the best method of physiologic monitoring necessary for the patient. Each lettered option may be used once, more than once, or not at all.

a. Central venous catheterization
b. Pulmonary artery catheterization
c. Blood-gas monitoring
d. Intracranial pressure monitoring
e. Arterial catheterization
f. Continuous ECG monitoring

98. A 74-year-old man has a 5-hour elective operation for repair of an abdominal aortic aneurysm. He had a small myocardial infarction 3 years earlier. In the ICU on the first postoperative day, he is hypotensive and is receiving dobutamine by continuous infusion.

99. A 62-year-old woman underwent a right carotid endarterectomy for symptomatic high-grade carotid artery stenosis. Postoperatively, her blood pressure is 202/105 mm Hg, and she is started on a nitroprusside infusion.

100. A comatose 28-year-old woman sustained a depressed skull fracture in an automobile collision. She has been unconscious for 6 weeks. Her vital signs are stable and she breathes room air. Following her initial decompressive craniotomy, she has returned to the operating room twice due to intracranial bleeding.

Questions 101 to 103

For each test, select the coagulation factor(s) whose functions are measured. Each lettered option may be used once, more than once, or not at all.

a. Factor II
b. Factor V
c. Factor VIII
d. Platelets
e. Fibrinogen

101. A patient is receiving oral warfarin to effect anticoagulation because of an artificial heart valve. Prothrombin time is 21 (INR = 2.3).

102. A patient with heparin-induced thrombocytopenia is placed on hirudin and undergoes assessment of his clotting function. Thrombin time is 30 seconds.

103. A patient is to undergo a coronary bypass. Bleeding time is 6 minutes.

Critical Care: Anesthesiology, Blood Gases, and Respiratory Care

Answers

50. The answer is c. (*Brunicardi, p 329.*) The patient had a sentinel bleed from a tracheoinnominate artery fistula, which carries a greater than 50% mortality rate. If the bleeding has ceased, then immediate fiberoptic exploration in the operating room is indicated. If the bleeding is ongoing, several stopgap measures can be attempted while preparing for median sternotomy in the operating room, including inflation of the tracheostomy balloon to attempt compression of the innominate artery, reintubation of the patient with an endotracheal tube, and removal of the tracheostomy and placement of the finger through the site with anterior compression of the innominate artery.

51. The answer is d. (*Brunicardi, p 332; Townsend, pp 617-618.*) There are multiple predictors that have been used to assess readiness for extubation. No single parameter is 100% predictive; attempted extubation should be based on correction of the underlying pathology, clinical status and hemodynamic stability, and a combination of the following parameters. The rapid shallow breathing index is the ratio of the respiratory rate to tidal volume. There is evidence to suggest that an index between 60 and 105 predicts successful extubation. The negative inspiratory force should be at least greater than −20 cm H_2O. The patient should be weaned to 5 cm H_2O PEEP before attempting extubation. The minute ventilation, which is the product of the tidal volume and respiratory rate, should be less than 10 L/min. The spontaneous respiratory rate should also be below 20 breaths per minute.

52. The answer is e. (*Brunicardi, pp 81-83.*) Whenever a hemolytic reaction caused by an incompatible blood transfusion is suspected, transfusion should be stopped immediately. A Foley catheter should be inserted and hourly urine output should be monitored. Renal damage caused by precipitation of hemoglobin in the renal tubules is the major serious consequence of hemolysis. This precipitation is inhibited in an alkaline environment and is promoted in an acid environment. Stimulating diuresis with mannitol and alkalinizing the urine with sodium bicarbonate intravenously are indicated procedures. Fluid and potassium intake should be restricted in the presence of severe oliguria or anuria.

53. The answer is b. (*Townsend, p 432.*) Nitrous oxide has a low solubility compared with other inhalation anesthetics; nitrous oxide is more soluble in blood than nitrogen and is the only anesthetic gas less dense than air. As a result of these properties, nitrous oxide may cause progressive distension of air-filled spaces during prolonged anesthesia. Since nitrous oxide diffuses into gas-filled compartments faster than nitrogen can diffuse out, its use can lead to worsened distention, which may be undesirable (eg, in an operation for intestinal obstruction).

54. The answer is a. (*Brunicardi, p 332.*) Adult respiratory distress syndrome has been called "shock lung" or "traumatic wet lung" and occurs under a variety of circumstances. The diagnosis can be made based on bilateral pulmonary infiltrates on chest x-ray, a PaO_2/FiO_2 ratio of less than 200, and pulmonary wedge pressures of less than 18 mm Hg (low filling pressures exclude the diagnosis of pulmonary edema). Three major physiologic alterations include (1) hypoxemia usually unresponsive to elevations of inspired O_2 concentration; (2) decreased pulmonary compliance, as the lungs become progressively stiffer and harder to ventilate; and (3) decreased functional residual capacity. Progressive alveolar collapse occurs owing to leakage of protein-rich fluid into the interstitium and the alveolar spaces with the subsequent radiologic picture of diffuse fluffy infiltrates bilaterally. Ventilatory abnormalities develop that result in shunt formation, decreased resting lung volume, and increased dead-space ventilation.

55. The answer is d. (*Brunicardi, pp 1748-1749.*) The curve depicted here plots the normal relationship of arterial PO_2 and percentage of hemoglobin saturation with other variables controlled at pH 7.4, $PaCO_2$ 40 mm Hg, temperature 37°C (98.6°F), and hemoglobin 15 g/dL. The only intervention listed that shifts the oxygen dissociation curve to the right to promote tissue oxygen uptake is to increase the $Paco_2$. Acidosis, a rise in $Paco_2$, and elevation of temperature all shift the curve to the right. Red blood cell organic phosphates, particularly 2,3-diphosphoglycerate (2,3-DPG), also affect the dissociation curve. Banked blood, being low in 2,3-DPG, shifts the curve to the left and therefore decreases tissue O_2 uptake. 2,3-DPG levels increase with chronic hypoxia. Chronic lung disease, therefore, results in a shift of the curve to the right, which enhances O_2 delivery to peripheral tissues. Acute anemia does not shift the curve but does lower the oxygen content of blood.

56. The answer is e. *(Brunicardi, pp 59-60.)* The patient is suffering from respiratory acidosis, caused by the accumulation of CO_2, and hypoxemia. Both disturbances can be resolved with endotracheal intubation and ventilatory support. Agitation can be an early sign of hypoxemia in an elderly patient and should never be ignored. Benzodiazepines such as Ativan in this patient will cause stupor and worsen his hypoxemia and respiratory acidosis. Bicarbonate should not be administered because buffer reserves are already adequate (serum bicarbonate is still 34 mEq/L based on the Henderson-Hasselbalch equation).

57. The answer is b. *(Townsend, pp 95-96.)* Dopamine has a variety of pharmacologic characteristics that make it useful in critically ill patients. At all doses, the diastolic blood pressure can be expected to rise; since coronary perfusion is largely a result of the head of pressure at the coronary ostia, coronary blood flow should be increased. In low doses (1-5 mg/[kg·min]), dopamine affects primarily the dopaminergic receptors. Activation of these receptors causes vasodilation of the renal and mesenteric vasculature and mild vasoconstriction of the peripheral bed, which thereby redirects blood flow to kidneys and bowel. At these low doses, the net effect on the overall vascular resistance may be slight. As the dose rises (2-10 mg/[kg·min]), β_1-receptor activity predominates and the inotropic effect on the myocardium leads to increased cardiac output and blood pressure. Above 10 mg/ (kg·min), α-receptor stimulation causes peripheral vasoconstriction, shifting of blood from extremities to organs, decreased kidney function, and hypertension.

58. The answer is d. *(Brunicardi, pp 81-83.)* The patient has TRALI or transfusion-related acute lung injury which manifests as respiratory distress, hypoxemia, and bilateral pulmonary infiltrates not due to volume overload.

The treatment of choice is respiratory support, including mechanical ventilation, as needed. The major risk factor for TRALI is transfusion of any plasma-containing blood products from multiparous female donors. Other complications of transfusions and their treatments include: (1) allergic reactions such as rash and fever—mild reactions are treated with an antihistamine; (2) transfusion-associated circulation overload (TACO) which occurs in patients with underlying heart failure who receive large volume transfusions—the treatment is administration of diuretics; and hemolytic reactions—diagnosis is made by a positive Coombs test and treatment is to stop the transfusion and identify the responsible antigen to prevent future reactions. There is no evidence that the patient has pneumonia or any other indication to perform bronchoscopy or to start antibiotics.

59. The answer is c. (*Brunicardi, pp 723-730.*) A ruptured abdominal aneurysm is a surgical emergency often accompanied by serious hypotension and vascular collapse before surgery and massive fluid shifts with renal failure after surgery. In this case, all the hemodynamic parameters indicate inadequate intravascular volume, and the patient is therefore suffering from hypovolemic shock. The low urine output indicates poor renal perfusion, while the high urine-specific gravity indicates adequate renal function with compensatory free-water conservation. The administration of a vasopressor agent would certainly raise the blood pressure, but it would do so by increasing peripheral vascular resistance and thereby further decrease tissue perfusion. The deleterious effects of shock would be increased. A vasodilating agent to lower the systemic vascular resistance would lead to profound hypotension and possibly complete vascular collapse because of pooling of an already depleted vascular volume. This patient's blood pressure is critically dependent on an elevated systemic vascular resistance. A diuretic would exacerbate the patient's existing volume depletion. To properly treat this patient, rapid fluid infusion and expansion of the intravascular volume must be undertaken. This can be easily done with lactated Ringer solution or blood (or both) until improvements in such parameters as the PCWP, urine output, and blood pressure are noted.

60. The answer is e. (*Townsend, pp 94-96.*) This patient has developed pump failure because of a combination of preexisting coronary artery occlusive disease and high preload following a fluid challenge; afterload remains moderately high as well because of systemic vasoconstriction in the presence of cardiogenic shock. Poor myocardial performance is reflected in the low cardiac output and high PCWP. Therapy must be directed at increasing cardiac output without creating too high a myocardial O_2 demand on the already failing heart. Administration of nitroglycerin could be expected to reduce both preload and afterload, but, if given without an inotrope, it would create unacceptable hypotension. Nitroprusside similarly would achieve afterload reduction but would result in hypotension if not accompanied by an inotropic agent. A β-blocker would act deleteriously by reducing cardiac contractility and slowing the heart rate in a setting in which cardiac output is likely to be rate-dependent. Dobutamine is a synthetic catecholamine that is becoming the inotropic agent of choice in cardiogenic shock. As a $β_1$-adrenergic agonist, it improves cardiac performance in pump failure both by positive inotropy and peripheral vasodilation. With minimal chronotropic effect, dobutamine only marginally increases myocardial O_2 demand.

61. The answer is d. *(Brunicardi, pp 1734-1740.)* Thoracic epidural narcotics have become an increasingly popular means of postoperative pain relief in thoracic and upper abdominal surgery. Local action on γ-opiate receptors ensures pain relief and consequent improvement in respiration without vasodilation or paralysis. The less lipid-soluble opiates are effective for long periods. Their slow absorption into the circulation also ensures a low incidence of centrally mediated side effects, such as respiratory depression or generalized itching. When these do occur, the intravenous injection of an opiate antagonist is an effective antidote. The locally mediated analgesia is not affected. One poorly understood side effect, which is apparently unrelated to systemic levels, is a profound reduction in gastric activity. This may be an important consideration after thoracic surgery when an early resumption of oral intake is anticipated.

62. The answer is c. *(Brunicardi, pp 346-353.)* The cardiac index is computed by dividing the cardiac output by the body surface area; the cardiac output is the product of the stroke volume and the heart rate (CI = CO/BSA; CO = SV × HR; therefore, CI = [SV × HR]/BSA). An increased heart rate will directly increase the cardiac output and cardiac index. The remaining choices will either decrease or not affect the stroke volume and consequently will not increase the cardiac index.

63. The answer is c. *(Brunicardi, p 1147-1148.)* The development of acute postoperative cholecystitis is an increasingly recognized complication of the severe illnesses that precipitate admissions to the ICU. The causes are obscure but probably lead to a common final pathway of gallbladder ischemia. The diagnosis is often extremely difficult because the signs and symptoms may be those of occult sepsis. Moreover, the patients are often intubated, sedated, or confused as a consequence of the other therapeutic or medical factors. Biochemical tests, though frequently revealing abnormal liver function, are nonspecific and nondiagnostic. Bedside ultrasonography is usually strongly suggestive of the diagnosis when a thickened gallbladder wall or pericholecystic fluid is present; nonvisualization of the gallbladder on a nuclear medicine (HIDA) scan can also be diagnostic. If diagnosis is delayed, mortality and morbidity are very high. Percutaneous drainage of the gallbladder is usually curative of acalculous cholecystitis and affords stabilizing palliation if calculous cholecystitis is present. Antibiotics without drainage are too cautious a choice for a patient with a potentially fatal complication. Operative intervention is indicated only if less invasive methods of treatment (percutaneous cholecystostomy tube) have failed, and ERCP is not indicated in the absence of ductal obstruction.

64. The answer is a. *(Townsend, pp 102-107.)* The case presented is most consistent with septic shock from a postoperative intra-abdominal abscess. In the early phase of septic shock, the respiratory profile is characterized by mild hypoxia with a compensatory hyperventilation and respiratory alkalosis. Hemodynamically, a hyperdynamic state is seen with an increase in cardiac output and a decrease in peripheral vascular resistance in the face of relatively normal central pressures. Initial therapy is aimed at resuscitation and stabilization. This includes fluid replacement and vasopressors as well as antibiotic therapy aimed particularly at gram-negative rods and anaerobes for patients with presumed intra-abdominal collections, especially after bowel surgery. Laparotomy and drainage of a collection is the definitive therapy but should await stabilization of the patient and confirmation of the presence and location of such a collection.

65. The answer is d. *(Moore, pp 1267-1268.)* PEEP improves oxygenation by increasing functional residual capacity by keeping the alveoli open at the end of expiration. Extravascular lung water is shifted from the alveolar to the interstitial space. The overall result is to increase surface area for diffusive exchange of gases. Potential negative effects of increased PEEP include alveolar overdistention resulting in barotraumas (pneumothoraces), decreased venous return and decreased cardiac output, and increased minute ventilation requirements due to increased dead-space ventilation.

66. The answer is c. *(Moore, pp 172-173.)* On physical examination, cardiac tamponade may manifest with Beck triad (systemic hypotension, jugular venous distention, and distant heart sounds). Also, the patient may have pulsus paradoxus, which is manifested by a decrease in systolic blood pressure by more than 10 mm Hg at the end of the inspiratory phase of respiration. On echocardiogram, there will be pericardial fluid and right atrial collapse. On Swan-Ganz monitoring, there will be equalization of pressures across the four chambers. The right atrial pressures and central venous pressure are increased and cardiac output is decreased.

67. The answer is c. *(Brunicardi, pp 629-633.)* The planned operation is a high-risk procedure. Clinical markers used to predict cardiac events during noncardiac surgery include the New York Heart Association functional classification and the Canadian Cardiovascular Society angina classification systems. Patients can be stratified as having major, intermediate, or mild predictors of having a cardiac event. Major predictors include unstable angina, recent myocardial infarction, decompensated congestive heart failure, significant arrhythmias, and severe valvular disease. Intermediate predictors include mild angina, prior myocardial infarction, compensated or prior congestive heart failure, diabetes, and renal insufficiency. Minor predictors include advanced age, abnormal electrocardiogram, irregular rhythm, poor functional capacity, prior stroke, and uncontrolled hypertension.

68. The answer is a. *(Townsend, pp 449-451.)* The maximal safe total dose of lidocaine administered to a 70-kg person is 4.5 mg/kg, or approximately 30 to 35 mL of a 1% solution. The addition of epinephrine to lidocaine, procaine, or bupivacaine not only doubles the duration of infiltration anesthesia, but increases the maximal safe total dose by one-third (eg, 7 mg/kg for lidocaine with epinephrine) by decreasing the rate of absorption of drug into the bloodstream. However, epinephrine-containing solutions should not be injected into tissues supplied by end arteries (eg, fingers, toes, ears, nose, penis). Hypersensitivity to local anesthetics is uncommon and occurs most prominently with anesthetics of the ester type (procaine, tetracaine). While small nerve fibers seem to be most susceptible to the action of local anesthetics, these agents act on any part of the nervous system and on every type of nerve fiber. CNS toxicity usually appears as stimulation followed by depression, probably because of an early selective depression of inhibitory neurons; with a massive overdose, all neurons may be depressed simultaneously.

69. The answer is d. *(Brunicardi, pp 107-108.)* The patient is in neurogenic shock as a result of a spinal cord injury. Neurogenic shock is characterized by loss of sympathetic tone peripherally as well as bradycardia owing to loss of the reflexive increase in heart rate in response to hypotension. Initial treatment is with fluid resuscitation followed by initiation of vasoconstrictors such as dopamine or phenylephrine. Hypovolemia caused by hemorrhage should also be ruled out in trauma patients.

70. The answer is d. *(Brunicardi, p 328.)* While other complications such as tension pneumothorax/hemothorax or arrhythmias can occur as a result of central venous catheter insertion, the scenario is most consistent with an air embolism, which can occur during central venous catheter placement or removal. The initial maneuvers when air embolism is suspected are to place the patient in a left lateral decubitus Trendelenburg (head-down) position and to aspirate the central venous catheter. Depending on the volume of air infused into the central venous catheter, symptoms can range from subclinical to fatal. Although thoracotomy may be necessary ultimately for treatment of an air embolism, immediate bilateral thoracotomy and aortic cross-clamping is not indicated. Decompression of the right chest with a needle or placement of a right chest tube would be appropriate maneuvers if a tension pneumothorax were suspected; a chest tube would be the treatment of choice for suspected hemothorax. Withdrawal of the central venous catheter or wire is appropriate if arrhythmias occur during line insertion.

71. The answer is a. *(Brunicardi, pp 1734-1739.)* The family history is suggestive of a pseudocholinesterase deficiency which prolongs the effects of succinylcholine, a depolarizing neuromuscular blocking agent, as well as of mivacurium, a non-depolarizing agent. Vecuronium, pancuronium, and cis-atracurium are other non-depolarizing agents that are not affected by this enzyme deficiency. Etomidate is used for rapid sequence induction and is not affected by pseudocholinesterase deficiency; etomidate does block steroid synthesis and has been associated with acute adrenal insufficiency, but the clinical relevance of the resultant insufficiency is controversial.

72. The answer is b. *(Mulholland, pp 149-153.)* This patient is having an anaphylactoid reaction with destabilization of the cardiovascular and respiratory systems. Anaphylactoid reactions are most commonly caused by iodinated contrast media, β-lactam antibiotics (eg, penicillin), and

Hymenoptera stings. Manifestations of anaphylactoid reactions include both lethal (bronchospasm, laryngospasm, hypotension, dysrhythmia) and nonlethal (pruritus, urticaria, syncope, weakness, seizure) phenomena. Epinephrine is the initial treatment for laryngeal obstruction and bronchospasm, followed by histamine antagonists (H_1 and H_2 blockers), aminophylline, and hydrocortisone. Vasopressors and fluid challenges may be given for shock. Conscious patients are usually stabilized with injected or inhaled epinephrine, while unconscious patients and those with refractory hypotension or hypoxia should be intubated.

73. The answer is e. *(Brunicardi, pp 81-83.)* Most transfusion reactions are hemolytic and are due to clerical errors that result in administration of blood with major (ABO) and minor antigen incompatibility. Intravascular hemolysis results in hemoglobinemia. Because haptoglobin binds hemoglobin via a receptor located on macrophages, serum haptoglobin levels are decreased; haptoglobin level less than 50 mg/dL is one criterion for a transfusion reaction. Additionally, hemoglobinuria with a free hemoglobin level greater than 5 mg/dL is another criterion. A positive Coombs test is diagnostic. Indirect hyperbilirubinemia and anemia may be seen in delayed transfusion reactions, which occur between 2 and 10 days after a transfusion. Delayed transfusion reactions can occur due to antibodies to Rh antigens and are characterized by extravascular hemolysis.

74. The answer is e. *(Mulholland, pp 167-168; Brunicardi, pp 128-129.)* Transfusion of 2 units of packed red blood cells will increase the patient's oxygen delivery the most. Mixed venous oxygen saturation reflects the difference between the oxygen delivered to the tissues and the oxygen taken up by the tissues. Oxygen delivery is the product of cardiac index and oxygen content of blood (CaO_2), the latter of which is determined primarily by hemoglobin (Hb) concentration. Oxygen saturation (SaO_2) and the partial pressure of oxygen (PaO_2) contribute much less. The formula for oxygen content (CaO_2) can be expressed as $CaO_2 = 1.36 \times Hb \times SaO_2/100 + 0.0031 \times PaO_2$. Since the patient's oxygen saturation is 100%, increasing his inspired oxygen concentration is unlikely to increase his oxygen delivery. Since the contribution of PaO_2 is so low, hyperbaric oxygen is also not the treatment of choice. Furthermore, transporting unstable patients to the hyperbaric chamber can be dangerous. Correction of the patient's anemia by the most expeditious manner, that is, transfusion of blood, is the treatment of choice.

75. The answer is c. (*Brunicardi, p 60.*) Because of the ease with which CO_2 diffuses across the alveolar membranes, $PaCO_2$ is a highly reliable indicator of alveolar ventilation. In this postoperative patient with respiratory acidosis and hypoxemia, the hypercarbia is diagnostic of alveolar hypoventilation. Acute hypoxemia can occur with pulmonary embolism, pulmonary edema, and significant atelectasis, but in all those situations the $PaCO_2$ should be normal or reduced, as the patient hyperventilates to improve oxygenation. The absorption of gas from the peritoneal cavity may transiently affect the $PaCO_2$, but should have no effect on oxygenation.

76. The answer is c. (*Townsend, pp 1484-1485.*) The serum albumin level provides a rough estimate of protein nutritional adequacy. The accuracy of this estimate is affected by the long half-life of albumin (3 weeks) and the vagaries of hemodilution. Prealbumin, which has a short half-life (2 days), may be a better indicator of his short-term nutritional status. The acute-phase serum proteins (such as C-reactive protein, haptoglobin, fibrinogen, and ferritin) also have a very short half-life (hours) and may also provide good short-term indications of nutritional status. Transferrin is one of these acute-phase proteins, but unfortunately its levels, too, are influenced by changes in intravascular volume and, along with the other acute-phase reactants, rise nonspecifically during acute illness. All the listed responses provide some useful information about nutrition and adequacy of replacement.

77. The answer is d. (*Brunicardi, p 332.*) The respiratory quotient (RQ) is the ratio of the rate of carbon dioxide production over the rate of oxygen uptake. An RQ of 0.75 to 0.85 is ideal. The RQ is dependent on the composition of nutritional support. An RQ of 0.7 indicates a diet comprised largely of lipids. An RQ of 1 or greater indicates a diet comprising primarily carbohydrates, which can impair weaning from the ventilator. Decreasing the carbohydrates in the enteral feeds would facilitate the patient's ventilator wean. Changing ventilator settings by decreasing the inspired concentration of oxygen or the rate may be indicated as part of the ventilator wean, but these will not affect the RQ.

78. The answer is e. (*Brunicardi, p 329.*) A rare but deadly complication of a tracheostomy is a tracheoinnominate artery fistula (TIAF); when suspected, the diagnosis should be confirmed or ruled out in the operating room. TIAFs can occur as early as 2 days after tracheostomy or as late as

2 months after the procedure. It is often associated with low placement of a tracheostomy (distal to the second and third tracheal rings). The patient may have a sentinel bleed in 50% of TIAF cases, followed by a very impressive bleed. If a sentinel bleed is suspected, the patient should be transported immediately to the operating room for bronchoscopic evaluation. Initial maneuvers for management of a TIAF include overinflation of the cuff on the tracheostomy or reintubation from above followed by removal of the tracheostomy and finger compression of the innominate artery against the sternum through the tracheostomy wound.

79. The answer is b. *(Brunicardi, pp 338-339.)* Shivering is the physiologic effort of the body to generate heat to maintain the core temperature. In healthy persons, shivering increases the metabolic rate by 3 to 5 times and results in increased O_2 consumption and CO_2 production. In critically ill patients, these metabolic consequences are almost always counterproductive and should be prevented with other means employed to correct systemic hypothermia. In the presence of vigorous shivering, O_2 debt in the muscles and lactic acidemia develop.

80. The answer is d. *(Townsend, pp 118-119.)* Von Willebrand disease is similar to true hemophilia in frequency of occurrence. It is being diagnosed more commonly today because of more reliable assays for factor VIII. This autosomal dominant disorder (recessive transmission can occur) is characterized by a diminution in factor VIII: C (procoagulant) activity. The reduction in activity is not as great as in classic hemophilia, and the clinical manifestations are more subtle. These manifestations are often overlooked until an episode of trauma or surgery makes them apparent. Treatment requires correcting the bleeding time and providing factor VIII R: WF (the von Willebrand factor). Only cryoprecipitate is reliably effective. High-purity factor VIII: C concentrates, effective in hemophilia, lack the von Willebrand factor and are consequently undependable.

81. The answer is e. *(Townsend, pp 2050-2051.)* ECMO is a form of cardiopulmonary support that is useful in the setting of potentially reversible pulmonary or cardiac disease. Treatment of meconium aspiration syndrome, sepsis, pneumonia, and congenital diaphragmatic hernia (pre- or postoperatively) are thus appropriate uses. The technique is also applicable in some circumstances as a bridge to cardiac or lung transplantation since the outlook for survival is quite good if the child can be maintained in a good physiological state until donor organs are available. Hypoplastic lungs do not have enough surface area to perform adequate gas exchange and are unlikely to mature to a point where they can sustain life. Babies with hypoplastic lungs will be bypass-dependent for life and consequently are not candidates for institution of ECMO therapy.

82. The answer is a. (*Moore, pp 383-384; Brunicardi, p 331.*) Bronchoscopy is indicated for aspiration pneumonitis if there is particulate matter in the tracheobronchial tree. Prophylactic antibiotics are not indicated after gross aspiration, which results in a chemical pneumonitis. Antibiotics are indicated only if pneumonia develops. Steroids and inhaled nitric oxide are not indicated for aspiration pneumonitis. High positive end-expiratory pressure is not required in patients unless respiratory failure develops.

83. The answer is c. (*Mulholland, pp 462-463.*) While findings such as fever, leukocytosis, purulent secretions, or a focal infiltrate on chest x-ray are suspicious for ventilator-associated pneumonia (VAP), quantitative cultures are diagnostic. Samples may be obtained using bronchoscopy with bronchoalveolar lavage (BAL). Greater than or equal to 10,000 colony-forming U/mL of a single organism is diagnostic for VAP. Empiric antibiotics may be initiated after cultures are obtained based on clinical suspicion, but antibiotic coverage should be narrowed or stopped once an organism is identified to minimize development of resistant organisms.

84. The answer is d. (*Brunicardi, pp 1750-1751.*) The cause of malignant hyperthermia is unknown, but it is associated with inhalational anesthetic agents and succinylcholine. It may develop in an otherwise healthy person who has tolerated previous surgery without incident. It should be suspected in the presence of a history of unexplained fever, muscle or connective tissue disorder, or a positive family history (evidence suggests an autosomal dominant inheritance pattern). In addition to fever during anesthesia, the syndrome includes tachycardia, increased O_2 consumption, increased CO_2 production, increased serum K^+, myoglobinuria, and acidosis. Rigidity rather than relaxation following succinylcholine injection may be the first clue to its presence. Treatment of malignant hyperthermia should include prompt conclusion of the operative procedure and cessation of anesthesia, hyperventilation with 100% O_2, and administration of intravenous dantrolene. The urine should be alkalinized to protect the kidneys from myoglobin precipitation. If reoperation is necessary, the physician should premedicate heavily, alkalinize the urine, and avoid depolarizing agents such as succinylcholine. Pretreatment for 24 hours with dantrolene is helpful; it is thought to act directly on muscle fiber to attenuate calcium release.

85. The answer is e. (*Moore, pp 1196-1197.*) Determination of CVP can be helpful in the overall hemodynamic assessment of the patient. This pressure can be affected by a variety of factors, including those of cardiac, noncardiac, and artifactual origin. Venous tone, right ventricular compliance, intrathoracic pressure, and blood volume all influence CVP. Vasoconstrictor drugs, positive-pressure ventilation (with and without PEEP), mediastinal compression, and hypervolemia all increase CVP. Acute pulmonary embolism, when clinically significant, elevates CVP by causing right ventricular overload and increased right atrial pressure. Sepsis, on the other hand, decreases CVP through both the release of vasodilatory mediators and the loss of intravascular plasma volume due to increased capillary permeability. Trends in CVP measurement are more reliable than isolated readings.

CVP, along with other hemodynamic parameters (see table below), can also be useful in differentiating septic shock from other etiologies of shock; shock is inadequate tissue perfusion. Septic shock has two phases: (1) a hypodynamic phase that is characterized by hypovolemia and myocardial depression and (2) a hyperdynamic phase that follows fluid resuscitation and is characterized by a normal to increased cardiac output.

	Hypovolemic Shock	Septic Shock– Hyperdynamic	Septic Shock– Hypodynamic	Neurogenic Shock	Cardiogenic Shock
Central venous pressure (CVP)	Decreased	Increased or decreased	Increased or decreased	Decreased	Increased
Cardiac output (CO)	Decreased	Increased	Decreased	Decreased	Decreased
Systemic vascular resistance (SVR)	Increased	Decreased	Increased	Decreased	Increased
Venous oxygen saturation (Svo_2)	Decreased	Increased	Increased or decreased	Decreased	Decreased

Modified, with permission, from Fauci AS, Kasper DL, Braunwald E, et al. Harrison's Principles of Internal Medicine, 17th ed. New York: McGraw-Hill; 2008: Table 270-4.

86. The answer is b. (*Mulholland, pp 181-182, 1543-1544.*) Cholesterol atheroembolism is a known complication of angiography or aortic manipulation during surgery and can result in lower extremity ischemia, acute myocardial infarction, ischemic bowel, and acute or chronic renal failure. Eosinophilia is strongly suggestive of cholesterol atheroembolization, and other laboratory findings include microscopic hematuria or proteinuria and elevated inflammatory mediators such as erythrocyte sedimentation rate. A fractional excretion of sodium (FENa) of greater than 1 suggests a renal cause of acute renal failure as opposed to prerenal causes such as hypovolemia or cardiogenic shock. Thoracic aortic dissections can result in acute renal failure if they involve the renal arteries and may present with hematuria and elevations in BUN and creatinine. However, aortic dissections are typically associated with significant chest pain.

87. The answer is d. (*Brunicardi, pp 1402-1403.*) Clinical manifestations of adrenocortical insufficiency include hyperkalemia, hyponatremia, hypoglycemia, fever, weight loss, and dehydration. There is excessive sodium loss in the urine, contraction of the plasma volume, and perhaps hypotension or shock. Classic hyperpigmentation is present in chronic Addison disease only. Addison disease may present in newborns as a congenital atrophy, as an insidious chronic state often caused by tuberculosis, as an acute dysfunction secondary to trauma or adrenal hemorrhage, or as a semiacute adrenal insufficiency seen during stress or surgery. In this last instance, signs and symptoms include nausea, lassitude, vomiting, fever, progressive salt wasting, hyperkalemia, and hypoglycemia. It may be confirmed by measurements of urinary Na$^+$ loss and absence of response to adrenocorticotropic hormone (ACTH).

88. The answer is c. (*Moore, p 412.*) Fat embolism syndrome is a relatively uncommon complication of long-bone fractures and is characterized by acute respiratory failure, altered mental status, and petechiae. Unfortunately, there are no reliable diagnostic tests, and management is supportive only. Pulmonary edema is unlikely in an otherwise healthy 19-year-old male without chest trauma or evidence of a cardiac contusion. Aspiration is unlikely in an awake patient with normal mental status. Pneumonias typically present with fever and/or leukocytosis, productive cough, and a new infiltrate on chest x-ray. Atelectasis in and of itself is not a cause for respiratory failure.

89. The answer is d. *(Moore, pp 189-194.)* Securing a stable airway is one of the most fundamental and important aspects of the management of the severely injured patient. The level of control required will vary from a simple oropharyngeal airway to tracheostomy, depending on the clinical situation. Full control of the airway should be secured in the emergency room if the patient is unstable. Endotracheal intubation will usually be the method chosen, but the physician should be prepared to do a tracheotomy if attempts at perioral or perinasal intubation are failing or are impractical because of maxillofacial injuries. The most dangerous period is just prior to and during the initial attempts to get control of the airway. Manipulation of the oronasopharynx may provoke combative behavior or vomiting in a patient already confused by drugs, alcohol, hypoxia, or cerebral trauma. The risk of aspiration is high during these initial attempts, and the physician should make no assumptions about the state of the contents of the patient's stomach. Antacids are recommended just prior to the intubation attempt, if feasible. Although steroids have been recommended in the past, they are no longer considered of value in the management of aspiration of acidic gastric juice. The best management requires prevention of the complication of aspiration. In a reasonably cooperative patient, awake intubation with topical anesthesia may help to prevent some of the risks of hypotension, arrhythmia, and aspiration associated with the induction of anesthesia. If awake intubation is inappropriate, then an alternative is rapid-sequence induction with a thiobarbiturate followed by muscle paralysis with succinylcholine. If elevated intracranial pressure is suspected, or if a penetrating eye injury exists, awake intubation is contraindicated.

90. The answer is c. *(Brunicardi, pp 127-128.)* Necrotizing skin and soft tissue infections may produce insoluble gases (hydrogen, nitrogen, methane) through anaerobic bacterial metabolism. While the term "gas gangrene" has come to imply clostridial infection, gas in tissues is more likely not to be caused by *Clostridium* species but rather to other facultative and obligate anaerobes, particularly streptococci. Though fungi have also been implicated, they are less often associated with rapidly progressive infections. Treatment for necrotizing soft tissue infections includes repeated wide debridement, with wound reconstruction delayed until a stable, viable wound surface has been established. The use of hyperbaric O_2 in the treatment of gas gangrene remains controversial, due to lack of proven benefit, difficulty in transporting critically ill patients to hyperbaric facilities, and the risk of complications. Antitoxin has neither a prophylactic nor a therapeutic role in the treatment of necrotizing infections.

91. The answer is a. (*Mulholland, pp 1777-1783; Brunicardi pp 784-789.*) The initial treatment for venous thromboembolism (VTE) which includes deep venous thromboses (DVTs) and pulmonary emboli (PEs) is systemic anticoagulation with either unfractionated heparin—by bolus and infusion—or low molecular weight heparins—by subcutaneous administration. Transition is then made to oral warfarin, which is a vitamin K antagonist. Warfarin is not the initial treatment because it requires several days to become therapeutic and proteins C and S (which are anticoagulants) are inhibited first resulting in a procoagulant state. Inferior vena cava (IVC) filters are indicated in patients for whom anticoagulation is contraindicated or in patients who develop recurrent VTE in the setting of adequate anticoagulation. Thrombolytic therapy and pulmonary embolectomy are typically reserved for patients with massive PEs with hemodynamic instability.

92. The answer is c. (*Brunicardi, pp 784-785.*) Heparin is reversed by the administration of protamine sulfate. Spontaneous retroperitoneal hemorrhage is a rare but potentially fatal complication of anticoagulation. Heparin is much more frequently associated with spontaneous retroperitoneal hemorrhage than are oral agents. Advanced patient age and poor regulation of coagulation times also increase the likelihood of bleeding complications. Most cases of retroperitoneal hemorrhage present with flank pain and signs of peritoneal irritation suggestive of an acute intra-abdominal process. CT scans are most useful in confirming the diagnosis and following the course of the bleeding. Successful management is usually nonoperative and consists of the discontinuation of anticoagulants, reversal of anticoagulation, possible transfusion of clotting factors, and repletion of intravascular volume with intravenous fluids. Warfarin inhibits synthesis of vitamin K–dependent clotting factors, whereas heparin potentiates antithrombin III activity. Aprotinin is a protease inhibitor that decreases the inflammatory and fibrinolytic response and is used in patients undergoing cardiopulmonary bypass surgery to reduce bleeding complications. Lepirudin is an anticoagulant that is used in patients who develop heparin-induced thrombocytopenia. Thrombin can be used topically as a hemostatic agent.

93. The answer is e. (*Brunicardi, pp 201-202; Mulholland, pp 220-221.*) The patient requires intubation because of suspicion of upper airway burns. Clinical suspicion should be increased given the singed nose hairs and facial burns. Intubation should be considered in the presence of posterior pharyngeal edema, mucosal sloughing, or carbonaceous sputum on direct laryngoscopy. Significant upper airway edema can result of upper airway burns, particularly 12 to 24 hours post-injury. Bronchoscopy can be used to evaluate for lower airway burn injuries, but would not change management in this patient given the high clinical suspicion for airway burn injuries and the need for intubation. Inhaled or intravenous steroids for airway burn injuries are not indicated in patients with large burns due to the increased risk of infections. Carbon monoxide poisoning is treated with 100% inhaled oxygen; hyperbaric oxygen is used in patients with neurologic symptoms and small burns as it reduces the half-life of carboxyhemoglobin. However, the risks outweigh the benefits in patients with large burns.

94. The answer is d. (*Brunicardi, pp 128-129.*) Early goal-directed therapy should be employed for patients with septic shock or severe sepsis. The tenets of resuscitation include intubation if hypoxic, fluid resuscitation to a central venous pressure target of 8 to 12 mm Hg if not intubated and infusion of vasopressors to maintain a mean arterial pressure of 65 mm Hg. Norepinephrine and dopamine are the vasopressors of choice; epinephrine vasoconstricts peripherally as well as increases cardiac contractility and is not a first-line agent for septic shock. Inotropes such as dobutamine have been used if oxygen delivery is low, but should not be used to push delivery to supranormal levels. Furthermore, cultures should be drawn immediately and empiric antibiotics initiated; if there is a surgical source of sepsis, then operative intervention for source control should be promptly performed after initial resuscitative efforts. Recombinant-activated protein C is indicated in patients with severe sepsis with a predicted high risk of mortality (ie, older age, increased severity of disease); this patient does not have evidence of end-organ dysfunction such as acute renal or respiratory failure at this time. The use of corticosteroids for septic shock is controversial, but should only be considered in the setting of shock nonresponsive to fluids and vasopressors.

95 to 97. The answers are 95-b, 96-e, 97-a. (*Brunicardi, pp 1734-1739.*) Nitrous oxide is a commonly used inhalation agent. Nitrous oxide is 30 times more soluble than nitrogen in the blood and enters a collection of trapped air at a rate faster than at which nitrogen leaves the collection. This leads to an increase in volume of trapped air such as loops of bowel leading to bowel distention. Succinylcholine, a depolarizing neuromuscular blocking agent, causes a rise in serum potassium of up to 1.0 mEq/L within a few minutes after administration. This is caused by efflux of potassium from the skeletal muscle at the neuromuscular junction. Patients with burns, trauma, severe infections, or neuromuscular disorders have a greater than normal potassium efflux that occasionally causes severe hyperkalemia. Morphine is a narcotic agent that interacts predominantly with the opioid receptor. Rapid intravenous injections of morphine may cause hypotension. Midazolam (Versed) is a benzodiazepine and is associated with acute respiratory depression, especially in the elderly. Pancuronium is a neuromuscular blocking drug that is associated with tachycardia.

98 to 100.   The answers are 98-b, 99-e, 100-d. (*Brunicardi, pp 346-351.*) This patient requires pulmonary artery catheter readings to allow his physicians to assess his volume status and need for ongoing inotropic support. Furthermore, the patient continues to be hypotensive and requires further investigation as to the etiology that would subsequently dictate treatment (volume, afterload reduction, etc). Central venous monitoring alone does not allow the physician to assess cardiac function.

A patient who is hypertensive after a carotid endarterectomy is at risk for hemorrhagic stroke and therefore requires aggressive blood pressure management, occasionally with a continuous infusion of nitroglycerin or nitroprusside. Beat-to-beat monitoring of the blood pressure is essential. A patient who has suffered blunt head trauma requiring repeated surgeries for intracranial bleeding will likely be monitored with an intracranial pressure device. Other indications for intracranial pressure monitoring include subarachnoid hemorrhage, hydrocephalus, postcraniotomy status, and Reye syndrome. Measurement of intracranial pressure (ICP) allows the physician to determine and optimize the cerebral perfusion pressure (which is the difference between the mean arterial pressure and the ICP).

101 to 103.   The answers are 101-a, 102-e, 103-d. (*Mulholland, pp 70-87.*) Prothrombin time measures the speed of coagulation in the extrinsic pathway. A tissue source of procoagulant (thromboplastin) with calcium is added to plasma. The test will detect deficiencies in factors II, V, VII, X, and fibrinogen and is used to monitor patients receiving Coumadin derivatives. However, even small amounts of heparin will artificially prolong the clotting time, so that accurate prothrombin times can be obtained only when the patient has not received heparin for at least 5 hours.

The intrinsic pathway is measured by the partial thromboplastin time. This test is sensitive for defects in the contact and intrinsic phases of coagulation (II, V, VIII, IX, X, XI, XII, fibrinogen) and is used to monitor the status of patients on heparin.

The bleeding time assesses the interaction of platelets and the formation of the platelet plug. Therefore it will pick up deficiencies in both qualitative and quantitative platelet function. Ingestion of aspirin within 1 week of the test will alter the result.

The thrombin time assesses qualitative abnormalities in fibrinogen and the presence of inhibitors to fibrin polymerization. A standard amount of fibrin is added to a fixed volume of plasma and clotting time is measured.

Skin: Wounds, Infections, and Burns; Hands; Plastic Surgery

Questions

104. A 45-year-old woman is seen with wasting of the intrinsic muscles of the hand, weakness, and pain in the wrist. Which of the following nerves has most likely been injured?

a. Ulnar nerve
b. Radial nerve
c. Brachial nerve
d. Axillary nerve
e. Median nerve

105. A 68-year-old woman presents with a pigmented lesion on the trunk. Upon further examination the lesion has an irregular border, darkening coloration, and raised surface. An incisional biopsy is performed and confirms a melanoma with a thickness of 0.5 mm. The patient is scheduled for a wide local excision of the melanoma in the operating room. Which of the following is the smallest margin recommended for excision?

a. 3 mm
b. 5 mm
c. 1 cm
d. 2 cm
e. 5 cm

106. A 25-year-old woman presents with a benign nevus on the right upper arm. She desires removal and undergoes a clean incision and then closure of the incision without complication. With regard to the healing process, which of the following cell types are the first infiltrating cells to enter the wound site, peaking at 24 to 48 hours?

a. Macrophages
b. Neutrophils
c. Fibroblasts
d. Lymphocytes
e. Monocytes

107. A 3-year-old boy is brought to the emergency room after spilling bleach onto his lower extremities. He is diagnosed with a chemical burn and all involved clothing are removed. In addition to resuscitation, which of the following is the most appropriate initial management of this patient?

a. Treatment of the burn wound with antimicrobial agents.
b. Neutralize the burn wound with weak acids.
c. Lavage of the burn wound with large volumes of water.
d. Wound debridement in the operating room.
e. Treatment of the burn wound with calcium gluconate gel.

108. A 35-year-old man with new diagnosis of Crohn disease presents with rapidly enlarging painful ulcerations on the lower extremities. Cultures of the lesion are negative, and skin biopsy reveals no evidence of malignancy. Which of the following is the most appropriate treatment option?

a. Surgical debridement of the wound with skin grafting
b. Local wound care with silver sulfadiazine
c. Topical corticosteroids
d. Systemic steroids and immunosuppressants
e. Saphenous vein stripping and compressive stockings

109. Following a weekend of snowmobiling, a 42-year-old man comes to the emergency department with pain, numbness, and discoloration of his right forefoot. You diagnose frostbite. Which of the following is the proper initial treatment?

a. Debridement of the affected part followed by silver sulfadiazine dressings
b. Administration of corticosteroids
c. Administration of vasodilators
d. Immersion of the affected part in water at 40°C-44°C (104°F-111.2°F)
e. Rewarming of the affected part at room temperature

110. A 63-year-old man with history of poorly controlled diabetes presents with right leg swelling and pain. The patient denies trauma to the leg and reports it was normal yesterday. Examination of the right lower extremity is significant for extreme tenderness to palpation, erythema, and edema extending up to the knee. X-ray of the right leg shows tissue swelling without gas or osteomyelitis. The patient's vital signs are normal and he is started on broad-spectrum IV antibiotics and insulin. An hour later the patient's heart rate increases to 125 beats per minute and the erythema has progressed to the thigh with new blister formation on the leg. Which of the following is the most appropriate next step in management?

a. Repeat x-ray of the right lower extremity
b. CT scan of the right lower extremity
c. MRI of the right lower extremity
d. Bone scan of the right lower extremity
e. Immediate surgical intervention with incision and direct visualization of potentially infected tissue

111. A 35-year-old woman undergoes an elective laparoscopic cholecystectomy for symptomatic cholelithiasis. Which of the following wound classes best describes her procedure?

a. Class I, Clean
b. Class II, Clean/contaminated
c. Class III, Contaminated
d. Class IV, Dirty
e. None of the above

112. A 65-year-old woman presents with a 1-cm lesion with a pearly border on her nose, and punch biopsy is consistent with a basal cell carcinoma. She is scheduled to undergo Mohs surgery. Which of the following is a benefit of Mohs surgery over wide local excision?

a. Mohs surgery results in a smaller cosmetic defect while obtaining negative margins circumferentially.
b. Mohs surgery offers a shorter operating time.
c. Mohs surgery can be performed on many different types of skin cancers.
d. Mohs surgery results in less recurrence and metastases.
e. Mohs surgery does not depend on intraoperative evaluation of specimen margins with frozen sections.

113. A 60-year-old woman presents with the skin lesion shown here. She reports a history of a burn injury to the hand while cooking a few years ago. She reports the wound has never healed completely. You are concerned about the skin lesion and perform a punch biopsy. Which of the following is the most accurate diagnosis given the patient's history?

a. Basal cell carcinoma
b. Malignant melanoma
c. Erythroplasia of Queyrat
d. Bowen disease
e. Marjolin ulcer

114. A 25-year-old man is brought to the emergency room after sustaining burns during a fire in his apartment. He has blistering and erythema of his face, left upper extremity, and chest. He also has circumferential frank charring of his right upper extremity with decreased capillary refill. He is agitated, hypotensive, and tachycardic. Which of the following is the most appropriate initial management of his wounds?

a. Topical antibiotics should be applied to the burn wounds.
b. Excision of facial and hand burns.
c. Escharotomy of the right upper extremity.
d. Excision of all third-degree burns.
e. Split-thickness skin grafts over the areas of third-degree burns.

115. A 24-year-old firefighter sustains 30% total body surface area (TBSA) burns to his torso, face, and extremities. His wounds are treated topically with silver nitrate. Which of the following complications is associated with use of this agent?

a. Hypernatremia
b. Metabolic acidosis
c. Hyperchloremia
d. Neutropenia
e. Hyponatremia

116. A 54-year-old man sees you because of a growth on his lower lip. He smokes tobacco, has a fair complexion, and works outdoors. The biopsy report confirms a carcinoma. Which of the following is the most common diagnosis for tumors involving the lips?

a. Squamous cell carcinoma
b. Basal cell carcinoma
c. Malignant melanoma
d. Keratoacanthoma
e. Verrucous carcinoma

117. A 40-year-old woman complains of mild, intermittent pain and paresthesias in her right wrist. She reports the pain is worse at night and with driving. On physical examination hyperflexion of the right wrist reproduces the paresthesia. With regard to her diagnosis, which of the following is the most appropriate initial treatment?

a. Ice pack to the affected wrist at nighttime
b. Heat pad to the affected wrist at nighttime
c. Wrist splint worn at nighttime
d. Surgical treatment with division of the flexor retinaculum
e. Surgical treatment with division of the extensor retinaculum

118. A 60-year-old diabetic man undergoes incision and drainage of an infected boil on his back. The wound is left open and packed daily. Week by week, the wound grows smaller and eventually heals. Which of the following terms describes the method of wound closure by the patient?

a. Primary intention
b. Secondary intention
c. Tertiary intention
d. Delayed primary closure
e. Delayed secondary closure

119. A 70-year-old man is concerned when his dentist finds a white patch on his oral mucosa during a routine examination. Proper management should include which of the following?

a. Excisional biopsy of all lesions
b. Application of topical antibiotics
c. Low-dose radiation therapy
d. Strict oral hygiene and avoidance of alcohol and tobacco
e. Application of topical chemotherapeutic agents

120. A 60-year-old man presents with a 6-mm basal cell carcinoma on the tip of his nose. He is scheduled to undergo excision of the tumor in the operating room with repair of the defect using skin and subcutaneous tissue from his earlobe. Which of the following terms most appropriately describes this form of reconstructive surgery?

a. Split-thickness graft
b. Full-thickness graft
c. Composite graft
d. Pedicle flap
e. Free flap

121. A 40-year-old woman undergoes an incisional biopsy of a pigmented lesion on her right thigh. Pathologic examination reveals malignant melanoma with a thickness of 3 mm. Findings on examination of the groin are normal. Which of the following is the most appropriate next step in her management?

a. Wide local excision of the melanoma with a 1-cm margin from the tumor, followed by radiation to the groin
b. Wide local excision of the melanoma with a 1-cm margin from the tumor and sentinel lymph node biopsy
c. Wide local excision of the melanoma with a 1-cm margin from the tumor and groin lymph node dissection
d. Wide local excision of the melanoma with a 2-cm margin from the tumor and sentinel lymph node biopsy
e. Wide local excision of the melanoma with a 2-cm margin from the tumor and groin lymph node dissection

122. A 22-year-old healthy African-American woman presents with a recurrent growth on her right thigh. She has a childhood history of a third-degree scald burn to the same area that did not require skin grafting. The growth was completely removed 2 years ago. On physical examination there is a 5 cm × 2 cm, raised, irregularly shaped purple lesion with a smooth top. Which of the following is the most likely diagnosis?

a. Angiosarcoma
b. Malignant melanoma
c. Squamous cell carcinoma
d. Kaposi sarcoma
e. Keloid

123. A 12-year-old boy is in a motor vehicle collision in which the car caught fire. He sustains significant inhalation injury and a circumferential burn without fractures or other soft tissue trauma to his left lower extremity during extrication from the burning vehicle. He is intubated and aggressively resuscitated in the intensive care unit. Which of the following is the most appropriate method of assessing for compartment syndrome of the left lower extremity?

a. X-ray of the left lower extremity
b. Doppler signals of the left lower extremity
c. Computed tomography (CT) scan of the left lower extremity
d. Magnetic resonance imaging (MRI) of the left lower extremity
e. Left lower extremity angiogram

124. During a bar brawl, a 19-year-old man sustains a 4-in laceration on his left arm from glass and presents to the emergency room the following morning, 10 hours later. He is neurovascularly intact and the wound is deep, extending down to fascia. Which of the following is the most appropriate management of the wound?

a. Closure of the skin only and administration of oral antibiotics for 1 week
b. Closure of the skin and subcutaneous tissue and administration of oral antibiotics for 1 week
c. A single dose of intravenous antibiotics and closure of the skin only
d. A single dose of intravenous antibiotics and closure of the skin and subcutaneous tissue
e. Local wound care without wound closure or antibiotics

125. A 59-year-old woman undergoes an exploratory laparotomy for peritonitis and is found to have perforated diverticulitis. She undergoes a sigmoid resection with an end colostomy. She is administered a third-generation cephalosporin within 1 hour prior to the incision and the antibiotic is continued postoperatively. One week later, she develops an intra-abdominal abscess, which is percutaneously drained. *Bacteroides fragilis* is isolated from the cultures. Which of the following statements regarding her perioperative antibiotic regimen is most accurate?

a. The preoperative dose of antibiotics should have been given closer to the time of incision.
b. The patient should have received several doses of antibiotics prior to laparotomy.
c. The patient should have received a first-generation cephalosporin.
d. The patient did not have adequate gram-negative coverage.
e. The patient did not have adequate anaerobic coverage.

126. A 30-year-old man with a history of Crohn disease develops an enterocutaneous fistula and is placed on total parenteral nutrition through a right subclavian central venous catheter. After 5 days, the patient develops a fever and leukocytosis; CT scan of the abdomen reveals no intra-abdominal abscess. The subclavian catheter insertion site is inspected and noted to be erythematous and painful. Blood cultures are positive. Which of the following organisms is the most likely cause of his fever?

a. Coagulase-positive staphylococci
b. Coagulase-negative staphylococci
c. Group A *Streptococcus*
d. *Enterococcus*
e. *Escherichia coli*

127. A 65-year-old man sustains a 50% TBSA burn while burning trash in the backyard. The patient is resuscitated with lactated Ringer (LR) solution using the Parkland formula and a weight of 80 kg. What is the rate of LR given in the first 8 hours?

a. 100 mL/h
b. 500 mL/h
c. 1000 mL/h
d. 5000 mL/h
e. 10,000 mL/h

128. A 67-year-old man presents to his primary care physician with a 1-cm skin lesion on his left forearm. On examination, it has a waxy appearance with rolled, pearly borders surrounding a central ulcer. Which of the following is the most appropriate management of this patient?

a. Mohs surgery
b. Curettage of the lesion
c. Electrodesiccation of the lesion
d. Laser vaporization of the lesion
e. Surgical excision

Questions 129 to 131

Match each lower extremity lesion with its correct etiology. Each lettered option may be used once, more than once, or not at all.

a. Ischemic ulcer
b. Venous stasis ulcer
c. Diabetic ulcer
d. Pyoderma gangrenosum
e. Marjolin ulcer

129. A 43-year-old man with a painless ulceration over the left medial malleolus with surrounding brawny induration.

130. A 69-year-old man with a history of diabetes mellitus with pain in the balls of his feet at night with an ulcer over the lateral aspect of his right fifth toe.

131. A 52-year-old woman with a history of diabetes mellitus with an ulcer on the plantar surface of her right heel.

Skin: Wounds, Infections, and Burns; Hands; Plastic Surgery

Answers

104. The answer is a. (*Townsend, pp 2154-2158.*) The ulnar nerve innervates 15 of the 20 intrinsic muscles of the hand. The musculocutaneous, radial, ulnar, and median nerves are all important to hand function. The musculocutaneous and radial nerves allow forearm supination; the radial nerve alone innervates the extensor muscles. The median nerve is the "eye of the hand" because of its extensive contribution to sensory perception; it also maintains most of the long flexors, the pronators of the forearm, and the thenar muscles.

105. The answer is c. (*Brunicardi, pp 415-416.*) The appropriate margin for wide excision of melanomas is dependent on the depth of the lesion. For thin lesions, less than or equal to 1 mm in depth (thickness), a 1-cm margin is adequate. For intermediate lesions (1-4 mm thick) a 2-cm margin is recommended, and thick (>4 mm) lesions benefit from a 2- to 3-cm margin of excision.

106. The answer is b. (*Brunicardi, pp 210-214.*) Wound healing is an overlapping sequence of inflammation, proliferation, and remodeling. The inflammatory phase is characterized by a rapid influx of neutrophils, followed in about 2 days by an influx of mononuclear cells. Derived from circulating monocytes, the macrophages act not only by phagocytosing debris and bacteria, but also by secreting numerous growth factors, including tumor necrosis factor (TNF), transforming growth factor, platelet-derived growth factor (PDGF), and fibroblast growth factor, which are essential to normal wound healing. Angiogenesis and collagen formation take place during the proliferative phase of wound healing. Fibroblasts, which enter the wound at about day 3, continue to proliferate with increasing collagen deposition. Throughout the proliferative phase, type III collagen predominates. Collagen content is maximal at 2 to 3 weeks, at which time the remodeling phase begins. Type III collagen, which is elastic fibrils, is gradually replaced by rigid fibrils, or type I collagen, at this time. During remodeling, collagen deposition and degradation reach a steady state, which may continue for up to 1 year.

107. The answer is c. *(Townsend, pp 582-583.)* Treatment of alkali chemical burns involves immediate removal of the alkali agent with large volumes of water lavage. Alkalis dissolve and unite with the proteins of the tissues to form alkaline proteinates which contain hydroxide ions. These ions cause further chemical reactions, penetrating deeper into the tissue. Attempts to neutralize the alkali with weak acids are not recommended because the heat released by neutralization reactions induces further injury. Operative debridement is indicated for particularly strong bases and takes place after resuscitation and lavage with large amounts of water. Tangential removal of affected areas is performed until the tissues removed are of normal pH. The wounds are then covered with antimicrobial agents or skin substitutes. Calcium gluconate is used to treat wounds exposed to hydrofluoric acid.

108. The answer is d. *(Brunicardi, pp 410-411.)* The patient has pyoderma gangrenosum, which is a rare cause of cutaneous ulcerations that can be associated with inflammatory bowel disease as well as other immune disorders. The mainstay of treatment is systemic steroids and immunosuppressants such as cyclosporine. Surgical debridement without medical therapy is not recommended, and local wound care alone or topical steroids are not therapeutic. Saphenous vein ligation and compressive stockings would be more appropriate treatment options in patients with venous stasis ulcers.

109. The answer is d. *(Moore, pp 1071-1072.)* Many methods of treating frostbite have been tried throughout the years. These include massage, warm-water immersion, and covering the affected area. Rapid warming by immersion in water slightly above normal body temperature (40°C-44°C, or 104°F-111.2°F) is the most effective method; however, because the frostbitten region is numb and especially vulnerable, it should be protected from trauma or excessive heat during treatment. Further treatment may include elevation to minimize edema, administration of antibiotics and tetanus toxoid, and debridement of necrotic skin as needed.

110. The answer is e. *(Brunicardi, pp 126-127.)* This patient's presentation is deeply concerning for a necrotizing soft tissue infection. The rapid progression of the erythema, bullae formation, and the tachycardia mandates immediate surgical intervention. During surgery an incision is made overlying the area of suspicion and the deep soft tissue, fascia, and underlying muscle are directly visualized. All affected areas are completely resected. Radiologic studies should not be undertaken in patients in whom the diagnosis is seriously considered as they delay surgical intervention and often provide confusing information.

111. The answer is b. (*Brunicardi, pp 123-124.*) Clean wounds are those in which no part of the respiratory, gastrointestinal, or genitourinary tract is entered. Examples include herniorrhaphy and breast surgery. Clean-contaminated wounds encompass those cases in which these systems are entered, but without evidence of active infection or gross spillage. Examples include elective cholecystectomy or elective colon resection with adequate bowel preparation. Contaminated wounds include open accidental wounds encountered early after injury, those with extensive introduction of bacteria into a normally sterile area of the body, or gross spillage of viscus contents such as from the intestine. Examples include penetrating abdominal trauma, large tissue injury, and enterotomy during bowel obstruction. Dirty wounds include traumatic wounds in which a significant delay in treatment has occurred and in which necrotic tissue is present, those created in the presence of purulent material, and those involving a perforated viscus accompanied by a high degree of contamination. Examples include perforated diverticulitis and necrotizing soft tissue infections.

112. The answer is a. (*Brunicardi, p 414.*) Mohs surgery describes a technique for resecting either basal or squamous cell carcinomas on the face or near the nose or eye in order to achieve the optimal cosmetic result. Resection of the tumor is performed in small increments with immediate frozen section analysis in order to ensure negative margins. The disadvantage of the Mohs technique is the longer time required. There is no difference in cure rate between Mohs surgery and wide local excision of a basal cell carcinoma. Wide local excision can be performed on all types of skin cancers.

113. The answer is e. (*Brunicardi, pp 413-414.*) The patient has squamous cell carcinoma. SCC occurs in people who have had chronic sun exposure, chronic ulcers or sinus tracts (draining osteomyelitis), or thermal injury called Marjolin ulcer. SCC is less common than basal cell carcinoma but is more devastating due to an increased rate of invasiveness and metastases. In situ SCC lesions are termed Bowen disease. In situ SCC tumors specific to the penis are referred to as erythroplasia of Queyrat.

114. The answer is c. *(Brunicardi, pp 204-205.)* Meticulous attention to deep circumferential burns is crucial in the management of burn patients. Progressive tissue edema may lead to progressive vascular and neurologic compromise. Because the blood supply is the initial system affected, frequent assessment of flow is vital, with longitudinal escharotomy performed at the first sign of vascular compromise. A low threshold should be maintained in performing an escharotomy in the setting of severely burned limbs. Burn wound management is characterized by early excision of areas of devitalized tissue, with the exception of deep wounds of the palms, soles, genitals, and face. Staged excision of deep partial-thickness or full-thickness burns occurs between 3 and 7 days after the injury. There are several proven advantages to early excision, including decreased hospital stay and lower cost. This is especially true of burns encompassing more than 30% to 40% of the total body surface area. In conjunction with early excision, topical antimicrobials such as silver sulfadiazine are extremely important in delaying colonization of the newly excised or fresh burn wounds. Permanent coverage through split-thickness skin grafting usually occurs more than 1 week after injury. Skin autograft requires a vascular bed and therefore cannot be placed over eschar.

115. The answer is e. *(Brunicardi, p 202.)* The 3 main topical agents used to treat burns include silver nitrate, silver sulfadiazine, and mafenide acetate. Complications of silver nitrate are electrolyte abnormalities (hyponatremia, hypokalemia, hypocalcemia, hypochloremia) and methemoglobinemia. The main complication with silver sulfadiazine is neutropenia; mafenide acetate causes metabolic acidosis secondary to inhibition of carbonic anhydrase.

116. The answer is a. *(Brunicardi, p 491.)* Squamous cell carcinoma of the lip is the most common malignant tumor of the lip and constitutes 15% of all malignancies of the oral cavity. The majority of lip malignancies present on the lower lip (88%-98%). Basal cell carcinomas occur much less frequently and affect the upper lip more often than the lower lip. Malignant melanoma, keratoacanthoma, and verrucous carcinoma also present in the upper lip, although much less frequently than SCC.

117. The answer is c. (*Townsend, p 2186.*) This patient has carpal tunnel syndrome. Signs and symptoms of carpal tunnel syndrome are related to the distribution of the median nerve. In many instances, symptoms are limited to nocturnal pain and paresthesias. Initial treatment of carpal tunnel syndrome includes use of wrist splints (at nighttime) and occasionally local corticosteroid injections. Ice packs or heating pads are not used to treat carpal tunnel syndrome. If conservative treatment of carpal tunnel syndrome is unsuccessful, surgical treatment may be required. Open and endoscopic techniques have been employed, both of which release adhesions of the median nerve and divide the transverse carpal ligament (flexor retinaculum).

118. The answer is b. (*Townsend, p 191.*) This patient's wound has healed by secondary intention. There are 3 types of wound closures: primary intention, secondary intention, and tertiary intention. In primary intention closures the edges of the wound are brought together and sealed immediately with simple suturing, skin graft placement, or flap at the end of the surgical procedure. Secondary intention closures involve leaving the wound open without active intent to seal the wound. The wound heals by re-epithelialization which results in contraction of the wound. This type of closure is generally reserved for highly contaminated wounds in which a primary intention repair would fail. Sometimes a contaminated wound is initially treated with repeated therapy (antibiotic, debridements, negative pressure dressing) until the infection is controlled and then it is closed with surgical interventions such as suturing, skin graft placement, or flap. This type of wound closure is called tertiary intention or delayed primary closure. A delayed secondary closure does not exist.

119. The answer is d. (*Townsend, pp 813-814.*) White patches in the oral cavity (leukoplakia) sometimes are incorrectly interpreted as a premalignant condition. Microscopic examination of leukoplakia may reveal hyperplasia, keratosis, or dyskeratosis, of which the last finding is the most serious because of its association with malignancy. Approximately 50% of all oral cancers occur in patients who have associated areas of hyperkeratosis and dyskeratosis. Only about 5% of patients with leukoplakia develop cancer. A suggested treatment protocol for patients with leukoplakia advocates a program of strict oral hygiene and avoidance of the source of irritants such as alcohol and tobacco. Biopsy is reserved only for those with thick lesions or those in whom the lesion does not resolve after avoidance therapy (to rule out malignancy). Radiation therapy is contraindicated.

120. The answer is c. *(Brunicardi, pp 1651-1656.)* A composite tissue graft contains tissue in addition to the epidermis and dermis. Depending on the donor site, it can contain subcutaneous fat, cartilage, and even muscle. This makes it ideal for deeper defects in which a partial-thickness or full-thickness skin graft would give a poor cosmetic outcome. A flap is a vascularized piece of tissue that is mobilized from its original site to another location. A free tissue flap involves severing the original blood supply with anastomosis to blood vessels in the recipient site. The remaining defect in this patient is too small to warrant the need for a flap.

121. The answer is d. *(Brunicardi, pp 415-416.)* The survival of patients with malignant melanoma correlates with the thickness of the lesion (Breslow). The current guidelines regarding wide local excision of the primary melanoma are as follows: melanomas measuring < 1 mm in thickness are resected with a 1-cm margin, melanomas 1-4 mm in thickness are resected with a 2-cm margin, melanomas measuring > 4 mm are resected with a 2- to 3-cm margin. Our patient has a melanoma with a thickness of 3 mm and therefore needs at least a 2-cm margin from the tumor during the resection. Lymph node dissection for melanoma is generally reserved for patients with a positive sentinel lymph node or clinically positive lymph nodes. The sentinel lymph node is the first node that drains a particular nodal basin and can be identified with preoperative injection of ^{99m}Tc sulfur colloid around the lesion and detection with a gamma counter intraoperatively and/or intraoperative injection of blue dye. If metastasis is identified in the sentinel lymph node, then a complete lymph node (LN) dissection is performed. This method helps identify patients who would benefit from a LN dissection while sparing others from an unnecessary operation. Sentinel lymph node biopsy is performed for lesions between 1 and 4 mm in thickness.

122. The answer is e. *(Brunicardi, pp 225-227, 413-414, 418.)* Keloids occur in areas of previous trauma to the skin (burns, surgery, piercings, tattoos) and represent an overexuberance of wound healing. Keloids are much more common in darker-pigmented ethnicities. Surgical excision alone of a keloid is associated with a high recurrence rate, and other adjunctive modalities that have been utilized include injection of steroids, radiation, external compression, and topical retinoids. Squamous cell carcinoma can develop in a previous burn scar or a sinus tract secondary to osteomyelitis. However, the description of the lesion along with the history of recurrence is consistent with a keloid. Although basal cell carcinoma, melanoma, and other malignancies can develop in a chronic wound, squamous cell carcinoma is the most common. The mainstay of treatment is surgical excision or amputation. Kaposi sarcoma usually presents as multifocal lesions on the extremities that may be associated with immunocompromised individuals, and the mainstay of therapy is radiation.

123. The answer is b. (*Townsend, p 569.*) Extremities at risk for compartment syndrome are identified by clinical examination. Patients complain of numbness and tingling along with increased pain in the digits. Arterial inflow can also be easily assessed with palpation of distal pulses or by determination of Doppler signals in the affected extremities. Compartment pressures can also be measured with a pressure of greater than 40 mm Hg being diagnostic. Compartment syndromes secondary to burns are a result of increased pressure secondary to tissue edema and lack of elasticity of the burnt skin (eschar), causing compression of the blood vessels. Imaging modalities such as x-ray, CT, MRI, or angiogram are not beneficial in the diagnosis of compartment syndrome.

124. The answer is e. (*Townsend, p 590.*) The wound should not be closed because the elapsed time to presentation was greater than 6 hours. Wounds that are dirty or contaminated (eg, animal bites), that are traumatically induced by a puncture, gunshot, or crush injury, or that are older than 6 hours should be left open. Prophylactic antibiotics have not been demonstrated to prevent wound infections.

125. The answer is e. (*Townsend, pp 265-267.*) Third-generation cephalosporins provide good coverage against most gram-negative bacteria, but have poor activity against anaerobic bacteria (eg, *B fragilis*). Clindamycin or metronidazole can be used in addition to a third-generation cephalosporin to provide anaerobic coverage. Other alternatives include a combination of a penicillin/β-lactamase inhibitor or a cefoxitin or cefotetan, both of which are second-generation cephalosporins. Prophylactic antibiotics against anaerobic organisms are indicated only in cases where they are likely to be encountered (eg, bowel cases). Prophylactic antibiotics should optimally be administered intravenously within 1 hour prior to incision. Continuation of postoperative antibiotics for more than 24 hours is indicated in patients with preexisting infection, for example, secondary to perforated viscera, but not after routine elective operations.

126. The answer is b. (*Townsend, pp 312-313.*) The most common organism in patients with nosocomial bacteremia is coagulase-negative *Staphylococcus*.

127. The answer is c. *(Brunicardi, p 200.)* The Parkland formula recommends 4 mL LR/kg for each percent TBSA burned over the first 24 hours, with one-half of the amount administered in the first 8 hours, and the remaining half over the next 16 hours.

$$4 \text{ mL/kg} \times 80 \text{ (kg)} \times 50\% \text{ TBSA} = 16,000$$
$$16,000/2 = 8000$$
$$8000 \text{ (mL)}/8 \text{ (hours)} = 1000 \text{ mL/h}$$

128. The answer is e. *(Brunicardi, pp 413-414.)* The patient's lesion has the classic appearance of a basal cell carcinoma. Basal cell carcinomas (BCCs) are the most common type of skin cancer. BCCs have a slow growth rate and commonly infiltrate locally but rarely metastasize. The nodulocystic or noduloulcerative type accounts for 70% of BCCs. Small lesions (< 2 mm) may be treated with curettage, electrodesiccation, or laser vaporization. However, these techniques destroy the tissue and eliminate the possibility of confirming the diagnosis or analyzing the margins. A surgical excision is the most appropriate method of resection given the size and location of this patient's lesion. Mohs surgery is reserved for managing tumors in aesthetic areas such as the eyelid, nose, or cheek.

129 to 131. The answers are 129-b, 130-a, 131-c. *(Townsend, pp 1376, 2009, 2148.)* Venous stasis ulcers are typically located over the medial malleolus, are painless, and may be associated with brawny induration. Treatment consists of leg elevation, compression stockings, local wound care, and occasionally surgical debridement. Ischemic ulcers are often associated with other symptoms of severe peripheral vascular disease such as rest pain, and are commonly located on the dorsum of the foot or the lateral first or fifth toes. Patients with ischemic ulcers should undergo urgent evaluation for lower extremity revascularization. Diabetic ulcers are often associated with trauma or pressure secondary to sensory neuropathy and typically occur on the plantar surface of the foot. Treatment should include optimization of the patient's blood sugars, protective shoe wear, and debridement of necrotic tissue. Pyoderma gangrenosum can be associated with underlying disorders such as inflammatory bowel disease, rheumatic heart disease, or malignancy. The lesions are painful ulcerations surrounded by erythema. Treatment consists primarily of corticosteroids and immunosuppressants. A Marjolin ulcer is a squamous cell carcinoma that arises in a chronic wound and is treated with surgical excision.

Trauma and Shock

Questions

132. A teenage boy falls from his bicycle and is run over by a truck. On arrival in the emergency room (ER), he is awake and alert and appears frightened but in no distress. The chest radiograph suggests an air-fluid level in the left lower lung field and the nasogastric tube seems to coil upward into the left chest. Which of the following is the next best step in his management?

a. Placement of a left chest tube
b. Thoracotomy
c. Laparotomy
d. Esophagogastroscopy
e. Diagnostic peritoneal lavage

133. A 10-year-old boy was the backseat belted passenger in a high-speed motor vehicle collision. On presentation to the ER, he is awake, alert, and hemodynamically stable. He is complaining of abdominal pain and has an ecchymosis on his anterior abdominal wall where the seatbelt was located. Which of the following is the best next step in his management?

a. Discharge him home without any other workup.
b. Discharge him home if his amylase level is normal.
c. Discharge him home if his abdominal plain films are negative for the presence of free air.
d. Discharge him home if an abdominal computed tomography (CT) scan is negative.
e. Observe him regardless of negative test results.

134. A 65-year-old man who smokes cigarettes and has chronic obstructive pulmonary disease falls and fractures the third, fourth, and fifth ribs in the left anterolateral chest. Chest x-ray is otherwise normal. Which of the following would be the most appropriate next step in his management?

a. Strapping the chest with adhesive tape
b. Admission to the hospital and treatment with oral analgesia
c. Tube thoracostomy
d. Placement of an epidural for pain management
e. Surgical fixation of the fractured ribs

135. A 36-year-old man who was hit by a car presents to the ER with hypotension. On examination, he has tenderness and bruising over his left lateral chest below the nipple. An ultrasound examination is performed and reveals free fluid in the abdomen. What is the most likely organ to have been injured in this patient?

a. Liver
b. Kidney
c. Spleen
d. Intestine
e. Pancreas

136. A 52-year-old man is pinned against a loading dock. The patient has a fractured femur, a pelvic fracture, a tender abdomen, and no pulses in the right foot with minimal tissue damage to the right leg. Angiography discloses a popliteal artery injury with obstruction. At surgery, the popliteal vein is also transected. His blood pressure is 85/60 mm Hg. Which of the following is the best management strategy for his vascular injuries?

a. Repair of the popliteal vein with simple closure
b. Repair of the popliteal vein with saphenous vein patch
c. Repair of the popliteal vein with a synthetic interposition graft
d. Ligation of the popliteal vein
e. Amputation of the right lower extremity above the knee

137. A 27-year-old man sustains a single gunshot wound to the left thigh. In the ER, he is noted to have a large hematoma of his medial thigh. He complains of paresthesias in his left foot. On examination, there are weak pulses palpable distal to the injury and the patient is unable to move his foot. Which of the following is the most appropriate initial management of this patient?

a. Angiography
b. Immediate exploration and repair in the operating room
c. Fasciotomy of the anterior compartment of the calf
d. Observation for resolution of spasm
e. Local wound exploration at the bedside

138. A 25-year-old woman arrives in the ER following an automobile accident. She is acutely dyspneic with a respiratory rate of 60 breaths per minute. Breath sounds are markedly diminished on the right side. Which of the following is the best first step in the management of this patient?

a. Take a chest x-ray.
b. Draw arterial blood for blood-gas determination.
c. Decompress the right pleural space.
d. Perform pericardiocentesis.
e. Administer intravenous fluids.

139. A 17-year-old adolescent boy is stabbed in the left seventh intercostal space, midaxillary line. He presents to the ER with a heart rate of 86 beats per minute, blood pressure of 125/74 mm Hg, and oxygen saturation of 98%. Breath sounds are equal bilaterally. Which of the following is the most appropriate next step in his workup?

a. Local exploration of the wound
b. Left tube thoracostomy
c. Diagnostic laparoscopy
d. CT scan of the abdomen
e. Echocardiography

140. Your hospital is conducting an ongoing research study involving the hormonal response to trauma. Blood is drawn regularly (with Institutional Review Board [IRB] approval) for various studies. Which of the following values are likely to be seen after a healthy 36-year-old man is hit by a bus and sustains a ruptured spleen and a lacerated small bowel?

a. Increased secretion of insulin
b. Increased secretion of thyroxine
c. Decreased secretion of vasopressin (antidiuretic hormone [ADH])
d. Decreased secretion of glucagon
e. Decreased secretion of aldosterone

141. A 29-year-old man sustained a gunshot wound to the right upper quadrant. He is taken to the operating room and, after management of a liver injury, is found to have a complete transection of the common bile duct with significant tissue loss. Which of the following is the optimal surgical management of this patient's injury?

a. Choledochoduodenostomy
b. Loop choledochojejunostomy
c. Primary end-to-end anastomosis of the transected bile duct
d. Roux-en-Y choledochojejunostomy
e. Bridging of the injury with a T tube

142. You evaluate an 18-year-old man who sustained a right-sided cervical laceration during a gang fight. Your intern suggests nonoperative management and observation. Which of the following is a relative, rather than an absolute, indication for neck exploration?

a. Expanding hematoma
b. Dysphagia
c. Dysphonia
d. Pneumothorax
e. Hemoptysis

143. Following blunt abdominal trauma, a 12-year-old girl develops upper abdominal pain, nausea, and vomiting. An upper gastrointestinal series reveals a total obstruction of the duodenum with a coiled spring appearance in the second and third portions. In the absence of other suspected injuries, which of the following is the most appropriate management of this patient?

a. Gastrojejunostomy
b. Nasogastric suction and observation
c. Duodenal resection
d. TPN (total parental nutrition) to increase the size of the retroperitoneal fat pad
e. Duodenojejunostomy

144. A 45-year-old man presents after a high-speed motor vehicle collision. He has a seatbelt sign across his neck and chest with an ecchymosis over his left neck. He is hemodynamically stable and neurologically intact. A CT angiogram shows a left carotid dissection. In the absence of other significant injuries, what is the next step in his management?

a. Antiplatelet therapy
b. Systemic anticoagulation with heparin
c. Neck exploration and left carotid artery repair
d. Neck exploration and left intra-extracranial bypass
e. Angiography and left carotid artery stenting

145. An 18-year-old man was assaulted and sustained significant head and facial trauma. Which of the following is the most common initial manifestation of increased intracranial pressure?

a. Change in level of consciousness
b. Ipsilateral (side of hemorrhage) pupillary dilation
c. Contralateral pupillary dilation
d. Hemiparesis
e. Hypertension

146. A 28-year-old man is brought to the ER for a severe head injury after a fall. He was intubated in the field for his decreased level of consciousness. He is tachycardic and hypotensive. On examination, he is noted to have an obvious skull fracture and his right pupil is dilated. Which of the following is the most appropriate method for initially reducing his intracranial pressure?

a. Elevation of the head of the bed
b. Saline-furosemide (Lasix) infusion
c. Mannitol infusion
d. Intravenous dexamethasone (Decadron)
e. Hyperventilation

147. A 45-year-old man was an unhelmeted motorcyclist involved in a high-speed collision. He was ejected from the motorcycle and was noted to be apneic at the scene. After being intubated, he was brought to the ER, where he is noted to have a left dilated pupil that responds only sluggishly. What is the pathophysiology of his dilated pupil?

a. Infection within the cavernous sinus
b. Herniation of the uncal process of the temporal lobe
c. Laceration of the corpus callosum by the falx cerebri
d. Occult damage to the superior cervical ganglion
e. Cerebellar hypoxia

148. A 31-year-old man is brought to the ER following an automobile accident in which his chest struck the steering wheel. Examination reveals stable vital signs and no evidence of respiratory distress, but the patient exhibits multiple palpable rib fractures and paradoxical movement of the right side of the chest. Chest x-ray shows no evidence of pneumothorax or hemothorax. Which of the following is the most appropriate initial management of this patient?

a. Intubation, mechanical ventilation, and positive end-expiratory pressure
b. Stabilization of the chest wall with sandbags
c. Stabilization with towel clips
d. Immediate operative stabilization
e. Pain control, chest physiotherapy, and close observation

149. A 30-year-old man is stabbed in the arm. There is no evidence of vascular injury, but he cannot flex his three radial digits. Which of the following structures has he most likely injured?

a. Flexor pollicis longus and flexor digitus medius tendons
b. Radial nerve
c. Median nerve
d. Thenar and digital nerves at the wrist
e. Ulnar nerve

150. Following a 2-hour firefighting episode, a 36-year-old fireman begins complaining of a throbbing headache, nausea, dizziness, and visual disturbances. He is taken to the ER, where his carboxyhemoglobin (COHb) level is found to be 31%. Which of the following is the most appropriate next step in his treatment?

a. Begin an immediate exchange transfusion.
b. Transfer the patient to a hyperbaric oxygen chamber.
c. Begin bicarbonate infusion and give 250 mg acetazolamide (Diamox) intravenously.
d. Administer 100% oxygen by mask.
e. Perform flexible bronchoscopy with further therapy determined by findings.

151. A 75-year-old man with a history of coronary artery disease, hypertension, and diabetes mellitus undergoes a right hemicolectomy for colon cancer. On the second postoperative day, he complains of shortness of breath and chest pain. He becomes hypotensive with depressed mental status and is immediately transferred to the intensive care unit. After intubation and placement on mechanical ventilation, an echocardiogram confirms cardiogenic shock. A central venous catheter is placed that demonstrates a central venous pressure of 18 mm Hg. Which of the following is the most appropriate initial management strategy?

a. Additional liter fluid bolus
b. Inotropic support
c. Mechanical circulatory support with intra-aortic balloon pump (IABP)
d. Cardiac catheterization
e. Heart transplant

152. An 18-year-old man climbs up a utility pole to retrieve his younger brother's kite. An electrical spark jumps from the wire to his metal belt buckle and burns his abdominal wall, knocking him to the ground. Which of the following should guide your treatment of this patient?

a. Injuries are generally more superficial than those from thermal burns.
b. Intravenous fluid replacement is based on the percentage of body surface area burned.
c. Electric burns often result in a transient traumatic optic neuropathy.
d. Evaluation for fracture of the other extremities and visceral injury is indicated.
e. Cardiac conduction abnormalities are unlikely.

153. A 22-year-old man is examined following a motor vehicle accident. He has a right knee dislocation which is reduced in the emergency room. He has palpable pedal pulses and is neurologically intact. Which of the following is an appropriate next step in his workup and management?

a. Measurement of ankle-brachial indices
b. Angiography of the right lower extremity
c. Prophylactic below-knee 4-compartment fasciotomies
d. Surgical exploration of the right popliteal artery
e. Observation with serial pulse checks

154. A 23-year-old, previously healthy man presents to the ER after sustaining a single gunshot wound to the left chest. The entrance wound is 3 cm inferior to the nipple and the exit wound is just below the scapula. A chest tube is placed that drains 400 mL of blood and continues to drain 50 to 75 mL/h during the initial resuscitation. Initial blood pressure of 70/0 mm Hg has responded to 2-L crystalloid and is now 100/70 mm Hg. Abdominal examination is unremarkable. Chest x-ray reveals a reexpanded lung and no free air under the diaphragm. Which of the following is the best next step in his management?

a. Admission and observation
b. Peritoneal lavage
c. Exploratory thoracotomy
d. Exploratory celiotomy
e. Local wound exploration

155. A patient is brought to the ER after a motor vehicle accident. He is unconscious and has a deep scalp laceration and one dilated pupil. His heart rate is 120 beats per minute, blood pressure is 80/40 mm Hg, and respiratory rate is 35 breaths per minute. Despite rapid administration of 2-L normal saline, the patient's vital signs do not change significantly. Which of the following is the most appropriate next step in the workup of his hypotension?

a. Neurosurgical consultation for emergent ventriculostomy to manage his intracranial pressure
b. Neurosurgical consultation for emergent craniotomy for suspected subdural hematoma
c. Emergent burr hole drainage at the bedside for suspected epidural hematoma
d. Administration of mannitol and hyperventilation to treat his elevated intracranial pressure
e. Abdominal ultrasound (focused assessment with sonography in trauma [FAST])

156. A 25-year-old man is involved in a gang shoot-out and sustains an abdominal gunshot wound from a .22 pistol. At laparotomy, it is discovered that the left transverse colon has incurred a through-and-through injury with minimal fecal soilage of the peritoneum. Which of the following is the most appropriate management of this patient?

a. A colostomy should be performed regardless of the patient's hemodynamic status to decrease the risk of an intraabdominal infection.
b. Primary repair should be performed, but only in the absence of hemodynamic instability.
c. Primary repair should be performed with placement of an intra-abdominal drain next to the repair.
d. Primary repair should be performed and intravenous antibiotics administered for 14 days.
e. The patient should undergo a 2-stage procedure with resection of the injured portion and reanastomosis 48 hours later when clinically stabilized.

157. A 34-year-old prostitute with a history of long-term intravenous drug use is admitted with a 48-hour history of pain in her left arm. She is tachycardic to 130 and her systolic blood pressure is 80 mm Hg. Physical examination is remarkable for crepitus surrounding needle track marks in the antecubital space with a serous exudate. The plain x-ray of the arm is shown here. Which of the following is the most appropriate next step in her management?

a. Treatment with penicillin G and close observation
b. MRI of the arm
c. CT scan of the arm
d. Surgical exploration and debridement
e. Hyperbaric oxygen therapy

158. A 47-year-old man is extricated from an automobile after a motor vehicle accident. He is hypotensive with a systolic blood pressure of 80. The patient has a steering wheel bruise on the anterior chest. His electrocardiogram (ECG) shows some premature ventricular complexes, and his cardiac isoenzymes are elevated. Which of the following is the best next test for evaluation for a blunt cardiac injury?

a. Measurement of serial creatinine phosphokinase and creatinine kinase (including the myocardial band) levels
b. Thallium stress test
c. Echocardiography
d. Single photon emission computed tomography (SPECT)
e. Multiple acquisition scans (MUGA)

159. A 70-year-old man presents to the ER with several fractures and a ruptured spleen after falling 20 ft. Which of the following will occur in response to the injury?

a. Decreased liver gluconeogenesis
b. Inhibition of skeletal muscle breakdown by interleukin 1 and tumor necrosis factor (TNF, cachectin)
c. Decreased urinary nitrogen loss
d. Hepatic synthesis of acute-phase reactants
e. Decreased glutamine consumption by fibroblasts, lymphocytes, and intestinal epithelial cells

160. A 36-year-old man sustains a gunshot wound to the left buttock. He is hemodynamically stable. There is no exit wound, and an x-ray of the abdomen shows the bullet to be located in the right lower quadrant. Which of the following is most appropriate in the management of his suspected rectal injury?

a. Barium studies of the colon and rectum
b. Barium studies of the bullet track
c. CT scan of the abdomen and pelvis
d. Angiography
e. Sigmoidoscopy in the ER

161. A 27-year-old man presents to the ER after a high-speed motor vehicle collision with chest pain and marked respiratory distress. On physical examination, he is hypotensive with distended neck veins and absence of breath sounds in the left chest. Which of the following is the proper initial treatment?

a. Intubation
b. Chest x-ray
c. Pericardiocentesis
d. Chest decompression with a needle
e. Emergent thoracotomy

162. A 48-year-old man sustains a gunshot wound to the right upper thigh just distal to the inguinal crease. He is immediately brought to the ER. Peripheral pulses are palpable in the foot, but the foot is pale, cool, and hypesthetic. The motor examination is normal. Which of the following statements is the most appropriate next step in the patient's management?

a. The patient should be taken to the operating room immediately to evaluate for a significant arterial injury.
b. A neurosurgical consult should be obtained and somatosensory evoked potential monitoring performed.
c. A fasciotomy should be performed prophylactically in the emergency room.
d. A duplex examination should be obtained to rule out a venous injury.
e. The patient should be observed for at least 6 hours and then reexamined for changes in the physical examination.

163. A 62-year-old woman is seen after a 3-day history of fever, abdominal pain, nausea, and anorexia. She has not urinated for 24 hours. She has a history of previous abdominal surgery for inflammatory bowel disease. Her blood pressure is 85/64 mm Hg, and her pulse is 136. Her response to this physiologic state includes which of the following?

a. Increase in sodium and water excretion
b. Increase in renal perfusion
c. Decrease in cortisol levels
d. Hyperkalemia
e. Hypoglycemia

164. A 20-year-old man presents after being punched in the right eye and assaulted to the head. On a facial CT scan, he is noted to have a blowout fracture of the right orbital floor. Which of the following findings mandates immediate surgical intervention?

a. A fracture 25% of the orbital floor
b. 1 mm of enophthalmos
c. Periorbital ecchymosis
d. Inability to move the right eye upward
e. Traumatic optic neuropathy

165. A 33-year-old woman is seen in the ER with severe rectal bleeding. She has a history of ulcerative colitis. Her blood pressure is 78/56 mm Hg, her pulse is 144, and she is pale and clammy. Which of the following responses is likely to occur after administration of Ringer lactate solution?

a. Increase in serum lactate concentration
b. Impairment of liver function
c. Improvement in hemodynamics by alleviating the deficit in the interstitial fluid compartment
d. Increase in metabolic acidosis
e. Increase in the need for blood transfusion

166. An 18-year-old high school football player is kicked in the left flank. Three hours later he develops hematuria. His vital signs are stable. A CT scan demonstrates a grade II renal injury based on the Urologic Injury Scale of the American Association for the Surgery of Trauma. Which of the following is the most appropriate treatment for this patient?

a. Resumption of normal daily activity excluding sports
b. Exploration and suture of the laceration
c. Exploration and wedge resection of the left kidney
d. Nephrostomy
e. Strict bed rest with serial hemoglobin levels

167. A 32-year-old man is in a high-speed motorcycle collision and presents with an obvious pelvic fracture. On examination, he has a scrotal hematoma and blood at his urethral meatus. Which of the following is the most appropriate next step in his management?

a. Placement of a Foley catheter
b. Cystoscopy
c. CT of the pelvis
d. Retrograde urethrogram
e. Nephrostomy tube placement

168. A 17-year-old adolescent boy sustains a small-caliber gunshot wound to the mid-epigastrium with no obvious exit wound. His abdomen is very tender; he is taken to the operating room and the bullet appears to have tracked through the stomach, distal pancreas, and spleen. The duct appears to have been injured. Which of the following is the best strategy for the management of this patient's pancreatic injury?

a. Drainage alone
b. Roux-en-Y pancreaticojejunostomy
c. Pancreaticoduodenectomy
d. Frey procedure
e. Distal pancreatectomy

169. A 22-year-old woman who is 4 months pregnant presents after a motor vehicle collision complaining of abdominal pain and right leg pain. She has an obvious deformity of her right femur. She is hemodynamically stable. Which of the following is the best next step in her management?

a. Observation with serial abdominal exams
b. Diagnostic peritoneal lavage
c. Plain film of the abdomen with a lead apron as a shield
d. Focused assessment with sonography for trauma (FAST) examination of the abdomen
e. MRI of the abdomen

170. The victim of a motor vehicle accident who was in shock is delivered to your trauma center by a rural ambulance service. On examination, his blood pressure is 80/60 mm Hg and he has an unstable pelvis. X-rays reveal a pelvic fracture. Chest x-ray is normal. FAST examination shows free fluid near the spleen. There are no major extremity deformities noted. A pelvic binder is placed. Which of the following statements is the best next step in the management of this patient?

a. Computed tomography of the chest
b. Computed tomography of the abdomen and pelvis
c. Angiography
d. Diagnostic peritoneal lavage
e. Exploratory laparotomy with pelvic packing

171. A radio transmission is received in your trauma unit stating that a victim of a motor vehicle collision is en route to your ER with no vital signs. The ambulance is 3 minutes away. As you formulate your plan, which of the following situations would constitute an indication for ER thoracotomy?

a. Massive hemothorax following blunt trauma to the chest
b. Blunt trauma to multiple organ systems with obtainable vital signs in the field, but none on arrival in the ER
c. Rapidly deteriorating patient with cardiac tamponade from penetrating thoracic trauma
d. Penetrating thoracic trauma and no signs of life in the field
e. Penetrating abdominal trauma and no signs of life in the field

172. A 22-year-old man sustains a gunshot wound to the abdomen. At exploration, an apparently solitary distal small-bowel injury is treated with resection and primary anastomosis. On postoperative day 7, small-bowel fluid drains through the operative incision. The fascia remains intact. The fistula output is 300 mL/day and there is no evidence of intra-abdominal sepsis. Which of the following is the most appropriate treatment strategy?

a. Early reoperation to close the fistula tract
b. Broad-spectrum antibiotics
c. Total parenteral nutrition
d. Somatostatin to lower fistula output
e. Loperamide to inhibit gut motility

173. A 26-year-old man complains of pelvic pain after a motorcycle collision. Physical and radiologic examinations confirm a pelvic fracture. Urologic workup reveals a normal urethrogram and an extraperitoneal bladder injury. Which of the following is the most appropriate treatment for his bladder injury?

a. Immediate surgical exploration and repair.
b. Placement of a permanent suprapubic tube
c. Catheter drainage followed by definitive repair after 2 weeks
d. Catheter drainage for 2 weeks followed by repeat imaging
e. Bilateral nephrostomy tubes

174. The patient shown in this chest x-ray film and contrast study was hospitalized after a car collision 2 days ago in which he suffered blunt trauma to the abdomen. He sustained several left rib fractures, but was hemodynamically stable. Which of the following is the appropriate next step in the patient's management?

a. Observation and serial abdominal exams
b. Immediate left posterolateral thoracotomy and repair of the injury
c. Immediate exploratory laparotomy and repair of the injury
d. Delayed left posterolateral thoracotomy and repair of the injury
e. Delayed exploratory laparotomy and repair of the injury

175. A 56-year-old woman sustains blunt abdominal trauma from an assault. Her blood pressure is 107/56 mm Hg and her pulse is 92. She complains of abdominal pain. She undergoes CT scanning of the abdomen and pelvis, which demonstrates a splenic injury. Which of the following would preclude an attempt at nonoperative management of the patient?

a. Presence of a subcapsular hematoma involving more than 25% of the surface area of the spleen
b. Presence of a subcapsular hematoma involving more than 50% of the surface area of the spleen
c. Evidence of a blush on CT scan
d. A red blood cell (RBC) count of 120,000/μL on diagnostic peritoneal lavage
e. Peritoneal signs on abdominal examination

176. A 49-year-old man was the restrained driver in a motor vehicle collision. He decelerated rapidly in order to avoid hitting another car and swerved into a ditch. He complains of chest pain. Which of the following findings on chest x-ray would be most suspicious for an aortic injury?

a. Multiple right-sided rib fractures
b. A left pulmonary contusion
c. A left pneumothorax
d. Widening of the mediastinum greater than 8 cm
e. Pneumomediastinum

177. A 29-year-old woman was hit by a car while crossing the street. She is hemodynamically unstable with a heart rate of 124 beats per minute and a systolic blood pressure of 82/45 mm Hg. The ultrasound machine is broken, and therefore a diagnostic peritoneal lavage (DPL) is performed. Which of the following findings on DPL is an indication for exploratory laparotomy in this patient?

a. Aspiration of 5 cc of gross blood initially
b. Greater than 50,000/μL red blood cells (RBCs)
c. Greater than 100,000/μL RBCs
d. Greater than 100/μL white blood cells (WBCs)
e. Greater than 250/μL WBCs

178. A 27-year-old construction worker falls about 30 ft from a scaffold. At the scene, he complains of inability to move his lower extremities. On arrival in the ER, he has a heart rate of 45 beats per minute and a blood pressure of 78/39 mm Hg. His extremities are warm and pink. His blood pressure improves with 1 L of crystalloid. A central venous catheter is placed for further resuscitation and his central venous pressure is 2 mm Hg. Which of the following is the best initial treatment strategy for improving his blood pressure?

a. Immediate celiotomy
b. Fluid resuscitation with crystalloids
c. Administration of O-negative blood
d. Administration of a peripheral vasoconstrictor
e. Administration of intravenous corticosteroids

179. A 22-year-old man undergoes an exploratory laparotomy after a gunshot wound to the abdomen. The patient has multiple injuries, including a significant liver laceration, multiple small-bowel and colon injuries, and an injury to the infrahepatic vena cava. The patient receives 35 units of packed RBCs, 15 L of crystalloid, 12 units of fresh-frozen plasma (FFP), and a 12 packs of platelets. The patient's abdomen is packed closed and he is taken to the intensive care unit for further resuscitation. Which of the following warrants a decompressive laparotomy?

a. Increased peak airway pressure
b. Increased cardiac output
c. Decreased systemic vascular resistance
d. Decreased plasma renin and aldosterone
e. Increased cerebral perfusion pressure

180. A 10-year-old girl is the unrestrained backseat passenger in a high-speed motor vehicle collision. She is intubated in the field for unresponsiveness and on presentation to the ER, her heart rate is 160 beats per minute, and her blood pressure is 60/35 mm Hg. She weighs 30 kg. Which of the following is the most appropriate recommendation for her fluid resuscitation?

a. Bolus 1 L of normal saline initially.
b. Bolus 1 L of 5% albumin initially.
c. Transfuse 300 cc of packed RBCs initially.
d. Bolus 600 cc of normal saline initially. Transfuse if no response.
e. Bolus 600 cc of normal saline initially followed by a repeat bolus. Transfuse if no response.

181. A 21-year-old woman sustains a stab wound to the middle of the chest. Upon arrival to the ER she has equal breath sounds, blood pressure of 85/46 mm Hg, distended neck veins, and pulsus paradoxus. Which of the following is the most appropriate management of this patient?

a. Emergent intubation and mechanical ventilation in the ER
b. Emergent pericardiocentesis in the ER
c. Emergent thoracotomy in the ER
d. Emergent pericardiocentesis or subxiphoid pericardial drainage after anesthetic induction in the operating room
e. Emergent pericardiocentesis or subxiphoid pericardial drainage under local anesthesia in the operating room

182. A 58-year-old man presents to the ER after falling 10 ft from a ladder. Examination reveals stable vital signs, no evidence of respiratory distress, and multiple right-sided rib fractures. Chest x-ray shows a hemothorax on the right side and a right tube thoracostomy is performed in the ER. Approximately 700 mL of blood is immediately drained with placement of the thoracostomy tube. Over the next 4 hours he continues to drain 300 mL/h after the original evacuation. Which of the following is the definitive treatment for this patient?

a. Platelets
b. Fresh-frozen plasma
c. Second tube thoracostomy
d. Thoracotomy in the operating room
e. Thoracotomy in the ER

183. A 65-year-old woman is involved in a motor vehicle collision and sustains multiple left-sided rib fractures. Upon presentation to the ER her vital signs are stable and she is in no respiratory distress. Chest x-ray reveals fractures of ribs 4 to 7 on the left side without evidence of hemothorax or pneumothorax. She is admitted for observation and a few hours later she develops shortness of breath. A repeat chest x-ray demonstrates a well-defined infiltrate in her left lung. What is the most likely diagnosis?

a. Pulmonary contusion
b. Pulmonary embolus
c. Pneumonia
d. Myocardial infarction
e. Cardiac tamponade

184. Following a head-on motor vehicle collision, a 21-year-old unrestrained passenger presents to the ER with dyspnea and respiratory distress. She is intubated and physical examination reveals subcutaneous emphysema and decreased breath sounds. Chest x-ray reveals cervical emphysema, pneumomediastinum, and a right-sided pneumothorax. What is the most likely diagnosis?

a. Tension pneumothorax
b. Open pneumothorax
c. Tracheobronchial injury
d. Esophageal injury
e. Pulmonary contusion

185. An intoxicated 22-year-old man is a restrained driver in a high-speed motor vehicle collision. Examination reveals normal vital signs, but the rest of the examination is unreliable secondary to the patient's intoxicated state from alcohol. Which of the following sole findings on a CT scan of the abdomen and pelvis mandates an exploratory laparotomy?

a. Free fluid in the pelvis
b. Pelvic fracture
c. Liver hematoma
d. Splenic hematoma
e. Renal hematoma

186. A 23-year-old man arrives in the ER after a motor vehicle collision. Examination reveals an unstable pelvis and blood at the urethral meatus. Which of the following studies would most accurately identify a urethral injury?

a. CT scan of the pelvis
b. Intravenous pyelogram
c. Stress cystogram
d. Antegrade urethrogram
e. Retrograde urethrogram

Questions 187 to 191

An 18-year-old woman is transported to your trauma unit after sustaining a side-impact collision on her side of the car. She is hypotensive and in respiratory distress, and has distended neck veins. For each immediately life-threatening injury of the chest, select the proper intervention. Each lettered option may be used once, more than once, or not at all.

a. Endotracheal intubation
b. Cricothyroidotomy
c. Subxiphoid window
d. Tube thoracostomy
e. Occlusive dressing

187. Laryngeal obstruction.

188. Open pneumothorax.

189. Flail chest.

190. Tension pneumothorax.

191. Pericardial tamponade.

Trauma and Shock

Answers

132. The answer is c. *(Townsend, pp 500-501.)* The patient has an acute diaphragmatic rupture, which occurs in about 4% of patients who sustain either blunt abdominal or chest trauma, and should be treated with immediate laparotomy, which allows both for examination of the intra-abdominal solid and hollow viscera for associated injuries and for adequate exposure of the diaphragm to allow secure repair. Because of the risk of vascular compromise of the contents of the hernia, exacerbated by the negative thoracic pressure, acute diaphragmatic rupture should be repaired immediately. Diagnosis may be difficult. The finding of an air-fluid level in the left lower chest, with a nasogastric tube entering it after blunt trauma to the abdomen, is diagnostic of diaphragmatic rupture with gastric herniation into the chest. Esophagogastroscopy is of limited value. CT scanning and MRI may be useful adjuncts, but neither can definitively rule out diaphragmatic rupture. Diagnostic peritoneal lavage is neither sensitive nor specific for diaphragmatic injuries, particularly in the absence of significant hemorrhage. Diaphragmatic repair can be accomplished via the left chest, but laparotomy is the procedure of choice for acute traumatic rupture for the stated reasons.

133. The answer is e. *(Townsend, pp 503-504.)* The presence of an abdominal wall ecchymosis from a seatbelt, or a "seatbelt sign," should raise suspicion for an enteric or mesenteric injury. Therefore, these patients should be observed closely for worsening abdominal pain, fevers, or signs of sepsis, even in the face of negative diagnostic tests. Serum amylase levels, plain films of the abdomen, abdominal CT scans, and DPL all have low sensitivity for small-bowel injuries. CT scan findings of free air, thickening of the small-bowel wall or mesentery, or free fluid in the absence of solid-organ injury should raise suspicion of a hollow viscus injury. DPL findings of a WBC count greater than 500/µL, an elevated amylase value, or detection of bile, bacteria, or food fibers should prompt exploratory laparotomy to rule out a bowel injury.

134. The answer is d. (*Townsend, pp 495-496*.) Patients with lower rib fractures may have associated abdominal injuries and should undergo appropriate evaluation (eg, ultrasound examination, CT scanning, or peritoneal lavage). Epidural catheters, continuous narcotic infusions, and patient-controlled analgesia are the most effective methods for ensuring pain control in hospitalized patients with rib fractures. Patients who are elderly, have multiple rib fractures, demonstrate ventilatory compromise, or have underlying respiratory problems (such as chronic obstructive pulmonary disease or smoking) are at increased risk for pulmonary complications (atelectasis, pneumonia, respiratory failure) and should be hospitalized. Patients with minor fracture injuries and no significant comorbidities may be managed at home with oral analgesics and appropriate instructions for coughing and deep breathing. Attempts to relieve pain by immobilization or splinting, such as strapping the chest, merely compound the problem of inadequate ventilation. Tube thoracostomy is indicated only if pneumothorax is diagnosed. Intercostal nerve blocks often provide prolonged periods of pain relief, but have been largely replaced by epidural catheters and intravenous narcotic administration. Rib fractures heal spontaneously, without need for surgical fixation.

135. The answer is c. (*Townsend, pp 502-504, 513-515*.) The spleen is the organ most likely to be damaged in blunt abdominal trauma, and splenic and liver injuries combined account for 75% of all blunt intra-abdominal injuries. The diagnosis of injuries resulting from blunt abdominal trauma is difficult; injuries are often masked by associated injuries. Thus, trauma to the head or chest, together with fractures, frequently conceals intra-abdominal injury. Apparently trivial injuries may rupture abdominal viscera in spite of the protection offered by the rib cage. Abdominal ultrasound (or FAST) is a rapid diagnostic test used to evaluate for free intraperitoneal fluid and has largely replaced DPL as the test of choice for evaluation for abdominal injury after blunt trauma. Abdominal CT scans are more specific than either ultrasound or DPL for hepatic, splenic, and renal injuries and can be performed in hemodynamically stable patients, who are candidates for nonoperative therapy.

136. The answer is d. (*Townsend, pp 542-544*.) Ligation rather than venous repair is the treatment of choice in hemodynamically unstable patients. However, the role of venous repair in hemodynamically stable patients with combined arterial and venous extremity injuries is controversial. Proximal veins should be repaired to avoid the sequelae of chronic venous insufficiency. Repairs can be performed primarily with suture closure, using saphenous vein patches, or using synthetic interposition grafts. Amputation may be necessary in the setting of extensive soft tissue and skeletal injuries in conjunction with the vascular injury.

137. The answer is b. *(Townsend, pp 542-544.)* Immediate exploration and repair is mandated for acute arterial insufficiency in the presence of neurologic symptoms. Exploration is indicated in the presence of "hard signs" such as expanding hematoma, pulsatile bleeding, audible bruit, palpable thrill, and evidence of absent distal pulses or evidence of distal ischemia. "Soft signs" include a hypotension/shock, history of hemorrhage at the scene of the injury, peripheral nerve deficit, stable hematoma, and proximity of the injury to a major vessel. The 5 Ps of acute arterial insufficiency include pain, paresthesias, pallor, pulselessness, and paralysis. In the extremities, the tissues most sensitive to anoxia are the peripheral nerves and striated muscle. The early developments of paresthesias and paralysis are signals that there is significant ischemia present, and immediate exploration and repair are warranted. The presence of palpable pulses does not exclude an arterial injury because this presence may represent a transmitted pulsation through a blood clot. When severe ischemia is present, the repair must be completed within 6 to 8 hours to prevent irreversible muscle ischemia and loss of limb function. Delay to obtain an angiogram or to observe for change needlessly prolongs the ischemic time. Fasciotomy may be required, but should be done in conjunction with and after reestablishment of arterial flow. Local wound exploration at the bedside is not recommended because brisk hemorrhage may be encountered without the securing of prior proximal and distal vascular control.

138. The answer is c. *(Townsend, pp 1671-1672.)* Tension pneumothorax is a life-threatening problem requiring immediate treatment. A lung wound that behaves as a ball or flap valve allows escaped air to build up pressure in the intrapleural space. This causes collapse of the ipsilateral lung and shifting of the mediastinum and trachea to the contralateral side, in addition to compression of the vena cava and contralateral lung. Sudden death may ensue because of a decrease in cardiac output, hypoxemia, and ventricular arrhythmias. To accomplish rapid decompression of the pleural space, a large-gauge needle should be passed into the intrapleural cavity through the second intercostal space at the midclavicular line just above the third rib. This may be attached temporarily to an underwater seal with subsequent insertion of a chest tube after the life-threatening urgency has been relieved. Tension pneumothorax produces characteristic x-ray findings of ipsilateral lung collapse, mediastinal and tracheal shift, and compression of the contralateral lung. Occasionally, adhesions prevent complete lung collapse, but the tension pneumothorax is evident because of the mediastinal displacement.

139. The answer is c. (*Townsend, pp 500-501, 502-504.*) Diaphragmatic or abdominal injuries should be suspected in patients with a penetrating injury below the nipples. Diagnostic laparoscopy is appropriate to evaluate for an abdominal injury in penetrating trauma to the thoracoabdominal transition area. CT scan has a low sensitivity for diagnosing abdominal injuries in the setting of penetrating trauma. Local wound exploration is contraindicated in penetrating trauma to the chest, given the risk of creating a pneumothorax. An immediate tube thoracostomy is indicated in patients with a suspected tension pneumothorax or in the hemodynamically unstable patient with a suspected pneumo- or hemothorax (eg, decreased breath sounds). In hemodynamically stable patients without clinical evidence of a pneumothorax, a chest x-ray should be obtained prior to tube thoracostomy. Echocardiography is appropriate for the evaluation for a pericardial effusion in the setting of a penetrating cardiac injury and should be performed for penetrating wounds between the clavicle and costal margin and medial to the midclavicular line.

140. The answer is a. (*Brunicardi, pp 16-20.*) Though the immediate release of catecholamines causes a transient drop in insulin levels, shortly thereafter there is a significant rise in plasma insulin levels in injured humans. Because of increased peripheral insulin resistance in conjunction with increased insulin production, the overall net effect after severe injury is that of hyperglycemia. Since injured patients are highly hypermetabolic, it might be expected that the activity of the thyroid hormones would be increased following injury. This is not the case, however, and increased levels of the thyroid hormones are not seen. Vasopressin (ADH) is regulated by serum osmolality. In the post-injury period, many factors are at play that provoke the excretion of vasopressin. Glucagon secretion is normal or increased after injury; not only are aldosterone levels elevated, but the diurnal fluctuations ordinarily seen are lost.

141. The answer is d. *(Moore, pp 654-656.)* Traumatic injury to the common bile duct must be considered in 2 separate categories. Complete transection of the common bile duct can be handled in many ways. If the patient is unstable and time is limited, simply placing a T tube in either end of the open common bile duct and staging the repair is the treatment of choice. In a stable patient with a transected bile duct and a loss of tissue, a biliary enteric bypass is preferred. This can be accomplished by Roux-en-Y choledochojejunostomy or cholecystojejunostomy. The jejunum is favored over the duodenum because a lateral duodenal fistula is avoided if the anastomosis leaks. For similar reasons, the defunctionalizing of the jejunal limb is also preferable. This can be accomplished by creating a Roux-en-Y limb of jejunum. Primary end-to-end repair of a completely transected common bile duct can be performed if there is no significant tissue loss and an anastomosis can be performed without significant tension. Primary repair under tension is associated with an increased likelihood of a subsequent stricture. Primary repair is the procedure of choice if the common bile duct is lacerated or only partially transected.

142. The answer is d. *(Townsend, pp 489-493.)* Acute signs of airway distress (stridor, hoarseness, dysphonia), visceral injury (subcutaneous air, hemoptysis, dysphagia), hemorrhage (expanding hematoma, unchecked external bleeding), and neurologic symptoms referable to carotid injury (stroke or altered mental status) or lower cranial nerve or brachial plexus injury require formal neck exploration. Pneumothorax would mandate a chest tube; the necessity for exploration would depend on clinical judgment and institutional policy. Additionally, all hemodynamically unstable patients with a penetrating neck wound should be explored, while management of asymptomatic, stable patients with neck injuries that penetrate the platysma is more controversial. In the past, treatment of asymptomatic, stable patients with zone II (between the lower border of the cricoid cartilage to the angle of the mandible) injuries was mandatory operative exploration. However, proponents for selective management of these patients argue that there is a high rate of negative explorations of the neck (40%-60%) and that serious injuries can be overlooked despite operative exploration. Furthermore, studies have demonstrated similar incidences of overall mortality with either selective or mandatory exploration. Stable patients with zone III (between the angle of the mandible and the skull), zone I (between the sternal notch and the lower border of the cricoid cartilage), or multiple neck wounds, should undergo initial angiography irrespective of the ultimate treatment plan. For zone II injuries, algorithms exist for nonoperative management of asymptomatic patients that employ observation alone or combinations of vascular and aerodigestive contrast studies and endoscopy.

143. The answer is b. (*Townsend, pp 505-506.*) Duodenal hematomas result from blunt abdominal trauma, and they should be managed initially with observation in patients not undergoing laparotomy to rule out other associated injuries. They present as a proximal bowel obstruction with abdominal pain and occasionally a palpable right upper quadrant mass. An upper gastrointestinal series is almost always diagnostic, with the classic coiled spring appearance of the second and third portions of the duodenum secondary to the crowding of the valvulae conniventes (circular folds) by the hematoma. Observation is the initial management strategy in patients with no other injuries, since the vast majority of duodenal hematomas resolve spontaneously. However, in patients undergoing immediate laparotomy for other associated injuries, duodenal exploration with drainage of the hematoma is indicated. Also, patients whose obstructive symptoms do not resolve after 2 weeks should undergo exploration and evacuation of the hematoma in order to rule out a perforation or injury to the head of the pancreas. Surgical bypass and duodenal resection are not indicated in the initial management of a duodenal hematoma.

144. The answer is b. (*Townsend, p 365; Moore, pp 473-475.*) Blunt carotid artery injuries should be treated with full systemic anticoagulation in the absence to any contraindications to prevent stroke. If anticoagulation is not feasible, antiplatelet therapy is an accepted second-line therapy. While surgery, intra-extracranial bypass, and stenting have all been used to treat carotid injuries, but none are the standard of care in the neurologically intact patient without any hard signs (eg, expanding hematoma, bruit, thrill, active bleeding). Ligation should be considered in an unstable patient with uncontrolled hemorrhage. Carotid artery injuries should be suspected in patients based on the mechanism of injury, associated injuries, and neurologic examination (eg, presence of a lateralizing neurologic deficit not explained by head CT).

145. The answer is a. (*Townsend, pp 485-487.*) Closed-head injuries may result in cerebral concussion owing to depression of the reticular formation of the brainstem. This type of injury is usually reversible. A characteristic symptom pattern occurs and it is initiated by progressive depression of mental status. Local bleeding and swelling (intracranial or extracranial) produce an increase in intracranial pressure. Patients may develop Cushing triad (hypertension, bradycardia, and irregular respirations) as a sign of increased intracranial pressure. Lateralizing signs (motor or pupillary) are relatively uncommon and are highly suggestive of focal intracranial lesions.

146. The answer is e. (*Townsend, pp 486-487.*) Emergency measures to reduce intracranial pressure include hyperventilation, mannitol infusion, and elevation of the head of the bed (reverse Trendelenburg position). However, in the face of inadequate volume resuscitation, osmotic diuresis with mannitol and placement of the patient in reverse Trendelenburg may exacerbate the patient's hypotension. CT scanning should be performed as soon as possible along with neurosurgical evaluation in order to determine the need for operative drainage or decompression.

147. The answer is b. (*Townsend, pp 485-487.*) Increasing intracranial pressure tends to displace brain tissue away from the source of the pressure; if the pressure is sufficient, herniation of the uncal process through the tentorium cerebri occurs. Pupillary dilation is caused by compression of the ipsilateral oculomotor nerve and its parasympathetic fibers. If the pressure is not relieved, the brainstem will herniate through the foramen magnum and cause death. Hypertension and bradycardia are preterminal events.

148. The answer is e. (*Townsend, pp 496-497.*) Management of flail chest consists of adequate analgesia, chest physiotherapy, and mechanical ventilation if respiratory compromise develops. Flail chest is diagnosed in the presence of paradoxical respiratory movement in a portion of the chest wall. At least 2 fractures in each of 3 adjacent rib or costal cartilages are required to produce this condition. The complications of flail chest are no longer believed to arise from this paradoxical motion, but rather the underlying pulmonary parenchymal injury with resultant hypoventilation can lead to atelectasis, pneumonia, and respiratory failure. Indications for mechanical ventilation include significant impedance to ventilation by the flail segment, large pulmonary contusion, an uncooperative patient (eg, owing to head injury), general anesthesia for another indication, and the development of respiratory failure. Chest stabilization with sandbags or towel clips is no longer used. Surgical stabilization is performed only if thoracotomy is to be performed for another indication.

149. The answer is c. *(Brunicardi, pp 1610-1616.)* The motor components of the median nerve maintain the muscular function of most of the long flexors of the hand as well as the pronators of the forearm and the thenar muscles. The median nerve is also an extremely important sensory innervator of the hand and is commonly described as the "eye of the hand" because the palm, the thumb, and the index and middle fingers all receive their sensation via the median nerve.

150. The answer is d. *(Brunicardi, pp 1104-1105.)* Carbon monoxide (CO) is the leading cause of toxin-related death in the United States. Tobacco smoke—particularly smoke released from the tip of the cigarette, which has 2.5 times more CO than inhaled smoke—produces a significant amount of the gas; nonsmokers working in closed quarters with smokers may have carboxyhemoglobin levels as high as 15%, easily enough to cause headache and some impairment of judgment. Firefighters are at particularly high risk for CO intoxication. The pathophysiology of CO poisoning is unclear. It is known to cause an adverse shift in the oxygen-hemoglobin dissociation curve, to cause direct cardiovascular depression, and to inhibit cytochrome a_3. Tissue hypoxia is the result. Treatment is directed toward increasing the partial pressures of O_2 to which the transalveolar hemoglobin is exposed. In most cases, administering 100% oxygen through a tightly fitted face mask will result in a serum elimination half-life of COHb of 80 minutes (compared with 520 minutes when breathing room air). In severe cases, where coma, seizures, or respiratory failure are present, the partial pressure of O_2 is increased by administering it in a hyperbaric chamber with an atmospheric pressure of 2.8. In this situation, the serum elimination half-life is reduced to 23 minutes. In any case, the oxygen therapy should continue until the COHb levels reach 10%.

151. The answer is b. *(Brunicardi, pp 105-106.)* Cardiogenic shock is a circulatory pump failure leading to substantial reduction in cardiac output and resulting tissue hypoxia in the setting of adequate intravascular volume. Acute myocardial infarction is the most common cause of cardiogenic shock. Treatment of cardiac dysfunction includes maintenance of adequate oxygenation and judicious fluid administration to avoid fluid overload and development of cardiogenic pulmonary edema. The patient in this scenario has evidence of volume overload based on the elevated central venous pressure; therefore, further fluid administration is contraindicated. Inotropic support is indicated when profound cardiac dysfunction exists to improve cardiac contractility and cardiac output. Dobutamine and dopamine are commonly used inotropes in cardiogenic shock. Patients who are refractory to inotropes may require mechanical circulatory support with an intra-aortic balloon pump. This balloon pump increases coronary blood flow by reduction in systolic afterload and augmentation of diastolic perfusion pressure. Cardiac catheterization and heart transplantation have no role in the management of cardiogenic shock.

152. The answer is d. *(Moore, p 1056.)* The treatment of electrical injury should be modified from that of thermal burns because tissue damage is much deeper than is apparent at first inspection. The heat generated is proportional to the resistance to the flow of current. Bone, fat, and tendons offer the greatest resistance. Therefore, the tissue deep within the center of an extremity may be injured while more superficial tissues are spared. For this reason, the quantification of fluid requirements cannot be based on the percentage of body surface area involved, as in the Parkland, Brooke, or Baxter formulas used to calculate fluid replacement after thermal burns. Massive fluid replacement is usually essential. A brisk urine output is desirable because of the likelihood of myonecrosis with consequent myoglobinuria and renal damage. As with deep thermal burns, debridement, skin grafting, and amputation of extremities may be required following electrical injury. However, fasciotomy is more frequently required than escharotomy with electrical injury because deep myonecrosis results in increased intracompartmental pressures and compromised limb perfusion. In addition, distant fractures may result, owing to vigorous muscle contraction during the accident or if subsequent falls occur. Cardiac or respiratory arrest may occur if the pathway of the current includes the heart or brain. An electrical current can also damage the pulmonary alveoli and capillaries and lead to respiratory infections, a major cause of death in these victims. Electrical burns can also result in cataract development even months after the injury, and therefore these patients require ophthalmologic follow-up.

153. The answer is a. *(Townsend, pp 427-428; Moore, pp 926-927.)* Popliteal arterial injuries are associated with knee dislocations because of the extreme force required to dislocate the joint. An ankle-brachial index (ABI) of greater than 0.9 is associated with a low risk for popliteal injury. If the ABI is less than 0.9, angiogram or CT angiogram is indicated. The ankle-brachial index is calculated as the ratio of the systolic pressure in the leg (the higher value between that of the posterior tibial artery and that of the dorsalis pedis artery) over the systolic pressure in the arm (the higher value between the right and left brachial artery pressure), measured with a Doppler and a manual blood pressure cuff. A popliteal injury can be present even in the absence of hard signs of arterial ischemia such as a diminished pulse, altered neurologic examination, expanding hematoma, pulsatile mass, or bruit/thrill. Popliteal artery injuries should be treated with operative repair after stabilization and external fixation of the knee. Fasciotomies should be considered after repair because compartment syndrome can occur from ischemia-reperfusion injury, particularly if the limb has been ischemic for more than 6 hours. Observation is reasonable in patients with ABI > 0.9 and no hard signs of arterial injury.

154. The answer is d. *(Townsend, pp 495-496, 500-504.)* Gunshot wounds to the lower chest are often associated with intra-abdominal injuries; any patient with a gunshot wound below the level of T4 should be subjected to abdominal exploration. The domes of the diaphragm are at the level of the nipples, and the diaphragm can rise to the level of T4 during maximal expiration. Exploratory thoracotomy is not automatically indicated because most parenchymal lung injuries will stop bleeding and heal spontaneously with tube thoracostomy alone. Indications for thoracic exploration for bleeding are 1500 mL of blood on initial chest tube placement or persistent bleeding at a rate of 200 mL/h for 4 hours or 100 mL/h for 8 hours. Peritoneal lavage is not indicated even when the abdominal examination is unremarkable. As many as 25% of patients with negative physical findings and negative peritoneal lavage will have significant intra-abdominal injuries in this setting. These injuries include damage to the colon, kidney, pancreas, aorta, and diaphragm. Local wound exploration is not recommended because the determination of diaphragmatic injury with this technique is unreliable.

155. The answer is e. *(Moore, pp 174-179.)* Except in the rare circumstance, hypotension in a trauma patient should be presumed to be secondary to hypovolemia and not the head injury. When cardiovascular collapse occurs as a result of rising intracranial pressure, it is generally accompanied by hypertension, bradycardia, and respiratory depression. On the other hand, loss of consciousness following head trauma should be assumed to be because of intracranial hemorrhage until proved otherwise. A thorough evaluation of the head-injured patient includes assessment for other potentially life-threatening injuries, including abdominal, thoracic, and pelvic hemorrhage. Appropriate workup should be initiated (chest and pelvic x-rays, abdominal evaluation with FAST examination or DPL). Rarely, a patient may have sufficient hemorrhage from a scalp laceration to cause hypotension, but caution should be used in attributing hypotension and tachycardia solely to such an injury.

156. The answer is b. (*Townsend, pp 508-509.*) Primary repair of traumatic colon injuries can be safely performed in the absence of risk factors such as gross fecal contamination, shock on presentation, multiple other injuries, or delayed intervention. Alternatives to primary repair include end colostomy with mucous fistula or Hartmann pouch and protection of a primary repair in the distal colon by formation of a proximal colostomy or ileostomy. A mucous fistula is when the proximal end of the distal colon is brought out as a stoma, in addition to the proximal end colostomy. The intent of a mucous fistula is to drain mucous and is typically created if there is an obstruction in the distal remaining colon or if there is a long segment of colon remaining. A Hartmann pouch is when the rectum or rectosigmoid is left as a blind pouch. There is no evidence that prolonged antibiotics greater than 24 hours in the setting of immediate repair or that placement of a drain reduces postoperative infectious complications.

157. The answer is d. (*Townsend, pp 307-309.*) Crepitus in a soft tissue infection implies anaerobic metabolism. Since human tissue cannot survive in an anaerobic environment, gas associated with an infection implies dead tissue and therefore a surgical infection. Necrotizing fasciitis is associated with high rates of morbidity and mortality and prompt surgical exploration is mandatory. While CT and MRI may be useful adjuncts in the diagnosis of necrotizing fasciitis, they should not be performed in unstable patients or patients in whom the diagnosis is likely. Treatment consists of prompt surgical debridement and intravenous antibiotics. Most of these infections are polymicrobial, although monomicrobial necrotizing soft tissue infections can be caused by group A beta-hemolytic *Streptococcus* or *Clostridium*. If the latter is suspected, high-dose penicillin G should be administered. Hyperbaric oxygen may be used as an adjunct; however, its efficacy has never been proven in clinical trials.

158. The answer is c. (*Moore, pp 578-583.*) Echocardiography provides a sensitive assessment of ventricular wall motion and ejection fraction after blunt chest trauma and is indicated in hemodynamically unstable patients, but is a poor predictor of the significant cardiac complications of pump failure and arrhythmia. On the other hand, although fewer than 10% of patients have an abnormal initial ECG, virtually all patients who develop cardiac complications display ECG abnormalities on arrival in the ER or within the first 24 hours. Nuclear medicine studies such as a thallium stress test, single photon emission computed tomography (SPECT), and multiple-acquisition scans (MUGA) add little value to the workup and/or management of patients with suspected blunt cardiac injury.

The spectrum of blunt cardiac injuries includes myocardial contusion, rupture, and internal (chamber and septal) disruptions such as traumatic septal defects, papillary muscle tears, and valvular tears. Myocardial contusions are by far the most common of these injuries. They usually occur in persons who sustain a direct blow to the sternum, as seen in a driver whose sternum is forcibly compressed by the steering column in a deceleration injury. They may have external signs of thoracic trauma, including sternal tenderness, abrasions, ecchymosis, palpable crepitus, rib fractures, or flail segments. Overall, fewer than 10% of patients have conduction abnormalities, dysrhythmias, or ischemic patterns on the initial ECG. Elevated cardiac isoenzyme levels are specific for myocardial injury, but they lack clinical significance in patients without ECG abnormalities or hemodynamic instability. Patients without evidence of ECG abnormalities on presentation and who are hemodynamically stable do not require extended ICU monitoring. Stable patients with possible myocardial contusions but with a normal ECG tracing may be placed on telemetry for 24 hours rather than monitored in an ICU.

159. The answer is d. (*Brunicardi, pp 16-40.*) Injury and sepsis result in accelerated protein breakdown with increased urinary nitrogen loss and increased peripheral release of amino acids. The negative nitrogen balance represents the net result of breakdown and synthesis (with breakdown increased and synthesis increased or diminished). Amino acids such as alanine are released by muscle and transported to the liver for incorporation into acute-phase proteins, including fibrinogen, complement, haptoglobin, and ferritin. The amino acids also undergo gluconeogenesis to glucose, which is utilized primarily by the brain and other glycolytic tissues such as peripheral nerves, erythrocytes, and bone marrow. Other tissues receive energy from fat in the form of fatty acids or ketone bodies during starvation following major trauma; this helps to conserve body protein. Glutamine is the most abundant amino acid in the blood, and its levels in muscle and blood decrease following injury and sepsis, as it is consumed rapidly by replicating fibroblasts, lymphocytes, and intestinal endothelial cells. The use of glutamine may decrease protein catabolism in the intestine and may help prevent atrophy of the gastrointestinal tract in starved and parenterally nourished patients. Along with the counter regulatory hormones (glucagon, epinephrine, cortisol), interleukin 1 appears to mediate muscle breakdown. Recent studies have indicated that TNF (also called cachectin because of the role it plays in muscle wasting in septic or oncologic patients) also may be a principal catabolic cytokine in the traumatized patient. This protein is secreted by macrophages and further affects metabolism by inducing secretion of interleukin 1 and inhibiting synthesis and activity of lipogenic enzymes.

160. The answer is c. (*Moore, pp 728-729.*) A CT scan should be routinely requested for suspected rectal perforation. The use of rectal contrast with water-soluble radiopaque medium such as Gastrografin is helpful when reconstructing a bullet trajectory. The use of barium is contraindicated because its spillage in the peritoneal cavity mixed with feces would increase the likelihood of subsequent intra-abdominal abscesses. Instrumentation of the bullet track is also contraindicated because of the risk of injury to adjacent structures (eg, bladder, ureters, iliac vessels). Angiography is not a sensitive method for demonstrating injury of the intestinal wall. Rigid sigmoidoscopy should be used if the CT scan is suggestive but ambiguous.

161. The answer is d. (*Moore, p 173.*) The patient has a tension pneumothorax caused by blunt trauma from the motor vehicle collision, which should be treated with emergent needle decompression. A tension pneumothorax develops when air continuously enters the pleural space from the lung or through the chest wall, cannot escape, and causes the lung to collapse. This air is under pressure and causes a shift of the mediastinum toward the opposite side with compression of the vena cava, leading to decreased venous return to the heart and hypotension. The diagnosis of a tension pneumothorax is a clinical one and should never wait for chest x-ray confirmation. This will delay lifesaving intervention with emergent needle decompression of the chest (14-gauge catheter-over-needle inserted into the second intercostal space in the midclavicular line). Hypotension and distended neck veins are also seen in cardiac tamponade, but breath sounds are usually symmetric. An emergent thoracotomy is not indicated for a tension pneumothorax.

162. The answer is a. (*Townsend, pp 542-544.*) The presence of ischemic changes following vascular trauma is an indication for emergency exploration and repair. Nonsurgical management of arterial trauma when distal pulses are palpable may lead to delayed sequelae of embolization, occlusion, secondary hemorrhage, false aneurysm, and traumatic arteriovenous fistula. The presence of palpable pulses does not reliably exclude significant arterial injury. Injuries that may be missed if exploration is not performed include lacerations and partial transections containing hematomas, intramural or intraluminal thromboses, and intimal disruptions or tears. Injury to motor nerves would be apparent on neurologic examination. Injury to bone would be diagnosed by x-ray. Adjacent venous injury, in the absence of an expanding hematoma, would not by itself mandate exploration because there are numerous collateral venous channels in the extremities.

Prophylactic fasciotomy is not routinely performed for all arterial injuries but is indicated in the presence of an ischemic period exceeding 4 to 6 hours, combined arterial and major venous injury, prolonged periods of hypotension, massive associated soft tissue trauma, and massive edema.

163. The answer is d. (*Townsend, pp 93-94.*) The biochemical changes associated with shock result from tissue hypoperfusion, endocrine response to stress, and specific organ system failure. During shock, the sympathetic nervous system and adrenal medulla are stimulated to release catecholamines. Renin, angiotensin, antidiuretic hormone, adrenocorticotropin, and cortisol levels increase. Resultant changes include sodium and water retention and an increase in potassium excretion, protein catabolism, and gluconeogenesis. Potassium levels rise as a result of increased tissue release, anaerobic metabolism, and decreased renal perfusion. If renal function is maintained, potassium excretion is high and normal plasma potassium levels are restored.

164. The answer is d. (*Moore, p 432.*) Blowout orbital fractures require immediate operative intervention in the event of extraocular muscle entrapment. Inability to move the eye upward suggests entrapment of the superior rectus muscle and mandates surgical release of the muscle. Patients with blowout fractures can have periorbital ecchymoses, pain, or diplopia. Surgery is indicated in patients with enophthalmos greater than 2 mm, diplopia on primary or inferior gaze, entrapment of extraocular muscles, or fracture greater than 50% of the orbital floor.

165. The answer is c. (*Townsend, p 100.*) Infusion of lactated Ringer solution, which is an isotonic fluid, is the initial management strategy for resuscitating patients with hypovolemic shock. However, if patients with hemorrhagic shock fail to respond to 2 L of isotonic fluids or if patients are predicted to require massive transfusion (> 10 units of packed red blood cells in 24 hours), blood should be administered. Use of this balanced salt solution helps correct the fluid deficit (in the extracellular, extravascular compartment), resulting from hypovolemic shock. Use of lactated Ringer may be sufficient for resuscitation in Class I (0%-15% total blood volume loss) or Class II (15%-30% total blood volume loss) hemorrhage. The patient in this scenario will likely require blood transfusion given her hypotension and tachycardia, indicating Class III (30%-40% total blood volume loss) or Class IV (> 40% total blood volume loss) hemorrhage. The lactate in lactated Ringer is metabolized to bicarbonate in the liver. Along with the hemodynamic improvement that follows volume restitution, liver function improves, lactate metabolism is improved, excess lactate levels drop, and metabolic acidosis improves.

166. The answer is e. *(Moore, pp 790-803.)* The organ injury scale utilizes 5 grades of injury, ranging from contusion or subcapsular hematoma (I) to shattered kidney or avulsion of the hilum (V). Grade II consists of a nonexpanding perirenal hematoma confined to the renal retroperitoneum or laceration less than 1 cm of parenchymal depth of renal cortex without urinary extravasation. Low-grade renal injuries can be managed nonoperatively with a high success rate. The patient is placed on strict bed rest for the first 24 to 72 hours with serial hemoglobins. If nonoperative management is successful, the patient is instructed to avoid significant physical exertion until follow-up imaging reveals adequate healing. Indications for renal exploration following injury include hemodynamic instability, ongoing hemorrhage requiring significant transfusion, or avulsion of the pedicle.

167. The answer is d. *(Moore, pp 805-806.)* If a urethral injury is suspected, a retrograde urethrogram should be performed before attempting to place a Foley catheter. If there is a urethral disruption, a suprapubic catheter should be placed. Urethral injuries can be associated with pelvic fractures, and suspicion of a urethral injury should be increased if any of the following signs are present: blood at the urethral meatus, a scrotal hematoma, or a free-floating prostate on rectal examination.

168. The answer is e. *(Moore, pp 713-716.)* While the majority of penetrating pancreatic injuries can be managed with simple drainage, injury to the major pancreatic duct to the left of the mesenteric vessels is effectively treated with a distal pancreatectomy. The high morbidity and mortality of pancreaticoduodenectomy for trauma limit its use to extensive blunt injuries to both pancreatic head and duodenum. For ductal injury in the region of the head of the pancreas (to the right of the mesenteric vessels), a Roux-en-Y limb of jejunum can be brought up and used to drain the transected duct. However small, all peripancreatic hematomas should be explored to search for pancreatic injury. Complications of pancreatic injury include fistula, pseudocyst, and abscess, but the cause of death in patients with pancreatic injury is most frequently exsanguination from associated injury to major vascular structures such as the splenic vessels, mesenteric vessels, aorta, or inferior vena cava. Frey procedure is used in chronic pancreatitis and involves removing part of the head of the pancreas, and it is not indicated for traumatic pancreatic injury.

169. The answer is d. (*Moore, pp 831-836.*) The goals in performing a diagnostic workup and managing a pregnant trauma patient are the same as those for any trauma patient. While radiologic imaging tests should be minimized, indicated tests should not be delayed or deferred because of concern of fetal exposure to radiation. FAST is the initial diagnostic modality of choice in a pregnant patient with abdominal trauma. While diagnostic peritoneal lavage can be used to evaluate the abdomen, it is invasive and has been largely replaced in centers by FAST. Plain films of the abdomen are not typically used in the workup of abdominal trauma patients. CT scanning can be performed in hemodynamically stable pregnant patients. MRI is not associated with ionizing radiation but is not typically rapidly available for use in evaluation of abdominal trauma.

170. The answer is e. (*Moore, pp 767-779.*) The patient is in hemorrhagic shock from an unstable pelvic fracture and a probable splenic injury. A formal pelvic binder or a bedsheet can be used to compress the pelvis to decrease pain, reduce the volume in the pelvis to reduce blood loss, and improve the patient's hemodynamics. However, use of a compressive device is a temporizing maneuver. In the hemodynamically unstable patient, choices for obtaining hemostasis include angiography with embolization or exploratory laparotomy with pelvic packing. The decision regarding which management strategy to use is dependent on suspicion of concomitant abdominal injuries (ie, favoring exploratory laparotomy) and the availability of angiography. External fixation can be performed at the bedside or in the operating room as well in the unstable patient. Computed tomography is not indicated in the unstable patient. Diagnostic peritoneal lavage may be useful in the setting of an equivocal focused assessment with sonography for trauma (FAST) examination.

171. The answer is c. (*Moore, pp 515-516.*) Although indications for thoracotomy in the ER are controversial, the procedure appears to be most beneficial when it is employed to (1) release cardiac tamponade in patients with penetrating thoracic trauma who are deteriorating too rapidly for a subxiphoid pericardial window to be created; (2) allow cross-clamping of the descending aorta in patients with intra-abdominal bleeding for whom other measures are not effective in maintaining blood pressure; or (3) allow effective internal cardiac massage in patients who arrive in the ER with faint or absent pulses and distant heart sounds, and for whom other resuscitative efforts are unsuccessful. By contrast, existing evidence suggests that patients who are unsalvageable and do not benefit from ER thoracotomy include (1) those with no vital signs (pulse, pupillary reaction, spontaneous respiration) in the field and (2) those with blunt trauma to multiple organ systems and absent vital signs on arrival in the ER.

172. The answer is c. (*Doherty, pp 639-641.*) In the absence of sepsis, patients with enterocutaneous fistulas should be treated initially nonoperatively with bowel rest, TPN, and correction of electrolyte abnormalities. Most enterocutaneous fistulas result from trauma sustained during surgical procedures. Irradiated, obstructed, and inflamed intestine is prone to fistulization. Complications of fistulas include fluid and electrolyte depletion, skin necrosis, and malnutrition. Fistulas are classified according to their location and the volume of output, because these factors influence prognosis and treatment. When the patient is stable, a small-bowel follow-through study can be obtained to determine (1) the location of the fistula, (2) the relation of the fistula to other hollow intra-abdominal organs, and (3) whether there is distal obstruction. Proximal small-bowel fistulas (from the stomach to mid-ileum) tend to produce a high output of intestinal fluid and are less likely to close with conservative management than are distal, low-output fistulas (distal ileum or colon). Small-bowel fistulas that communicate with other organs (eg, bladder) may need aggressive surgical repair because of the risk of associated infections. A mnemonic for recalling reasons why a fistula may remain open is "FRIENDS" (foreign bodies, radiation, inflammation/infection, epithelialization, neoplasm, distal obstruction, and steroids). When these poor prognostic factors for stabilization and spontaneous closure are observed, early surgical intervention must be undertaken. The patient in the question, however, appears to have a low-output, distal enterocutaneous fistula. Antispasmodic drugs have not been proved effective; somatostatin has been used with mixed success in the setting of high-output fistulas. There is no indication for antibiotics in the absence of sepsis. TPN is given to maintain or restore the patient's nutritional balance while minimizing the quantity of dietary fluids and endogenous secretions in the gastrointestinal tract. Initial TPN therapy is warranted to allow for spontaneous closure of a low-output distal fistula, but often these patients can be subsequently placed on a low-residue diet. Should conservative management fail, surgical closure of the fistula is performed.

173. The answer is d. (*Moore, pp 804-805.*) The management of bladder injuries is dependent on its location and concomitant injuries. Extraperitoneal bladder injuries can be treated with initial catheter drainage followed by repeat imaging to confirm healing. Surgical repair for extraperitoneal bladder injuries is indicated at the time of internal fixation of the pelvis to prevent infection of the hardware, if there is a need for operative repair of the rectum and/or vagina, if exploratory laparotomy is indicated for other reasons, and if there is an injury to or avulsion of the bladder neck. Intraperitoneal bladder injuries are repaired surgically. A suprapubic catheter is not indicated in the setting of a normal urethrogram, but is indicated if there is a displaced urethral injury. Bilateral nephrostomy tubes are not indicated in the setting of a bladder injury.

174. The answer is c. (*Moore, pp 623-633.*) The film shows a left diaphragmatic injury with the splenic flexure of the colon visualized in the left chest. All such injuries require repair once the diagnosis is made and the patient has been stabilized. The treatment of an acute traumatic diaphragmatic injury is via an abdominal approach (ie, an exploratory laparotomy or diagnostic laparoscopy) so as to rule out associated intra-abdominal injuries. Missed injuries lead to problems with herniation and bowel strangulation with sufficient frequency whose repair should not be delayed. The treatment of chronic traumatic diaphragmatic injury, which may occur due to a missed diagnosis, is either via a thoracic or an abdominal approach. Traumatic injuries to the diaphragm are associated with both blunt and penetrating trauma. The spleen, kidneys, intestines, and liver are the most frequently injured abdominal organs in blunt trauma; the diaphragm is the least.

175. The answer is e. (*Moore, pp 666-672.*) Nonoperative management of a splenic injury is contraindicated if the physical examination is suggestive of an associated injury, requiring operative intervention such as a blunt intestinal injury. The severity of the splenic injury can be graded based on the CT scan, but the grade of splenic injury does not always correlate to the need for operative intervention. Therefore, even the presence of a grade V injury (completely shattered spleen or hilar vascular injury) does not preclude a trial of nonoperative therapy. However, the opposite may also be true in that an apparently minor injury on CT scan may be much more significant on exploration. There may be a role for angiographic embolization of the splenic artery in the presence of a blush on CT scan, and there is evidence to suggest that the presence of a blush decreases the likelihood of success with nonoperative management. Patients who are hemodynamically unstable or who demonstrate clinical deterioration should undergo exploratory laparotomy. Although an RBC count greater than 100,000/μL constitutes a positive DPL in blunt abdominal trauma, a positive DPL in and of itself (ie, in a hemodynamically stable patient) does not require exploratory laparotomy.

176. The answer is d. (*Moore, pp 590-595.*) There are multiple findings on chest x-ray that are suggestive of a thoracic aortic injury, such as widening of the mediastinum more than 8 cm (because of the presence of a mediastinal hematoma), loss of the aortic knob, deviation of the nasogastric tube in the esophagus, depression of the left mainstem bronchus, an apical cap (apical pleural hematoma), sternal or scapular fracture, multiple left-sided rib fractures, and massive left hemothorax. However, a normal chest x-ray does not rule out a diagnosis of a thoracic great vessel injury. If clinical suspicion is high, then further diagnostic workup should be pursued. Aortography, CT angiography, and transesophageal echocardiography may establish the diagnosis. Traumatic aortic injuries are deceleration injuries because of differential forces to the fixed and mobile parts of the thoracic aorta; most aortic injuries are located near the ligamentum arteriosus.

177. The answer is c. (*Moore, pp 608-609.*) A positive DPL or a positive ultrasound examination in the hemodynamically unstable patient mandates exploratory laparotomy. A positive DPL for blunt abdominal trauma is characterized by aspiration of 10 cc of gross blood initially or more than 100,000/μL RBC, more than 500/μL WBC, or elevated amylase, bilirubin, or alkaline phosphatase.

178. The answer is b. (*Moore, p 224.*) The patient is in neurogenic shock secondary to a spinal cord injury. In patients with cervical or thoracic injuries, loss of sympathetic regulation results in loss of vasomotor tone and hypotension. Patients with neurogenic shock are warm and pink, as opposed to patients who are hypovolemic, and who are cold and clammy. Because of loss of the reflexive tachycardic response to hypotension, these patients are usually also bradycardic. Treatment is with fluid resuscitation initially and vasoconstrictors after the intravascular volume have been restored. Central venous pressure (CVP) is used to assess right ventricular function and systemic fluid status. Normal CVP is 2 to 6 mm Hg. The patient in this scenario has a low CVP suggesting intravascular volume depletion. Therefore, the patient requires further fluid resuscitation.

179. The answer is a. (*Moore, pp 858-860.*) There are multiple sequelae of increased abdominal pressure or abdominal compartment syndrome. Compartment syndrome results in increased peak airway pressures, decreased venous return and decreased cardiac output, increased systemic vascular resistance, decreased renal blood flow and glomerular filtration rate, and decreased portal venous flow with decreased liver function. Because of decreased venous return, the intracranial pressure increases and cerebral perfusion pressure decreases. Treatment requires decompressive laparotomy.

180. The answer is e. (*Moore, pp 989-990.*) Initial management should consist of isotonic crystalloid resuscitation with either normal saline or lactated Ringer at a dose of 20 mL/kg body weight (800 mL). If the patient transiently responds, a second bolus should be administered. If the patient has a sustained response, fluids can be decreased to maintenance. If the patient does not respond, the bolus should be repeated and then blood transfusion initiated.

181. The answer is e. (*Moore, p 356.*) The clinical presentation is consistent with cardiac tamponade. In most cases of trauma-related cardiac tamponade, patients need surgical exploration to relieve the tamponade and repair the wound in the heart that caused it. It is advisable to perform pericardiocentesis or subxiphoid pericardial drainage under local anesthesia before anesthetic induction in these unstable patients. Cardiac tamponade is a reversible cause of shock that occurs when fluid or blood accumulates between the pericardium and the heart. If the pericardial fluid develops under significant pressure, filling of the heart cannot occur during diastole, and the amount of blood ejected during systole decreases. Cardiac tamponade is mainly seen in patients with penetrating trauma in proximity to the sternum. The diagnosis should be considered in patients with pulsus paradoxus, which is a greater than 10-mm Hg fall in arterial systolic blood pressure with inspiration. Echocardiography is the preferred diagnostic tool for identification of fluid or blood in the pericardium.

182. The answer is d. *(Moore, pp 173-174.)* The recommended guidelines for a thoracotomy in patients with a hemothorax are greater than or equal to 1500 mL of immediate drainage of blood through the thoracostomy tube after placement or greater than 200 mL/h of continuous drainage of blood for several hours after the original evacuation. The patient's physiology and blood transfusion requirements should also factor into a decision for operative intervention.

183. The answer is a. *(Moore, p 542.)* Pulmonary contusion is hemorrhage and edema of the lung parenchyma without parenchymal disruption. It occurs more frequently after blunt chest trauma and radiologic findings may not be present on admission, developing several hours after the initial injury. The management of pulmonary contusion is almost entirely supportive with maintenance of good oxygenation and adequate pulmonary toilette. Patients with persistent low PaO_2 levels who do not respond to supplemental oxygen, pulmonary toilette, and pain control should be intubated and mechanically ventilated. The findings of rib fractures and an underlying well-defined infiltrate are less supportive of the diagnosis of pulmonary embolus, pneumonia, myocardial infarction, or cardiac tamponade.

184. The answer is c. *(Moore, pp 553-557.)* Tracheobronchial injuries are uncommon and can occur with blunt or penetrating trauma. Blunt injuries to the tracheobronchial tree occur after direct compression of the airway with a closed glottis or after decelerating injuries causing partial or complete avulsion of the right mainstem bronchus from the carina or tracheal lacerations. Patients may present with pneumothorax, subcutaneous emphysema, pneumomediastinum, hemoptysis, and respiratory distress. Small injuries usually heal spontaneously with supportive care but are associated with late complications such as stricture formation at the site of injury and recurrent pulmonary infection. More extensive wounds are primarily repaired in the operating room. The patient does not have physical examination findings of a sucking chest wound to support an open

pneumothorax. A tension pneumothorax would not involve air in the subcutaneous space or mediastinum. An esophageal injury would not present
with the large amount of emphysema or respiratory distress. A pulmonary
contusion is not associated with a pneumothorax.

185. The answer is a. (*Moore, pp 686-688, 693.*) Free fluid in the abdomen or pelvis in the absence of solid-organ injury warrants an exploratory
laparotomy to evaluate for small-bowel or mesenteric injury. DPL to evaluate the fluid for WBCs, amylase levels, or bacteria on Gram stain could
be performed alternatively. However, DPL is being used less frequently
because of its invasiveness. Furthermore, the lavage WBC count was found
to be nonspecific for hollow viscus injuries. Findings seen on CT scan
suggestive of small-bowel injury include bowel wall thickening, pneumoperitoneum, mesenteric fat streaking, and extravasation of either luminal
or vascular contrast. Exploratory laparotomy is not indicated in solid-organ
injury (liver, spleen, kidney) in patients with hemodynamic stability and
no evidence of contrast extravasation. A pelvic fracture requires internal or
external fixation if it is unstable.

186. The answer is e. (*Moore, pp 796-799.*) A retrograde urethrogram is
essential for diagnosis of a urethral injury. A Foley catheter is inserted into
the distal urethra and minimally inflated. This is followed by instillation
of 30 mL of water-soluble contrast and a plain radiograph is obtained. No
attempt at insertion of a bladder catheter should be made until a negative
retrograde urethrogram is obtained to avoid further damaging a urethral
injury. A stress cystogram is useful in diagnosing a bladder injury. An intravenous pyelogram is obtained to evaluate the kidneys, ureter, and bladder.
A CT scan of the pelvis does not evaluate the urethra.

187 to 191. The answers are 187-b, 188-e, 189-a, 190-d, 191-c.
(*Moore, pp 532-538, 553-560, 569-572.*) Flail chest describes the paradoxical motion of the chest wall that occurs when consecutive ribs are broken
in more than 1 place, usually following blunt trauma to the thorax. Respiratory distress may ensue when the noncompliant flail segment interferes
with generation of adequate positive and negative intrathoracic pressure
needed to move air through the trachea. In addition, a blow sufficiently
violent to cause a flail chest may also contuse the underlying pulmonary
parenchyma, which compounds the respiratory distress. Treatment consists
of pain control and treatment of the underlying pulmonary contusion.

Airway obstruction denotes partial or complete occlusion of the tracheobronchial tree by foreign bodies, secretions, or crush injuries of the upper respiratory tract. Patients may present with symptoms ranging from cough and mild dyspnea to stridor and hypoxic cardiac arrest. An initial effort should be made to digitally clear the airway and to suction visible secretions; in selected stable patients, fiberoptic endoscopy may be employed to determine the cause of obstruction and to retrieve foreign objects. Unstable patients whose airways cannot be quickly reestablished by clearing the oropharynx must be intubated. An endotracheal intubation may be attempted, but cricothyroidotomy is indicated in the presence of proximal obstruction or severe maxillofacial trauma.

Blunt or penetrating trauma to the pericardium and heart will result in pericardial tamponade when fluid pressure in the pericardial space exceeds central venous pressure and thus prevents venous return to the heart. The result is shock, despite adequate volume and myocardial function. The treatment is pericardial decompression. A subxiphoid, supradiaphragmatic incision and creation of a pericardial window, ideally performed in the operating room, provides a rapid, safe means of confirming the diagnosis of tamponade and of relieving venous obstruction. If bleeding is encountered on opening the pericardial window, a sternotomy should be performed.

Tension pneumothorax occurs when a laceration of the visceral pulmonary pleura acts as a one-way valve that allows air to enter the pleural space from an underlying parenchymal injury but not to escape. Increasing intrapleural pressure causes collapse of the ipsilateral lung, compression of the contralateral lung due to mediastinal shift toward the opposite hemithorax, and diminished venous return. Treatment consists of relieving the pneumothorax. This is best accomplished via tube thoracostomy.

Open pneumothorax occurs when a traumatic defect in the chest wall permits free communication of the pleural space with atmospheric pressure. If the defect is larger than two-thirds of the tracheal diameter, respiratory efforts will move air in and out through the defect in the chest wall rather than through the trachea. The immediate treatment is placement of an occlusive dressing over the defect; subsequent interventions include placement of a thoracostomy tube (preferably through a separate incision), formal closure of the chest wall, and ventilatory assistance if needed.

Transplants, Immunology, and Oncology

Questions

192. A 43-year-old man with a gangrenous gallbladder and gram-negative sepsis agrees to participate in a research study. An assay of tumor necrosis factor (TNF) is performed. Which of the following is the origin of this peptide?

a. Fibroblasts
b. Damaged vascular endothelial cells
c. Monocytes/macrophages
d. Activated T lymphocytes
e. Activated killer lymphocytes

193. A 49-year-old man who underwent liver transplantation 5 years ago for alcoholic cirrhosis presents with a gradually increasing bilirubin level. He undergoes a liver biopsy, which demonstrates a paucity of bile ducts. Which of the following is his best option for treatment?

a. Increase his immunosuppression
b. Administration of a monoclonal antibody against T cells
c. Exploratory laparotomy with hepatic arterial reconstruction
d. Exploratory laparotomy with thrombectomy of the portal vein
e. Retransplantation

194. A 52-year-old woman in renal failure is listed as a transplant candidate. In order to assess the propriety of the transplant, which of the following combinations represents how a cross-match is performed?

a. Donor serum with recipient lymphocytes and complement
b. Donor lymphocytes with recipient serum and complement
c. Donor lymphocytes with recipient lymphocytes
d. Recipient serum with a known panel of multiple donor lymphocytes
e. Recipient serum with donor red blood cells and complement

195. A 39-year-old woman presents with generalized malaise and lymphadenopathy. Biopsy of a supraclavicular lymph node reveals non-Hodgkin lymphoma. Forty-eight hours after initiation of chemotherapy, she develops a high-grade fever and her laboratory studies demonstrate hyperkalemia, hyperphosphatemia, and hypocalcemia. Which of the following cells mediate this syndrome?

a. Macrophages
b. Cytotoxic T lymphocytes
c. Natural killer cells
d. Polymorphonuclear leukocytes
e. Helper T lymphocytes

196. A 33-year-old diabetic man receives a renal allograft. The physicians choose cyclosporine as one of the antirejection medications. Which of the following functions does cyclosporine A primarily inhibit?

a. Macrophage function
b. Antibody production
c. Interleukin 1 production
d. Interleukin 2 production
e. Cytotoxic T-cell effectiveness

197. A 24-year-old woman presents with lethargy, anorexia, tachypnea, and weakness. Laboratory studies reveal a BUN of 150 mg/dL, serum creatinine of 16 mg/dL, and potassium of 6.2 mEq/L. Chest x-ray shows increased pulmonary vascularity and a dilated heart. Which of the following is the most appropriate management of this patient?

a. Emergency kidney transplantation
b. Creation and immediate use of a forearm arteriovenous fistula
c. Placement of a catheter in the internal jugular vein and initiation of hemodialysis
d. A 100-g protein/day diet
e. Renal biopsy

198. A hypertensive 47-year-old man is proposed for kidney transplantation. He is anemic but is otherwise functional. Which of the following would preclude renal transplantation?

a. Positive cross-match
b. Donor blood type O
c. Two-antigen HLA match with donor
d. Blood pressure of 180/100 mm Hg
e. Hemoglobin level of 8.2 g/dL

199. A 56-year-old woman is undergoing a cadaveric renal transplant. After revascularization of the transplanted kidney, the transplanted renal parenchyma becomes swollen and blue. The surgeon suspects hyperacute rejection. What is the treatment of choice for this patient?

a. There is no therapy for hyperacute rejection
b. Systemic anticoagulation
c. Catheter-directed anticoagulation into the renal artery
d. Intravenous steroids
e. Intravenous steroids and cyclosporine

200. A 57-year-old man has end-stage heart failure due to atherosclerosis. His cardiologist refers him for evaluation for heart transplantation. Which of the following is an absolute contraindication for heart transplantation?

a. Cirrhosis
b. Age over 65
c. Diabetes without end-organ damage
d. Reversible high pulmonary vascular resistance
e. History of colon cancer resected 5 years ago with no evidence of recurrence

201. A 47-year-old man with hypertensive nephropathy develops fever, graft tenderness, and oliguria 4 weeks following cadaveric renal transplantation. Serum creatinine is 3.1 mg/dL. A renal ultrasound reveals mild edema of the renal papillae but normal flow in both the renal artery and the renal vein. Nuclear scan demonstrates sluggish uptake and excretion. Which of the following is the most appropriate next step?

a. Performing an angiogram
b. Decreasing steroid and cyclosporine dose
c. Beginning intravenous antibiotics
d. Performing renal biopsy, steroid boost, and immunoglobulin therapy
e. Beginning FK 506

202. Approximately 6 weeks following a kidney transplant, a 59-year-old woman develops fever, malaise, and myalgias and is found to have a cytomegalovirus (CMV) infection. Which of the following is a potential sequela of CMV infection?

a. Pyelonephritis
b. Gastrointestinal (GI) ulceration and hemorrhage
c. Cholecystitis
d. Intra-abdominal abscess
e. Parotitis

203. A 55-year-old man presents with worsening cirrhosis. After evaluation by a hepatologist, he presents for evaluation for hepatic transplantation. He is informed that prioritization for transplantation is based on the Model of End-stage Liver Disease (MELD) score, and that patients with higher MELD scores have a greater benefit from transplantation. Which of the following contributes to the MELD score?

a. Platelet count
b. Total bilirubin
c. Albumin
d. Encephalopathy
e. Ascites

204. A young woman who has received a transplant has posttransplant fever and malaise. Graft-versus-host disease (GVHD) is diagnosed. This has occurred most commonly with the transplantation of which of the following?

a. Kidney
b. Lung
c. Heart
d. Bone marrow
e. Pancreas

205. A brain-dead potential donor has become available. You must plan for the dispersal of the thoracic organs. Which of the following will necessitate a heart-lung transplant?

a. Primary pulmonary hypertension
b. Cystic fibrosis
c. End-stage emphysema
d. Idiopathic dilated cardiomyopathy with long-standing secondary pulmonary hypertension
e. End-stage pulmonary fibrosis secondary to sarcoidosis

206. A 35-year-old man who has had type 1 diabetes for many years undergoes a pancreas transplant with enteric drainage (connection of the donor duodenum to the recipient jejunum). Postoperatively, he has increased pain near his pancreas transplant. Which of the following should be performed to confirm a diagnosis of rejection?

a. Percutaneous biopsy of the transplanted pancreas
b. Measurement of serum amylase levels
c. Measurement of serum lipase levels
d. Measurement of urinary amylase levels
e. Determination of the ratio of the level of urinary amylase to serum amylase

207. A 55-year-old woman who has end-stage liver disease is referred to a hepatologist for evaluation. Which of the following would prevent her from being a transplantation candidate?

a. Use of alcohol 3 months ago
b. Two 2-cm hepatocellular carcinomas (HCCs) in the right lobe of the liver
c. A 4-cm hepatocellular carcinoma in the right lobe of the liver
d. Development of hepatorenal syndrome requiring hemodialysis
e. History of breast cancer 5 years ago with no evidence of disease currently

208. A kidney transplant recipient presents with severe acute rejection that does not respond to steroid treatment. Administration of which of the following agents is the best step in her management?

a. Cyclosporine
b. Tacrolimus
c. Azathioprine
d. Muromonab-CD3
e. Sirolimus

209. A 19-year-old college student presents with a testicular mass, and after treatment he returns for regular follow-up visits. Which of the following is the most useful serum marker for detecting recurrent disease after treatment of nonseminomatous testicular cancer?

a. Carcinoembryonic antigen (CEA)
b. Human chorionic gonadotropin (hCG)
c. Prostate-specific antigen (PSA)
d. CA125
e. p53 oncogene

210. An edentulous 72-year-old man with a 50-year history of cigarette smoking presents with a nontender, hard mass in the lateral neck. Which of the following is the best diagnostic test for establishing a diagnosis of malignancy?

a. Fine-needle aspiration cytology
b. Bone marrow biopsy
c. Nasopharyngoscopy
d. Computed tomography (CT) scan of the head and neck
e. Sinus x-ray

211. A 49-year-old woman undergoes surgical resection of a malignancy. The family asks about the prognosis. The histopathology is available for review. For which of the following malignancies does histologic grade best correlate with prognosis?

a. Lung cancer
b. Melanoma
c. Colonic adenocarcinoma
d. Hepatocellular carcinoma
e. Soft tissue sarcoma

212. A mother notices an abdominal mass in her 3-year-old son while giving him a bath. There is no history of any symptoms, but the boy's blood pressure is elevated at 105/85 mm Hg. Metastatic workup is negative and the patient is explored. The mass shown here is found within the left kidney. Genetic testing reveals deletion of 2 genes on chromosome band 11p13. Which of the following anomalies in addition to the identified tumor is associated with these chromosomal deletions?

a. Cardiac anomalies
b. Hemihypertrophy
c. Hypoglycemia
d. Macroglossia
e. Aniridia

213. An 11-year-old girl presents to your office because of a family history of medullary carcinoma of the thyroid. Physical examination is normal. Which of the following tests should you perform?

a. Urine vanillylmandelic acid (VMA) level
b. Serum insulin level
c. Serum gastrin level
d. Serum glucagon level
e. Serum somatostatin level

214. A 37-year-old woman has developed a 6-cm mass on her anterior thigh over the past 10 months. The mass appears to be fixed to the underlying muscle, but the overlying skin is movable. Which of the following is the most appropriate next step in her management?

a. Above-knee amputation
b. Excisional biopsy
c. Incisional biopsy
d. Bone scan
e. Abdominal CT scan

215. A 50-year-old man is incidentally discovered to have a low-grade mucosa-associated lymphoid tissue (MALT) lymphoma on biopsy of the stomach during esophagogastroduodenoscopy for dyspepsia. CT scans of the chest, abdomen, and pelvis demonstrate no evidence of enlarged regional lymph nodes or distant metastases. Which of the following is the initial treatment of choice?

a. Total gastrectomy with esophagojejunostomy
b. Total gastrectomy with esophagojejunostomy and adjuvant chemotherapy
c. Chemotherapy
d. Steroids
e. Antibiotics

216. A 33-year-old woman seeks assistance because of a swelling of her right parotid gland. Biopsy is performed and reveals acinar carcinoma. You consent the patient for resection and inform her that at the very least, she will require superficial parotidectomy. Which of the following intraoperative findings would require sacrifice of the facial nerve?

a. Invasion of the deep lobe of the parotid.
b. Invasion of the lateral lobe of the parotid.
c. Proximity of the carcinoma to the facial nerve.
d. Encasement of the facial nerve by carcinoma.
e. The facial nerve should always be preserved regardless of intraoperative findings.

217. A 42-year-old man is undergoing chemotherapy after resection of a cecal adenocarcinoma with positive lymph nodes. You are asked to see him regarding a potential surgical complication. Which of the following potentially operable complications is a common occurrence among patients receiving systemic chemotherapy?

a. Acute cholecystitis
b. Perirectal abscess
c. Appendicitis
d. Incarcerated femoral hernia
e. Diverticulitis

218. A 28-year-old medical student seeks your attention because of a testicular mass. Biopsy is consistent with pure seminoma. There is no evidence of enlarged retroperitoneal lymph nodes on CT scan. Which of the following is the best treatment strategy for this patient?

a. Orchiectomy alone
b. Orchiectomy followed by chemotherapy
c. Orchiectomy with retroperitoneal lymph node dissection
d. Orchiectomy with retroperitoneal lymph node dissection followed by external beam radiation
e. Orchiectomy followed by external beam radiation to the retroperitoneal lymph nodes

219. A 25-year-old woman with end-stage renal disease is exploring the benefits of renal transplantation. Which of the following is an advantage of dialysis over renal transplantation?

a. Better patient survival
b. More cost-effective longterm
c. Improved quality of life
d. No need for lifelong immunosuppression
e. More cost-effective if the renal transplant functions for more than 2 years

220. A 30-year-old previously healthy man presents with refractory hypertension on four medications. Urinalysis is positive for metanephrines. He was adopted as an infant and therefore does not know his family history. Which of the following inherited syndromes is not associated with this disease?

a. MEN2A
b. MEN2B
c. von Hippel-Lindau disease
d. Neurofibromatosis I
e. Neurofibromatosis II

221. A 24-year-old man whose father was just diagnosed with colon cancer presents to his family physician to discuss screening colonoscopy. His physician suspects that he has hereditary nonpolyposis colon cancer (HNPCC) or Lynch syndrome and recommends screening colonoscopy beginning at age 25. Which of the following is most supportive of a clinical diagnosis of HNPCC?

a. A father with colon cancer at 52 years of age
b. A father and an uncle (same side of the family) with colon cancer
c. A father and grandfather (same side of the family) with colon cancer
d. A father and 2 uncles (same side of the family) with colon cancer
e. A father, uncle, and grandfather (same side of the family) with colon cancer at 50 years of age

222. A 53-year-old woman presents with bright red blood per rectum, increased abdominal distention, and weight loss. She is found to have a large fungating mass 8 cm from the anal verge. No other lesions are identified. Biopsy is consistent with invasive rectal adenocarcinoma. Endorectal ultrasound shows invasion of the tumor into the perirectal fat and multiple enlarged lymph nodes. CT scans of the chest, abdomen, and pelvis do not show any metastases. She would like to preserve her sphincter if possible. Which of the following is the best treatment option for this patient given her preferences?

a. Abdominoperineal resection
b. Neoadjuvant chemoradiation followed by low anterior resection
c. Neoadjuvant chemoradiation followed by abdominoperineal resection
d. Transanal excision followed by adjuvant chemoradiation
e. Neoadjuvant chemoradiation followed by transanal excision

223. A 35-year-old woman presents with a right breast mass. You perform a thorough history and physical examination as well as a core biopsy of the right breast mass. In which of the following circumstances would a sentinel lymph node biopsy be indicated?

a. The core biopsy is consistent with ductal carcinoma in situ without comedo necrosis for which the patient desires partial mastectomy only.
b. The core biopsy is consistent with ductal carcinoma and the patient has a positive pregnancy test.
c. The core biopsy is consistent with ductal carcinoma and the patient desires partial mastectomy.
d. The core biopsy is consistent with ductal carcinoma and the patient has palpable axillary lymph nodes.
e. The core biopsy is consistent with ductal carcinoma and the patient has a bone scan suspicious for metastasis.

224. A patient requires both cardiac and renal transplantation. Preparation for the procedures has begun. How do cardiac allografts differ from renal allografts?

a. Cardiac allografts are matched by HLA tissue typing and renal allografts are not.
b. Cardiac allografts can tolerate a longer period of cold ischemia than renal allografts.
c. One-year graft survival for cardiac allografts is substantially lower than that for renal allografts.
d. Cardiac allografts are matched only by size and ABO blood type.
e. Cyclosporine is a critical component of the immunosuppressive regimen for cardiac allografts but not renal allografts.

225. A patient with colon cancer has a mass in the upper lobe of his left lung 2.5 years following resection of his colon cancer and subsequent 12 months of chemotherapy. His CEA level is rising. Which of the following predicts a 5-year survival rate of greater than 20% following resection of pulmonary metastases?

a. Other organ metastases are present.
b. Lung lesions are solitary.
c. Local tumor recurrence is found.
d. The tumor doubling time is less than 20 days.
e. The patient has received prior chemotherapy.

226. A 61-year-old man undergoes upper endoscopy for evaluation of weight loss and is identified to have a submucosal mass in the stomach. Biopsy is consistent with a gastrointestinal stromal tumor (GIST). Workup reveals the presence of liver metastases. Which of the following is the best initial treatment for this patient?

a. Tyrosine kinase inhibitor (Imatinib)
b. Monoclonal antibody against interleukin-2 receptor (Daclizumab)
c. Monoclonal antibody against tumor necrosis factor α (Infliximab)
d. Monoclonal antibody against vascular endothelial growth factor A (Bevacizumab)
e. Monoclonal antibody against epidermal growth factor receptor (Cetuximab)

227. A 57-year-old woman develops bony metastases 1 year after right modified radical mastectomy for breast cancer. The tumor was estrogen receptor-negative, progesterone receptor-negative, and Her-2/neu positive. Which of the following agents is indicated for treatment of her metastatic disease?

a. Antiestrogen (Tamoxifen)
b. Selective estrogen receptor modulator (Raloxifene)
c. Monoclonal antibody (Trastuzumab)
d. Aromatase inhibitor (Anastrozole)
e. 5-fluorouracil

228. A 42-year-old man is diagnosed with an osteosarcoma. His family history is significant for a 37-year-old sister with breast cancer and an uncle with adrenocortical carcinoma. His family physician suspects that he may have Li-Fraumeni syndrome and suggests genetic testing. Which of the following genes is most likely to be mutated if he has the syndrome?

a. Adenomatous polyposis coli (APC) gene
b. RET
c. p53
d. Phosphatase and tensin homologue (PTEN)
e. p16

229. A patient with a solid malignancy discusses chemotherapy with his oncologist. He is interested in the risks of the treatment. What is the primary toxicity of doxorubicin (Adriamycin)?

a. Cardiomyopathy
b. Pulmonary fibrosis
c. Peripheral neuropathy
d. Uric acid nephropathy
e. Hepatic dysfunction

230. A 22-year-old woman has a known family history of breast cancer in her first-degree relatives. She undergoes genetic testing and is found to be a BRCA1 mutation carrier. She does not currently desire bilateral prophylactic mastectomy. Which of the following is the next best option to manage her risk for breast cancer?

a. Mammography every 6 months starting at age 25
b. Mammography every 6 months starting at age 35
c. Mammography every 12 months starting at age 25
d. Mammography every 12 months starting at age 35
e. Tamoxifen for chemoprevention

231. A 56-year-old woman is undergoing chemotherapy. She presents today with complaints of burning on urination and bloody urine. Which of the following agents causes hemorrhagic cystitis?

a. Bleomycin
b. 5-fluorouracil
c. Cisplatin
d. Vincristine
e. Cyclophosphamide

232. A 38-year-old woman who underwent a cadaveric renal transplant 8 years ago presents with fevers, fatigue, and weight loss. Evaluation included CT scans of the head, neck, chest, abdomen, and pelvis; she is noted to have diffuse lymphadenopathy and pulmonary nodules. A biopsy and histologic examination of a lymph node is performed. Which of the following viruses is most likely to be present in the lymph node?

a. Cytomegalovirus
b. Human papillomavirus
c. Human herpesvirus 8
d. Epstein-Barr virus
e. Coxsackie virus

233. A 41-year-old man underwent a successful living-related kidney transplantation 1 year ago with good results. Preoperatively, he was noted to have an elevated calcium level; posttransplantation, he continues to have elevated calcium levels and associated symptoms. Which of the following is the most appropriate next step in management?

a. ^{99m}Tc sestamibi scanning
b. Ultrasound of the neck
c. CT scan of the neck and mediastinum
d. Total parathyroidectomy with autotransplantation of a portion of a gland into the forearm
e. Measurement of urinary calcium levels

234. A 53-year-old man presents with constipation and a 20-lb weight loss over the course of 6 months. Colonoscopy reveals a fungating mass in the sigmoid colon; biopsy is consistent with adenocarcinoma. His metastatic workup is negative. A CEA level is obtained and is 4-fold greater than normal. Which of the following is the appropriate use of this test?

a. As an indication for neoadjuvant chemotherapy
b. As an indication for postoperative radiation therapy
c. As an indication for preoperative PET scanning
d. As an indication for a more aggressive sigmoid resection
e. As a baseline measurement prior to monitoring postoperatively for recurrence

Questions 235 to 237

For each stage in the patient's treatment, select the appropriate next step. Each lettered option may be used once, more than once, or not at all.

a. Left hemicolectomy
b. Right hemicolectomy
c. Subtotal colectomy
d. Total colectomy
e. Hepatic resection
f. External beam irradiation
g. 5-fluorouracil and leucovorin
h. External beam irradiation and chemotherapy
i. Abdominal MRI
j. No further treatment

235. A 65-year-old man presents to his primary care physician with complaints of intermittent constipation and is found to have microcytic anemia. Colonoscopy reveals a fungating mass in the proximal sigmoid colon with no other synchronous lesions. Biopsy of the mass confirms adenocarcinoma.

236. The patient undergoes surgery and recovers uneventfully. Pathology of the resected specimen is reported as T3, N1 with negative surgical margins.

237. At 6-month follow-up, an abdominal CT scan shows a 2-cm isolated lesion in the right lobe of the liver. Repeat colonoscopy shows no evidence of recurrent or metachronous lesions. Chest x-ray and bone scan are normal.

Questions 238 to 241

A 32-year-old man with diabetic nephropathy undergoes an uneventful renal transplant from his sister (2-haplotype match). His immunosuppressive regimen includes azathioprine, steroids, and cyclosporine. For each development in the postoperative period, select the most appropriate next step. Each lettered option may be used once, more than once, or not at all.

a. Begin gancyclovir.
b. Administer steroid boost.
c. Withhold steroids.
d. Decrease cyclosporine.
e. Increase cyclosporine.
f. Decrease azathioprine.
g. Obtain renal ultrasound.
h. Begin broad-spectrum antibiotics.

238. On postoperative day 3 the patient is doing well, but you notice on his routine laboratory tests that his white blood cell count is 2.0.

239. The patient's WBC count gradually returns to normal, but on postoperative day 7 he develops a fever of 39.4°C (103°F) and a nonproductive cough. A chest x-ray reveals diffuse interstitial infiltrates, and a buffy coat is positive for viral inclusions.

240. The patient recovers from this illness and is discharged home on postoperative day 18. At 3-month follow-up he is doing well, but you notice that his creatinine is 2.8 mg/dL. He has no fever, his graft is not tender, and his renal ultrasound is normal.

241. Six months following his transplant, the patient begins to develop fever, malaise, and pain of the right lower quadrant. On palpation, the graft is tender. Chest x-ray and urine and blood cultures are normal. Renal ultrasound shows an edematous graft.

Transplants, Immunology, and Oncology

Answers

192. The answer is c. (*Mulholland, pp 108-112.*) TNF is a peptide hormone produced by endotoxin-activated monocytes/macrophages and has been postulated to be the principal cytokine mediator in gram-negative shock and sepsis-related organ damage. Biologic actions of TNF include polymorphonuclear neutrophil (PMN) activation and degranulation; increased nonspecific host resistance; increased vascular permeability; lymphopenia; promotion of interleukins 1, 2, and 6; capillary leak syndrome; microvascular thrombosis; anorexia and cachexia; and numerous other protective and adverse effects in sepsis. Its role in sepsis provides a fertile field for research in critical care.

193. The answer is e. (*Brunicardi, pp 274-275.*) Chronic rejection is a late complication that manifests months to years after transplantation and is characterized by a paucity of bile ducts on biopsy due to immune-mediated injury to the biliary epithelium—the "vanishing bile duct syndrome." Treatment options are limited, and the best option for treatment is retransplantation. Portal venous thrombosis that occurs early after transplantation should be treated with exploratory laparotomy and thrombectomy, but late portal venous thrombosis does not necessitate operative intervention due to the formation of collaterals. Hepatic arterial thrombosis (HAT), when detected early, should be treated with reexploration and thrombectomy with revision of the anastomosis. A late sequela of HAT is biliary strictures secondary to ischemia.

194. The answer is b. (*Mulholland, p 506.*) The purpose of a cross-match is to determine whether the recipient has circulating antibodies against donor HLA antigens. Such antibodies do not occur naturally, but rather are the result of prior sensitization during pregnancy, blood transfusions, or previous transplantation. A complement-dependent lymphocytotoxicity cross-match is performed by adding recipient serum and complement to donor cells (T cells, B cells, or monocytes). If specific antidonor antibodies are present, antibody binding results in complement fixation and cell lysis. This is detected by addition of a vital dye, which is taken up by the damaged cell membrane, resulting in a positive cross-match. If a positive cross-match is detected to donor T cells (HLA class I), transplantation will result in hyperacute rejection.

195. The answer is b. (*Brunicardi, p 265.*) The patient is manifesting symptoms of tumor lysis syndrome, which is mediated by cytotoxic T cells. Hyperkalemia and hyperphosphatemia are a result of tumor cell lysis, and hypocalcemia is a result of precipitation of phosphate and calcium. Unlike the granulocyte line, T lymphocytes express the T-cell receptor. This receptor imparts antigen specificity to T cells. The helper T cell, when stimulated by interleukin 1 and antigens, produces various lymphokines that ultimately produce effector cells. One of these effector cells is the cytotoxic T cell, which kills cells that express specific antigens, including viral, tumor, and nonbiologic antigens. Macrophages and natural killer cells have some tumoricidal activity; however, this is not specific for tumors.

196. The answer is d. (*Mulholland, p 584.*) Cyclosporine is a highly effective immunosuppressive agent produced by fungi. It is more specific than the anti-inflammatory agents such as steroids or the antiproliferative agents such as azathioprine. The effectiveness of cyclosporine in preventing allograft rejection is related to its ability to inhibit interleukin 2 production. Without interleukin 2 from helper T cells, there is no clonal expansion of alloantigen-directed cytotoxic T cells and no stimulation of antibody production by B cells.

197. The answer is c. (*Townsend, pp 692-693.*) Hemodialysis, rather than management by dietary manipulation alone, should be considered for patients with stage 5 kidney disease defined as an estimated glomerular filtration rate of less than 15 mL/min/1.73 m^2 or earlier in patients with complications due to renal failure according to National Kidney Foundation guidelines. These complications include hyperkalemia, congestive heart failure, peripheral neuropathy, severe hypertension, pericarditis, bleeding, and severe anemia. The uremic hyperkalemic patient in congestive heart failure may require emergency dialysis in addition to the standard conservative measures, which include (1) limitation of protein intake to less than 60 g/day and restriction of fluid intake and (2) reduction in elevated serum potassium levels by insulin-glucose or sodium polystyrene sulfonate (Kayexalate) enema treatment. Arteriovenous fistulas require several weeks to months to develop adequate size and flow. While awaiting maturation, temporary dialysis can be satisfactorily performed using a catheter placed in a central vein. Renal biopsy would be performed in an attempt to obtain a diagnosis of the underlying renal disease. Patients who are acceptable candidates for kidney transplantation usually should undergo this form of treatment, after they are stabilized, rather than chronic hemodialysis, the mortality for which is now higher than for transplantation. Despite adequate dialysis, problems of neuropathy, bone disease, anemia, and hypertension remain difficult to manage. Compared with chronic dialysis, transplantation restores more patients to happier and more productive lives.

198. The answer is a. (*Townsend, pp 693-694.*) A positive cross-match means that the recipient has circulating antibodies that are cytotoxic to donor-strain lymphocytes. This incompatibility, which almost always leads to an acute humoral rejection of the graft, precludes transplantation. Blood type matching prior to organ allograft is similar to cross-matching prior to transfusion; O is the universal donor and AB the universal recipient. Minor blood group factors do not appear to act as histocompatibility antigens. Matching of HLA antigens in cadaveric renal transplants may improve graft survival, but the impact is relatively minor. While attempts are made to pair recipient and donor by tissue typing, a 2-antigen match is perfectly acceptable and even 0-antigen matches can be transplanted with good results. Neither hypertension nor anemia is a contraindication to transplantation; indeed, hypertension may be cured or ameliorated following successful transplantation. Patients with end-stage renal failure generally are anemic and can be transfused, if necessary, intraoperatively or postoperatively. Anemia generally also improves following transplantation because of increased erythropoietin production by the graft.

199. The answer is a. (*Townsend, p 713; Mulholland, pp 509-510.*) Hyperacute rejection is refractory to immunosuppressive or anticoagulant therapy and inevitably leads to rapid destruction of the transplanted kidney. Hyperacute rejection occurs within minutes after transplantation and is mediated primarily by preformed antibody. It usually occurs during surgery after the clamps are released from the vascular anastomosis and the recipient's antibodies are exposed to the donor's passenger lymphocytes and kidney tissue. Typically, the kidney will become swollen and bluish. Intraoperative biopsies of the transplanted kidney should be performed to evaluate for signs of hyperacute rejection such as extensive intravascular deposits of fibrin and platelets and intraglomerular accumulation of polymorphonuclear leukocytes, fibrin, platelets, and red blood cells. The intravascular coagulation rarely results in a systemic coagulopathy. Careful cross-matching can test for cytotoxic antibodies and prevent hyperacute rejections.

200. The answer is a. (*Mulholland, pp 566-567.*) Cardiac transplantation is a treatment modality for selected patients with end-stage cardiac failure without any lower-risk options for treatment. Selection of recipients is dependent primarily on the coexistence of noncardiac comorbidities that are likely to limit survival, limit administration of immunosuppression, or increase the risk of potentially fatal infection with immunosuppression. Contraindications to cardiac transplantation include high pulmonary vascular resistance (irreversible, on maximal medical therapy), irreversible renal insufficiency, diabetes with end-organ damage, symptomatic extravascular disease, current or recent malignancy (< 2 years), noncardiac comorbidity that would limit survival (eg, cirrhosis, symptomatic chronic obstructive pulmonary disease), active infection, active peptic ulcer disease, high risk for inability to comply with the medical regimen. The other answers listed are all relative contraindications: age over 65, reversible high pulmonary vascular resistance, established renal failure, diabetes without end-organ damage, asymptomatic extravascular disease, remote malignancy without evidence of recurrence (> 4 years), noncardiac comorbidity that might limit survival, and possible difficulty with compliance with medical regimen.

201. The answer is d. (*Mulholland, pp 510-511.*) The patient is experiencing an acute rejection episode. Acute rejection typically occurs between 1 week and 3 months posttransplantation and is characterized by an increasing creatinine, decreased urine output, and possible fevers or tenderness over the graft. Diagnosis is confirmed with a biopsy of the graft, and treatment includes high-dose steroids and an anti–T-cell antibody (eg, OKT3, which is a murine monoclonal antibody to the human CD3 complex).

202. The answer is b. (*Mulholland, pp 540-541, 586.*) The most common posttransplantation viral infections are DNA viruses of the herpesvirus family and include cytomegalovirus (CMV), Epstein-Barr virus (EBV), herpes simplex virus, and varicella zoster virus. CMV infections may occur as either primary or reactive infections and have a peak incidence at about 6 weeks after transplant. The classic signs include fever, malaise, myalgia, arthralgia, and leukopenia. CMV infection can affect several organ systems and result in pneumonitis; ulceration and hemorrhage in the stomach, duodenum, or colon; hepatitis; esophagitis; retinitis; encephalitis; or pancreatitis. The risk of developing posttransplant CMV depends on donor-recipient serology, with the greatest risk in seronegative patients who receive organs from seropositive donors. Pyelonephritis, cholecystitis, intra-abdominal abscesses, and parotitis are caused by bacterial infections or GI perforation and not primarily by CMV infection.

203. The answer is b. *(Townsend, pp 707-708.)* The Model for End-stage Liver Disease (MELD) score enables liver allocation to be based on objective variables: total bilirubin, international normalized ratio, and creatinine. The MELD score is a statistical model employed for adult patients that has been shown to have a high predictive capacity in identifying patients with end-stage liver disease at greatest risk of mortality within 3 months. The MELD score was part of a new system put into place by the United Network for Organ Sharing for liver allocation which did not suffer from emphasis on waiting time and subjective clinical parameters (degree of ascites or encephalopathy).

204. The answer is d. *(Mulholland, p 1204.)* Donor-type lymphoid cells transplanted within a graft may recognize the host's tissue as foreign and mount an immune response against the host. This response, termed GVHD, is common in bone marrow transplantation and is an important source of morbidity and mortality. Treatment requires more aggressive immunosuppression. Current clinical practice includes depletion of lymphocytes from the marrow graft in order to prevent the development of GVHD. GVHD has been documented following liver transplantation, presumably because of the large amount of lymphoid tissue in the donor liver. GVHD has not been described following heart, lung, pancreas, or kidney transplantation.

205. The answer is d. *(Mulholland, pp 578-579.)* Many causes of end-stage lung disease have been appropriately treated with lung transplantation. Whether 1 lung or both lungs are replaced at the time of transplantation depends on recipient factors. Patients with restrictive processes such as primary pulmonary fibrosis do well with a single lung transplant. For patients with primary pulmonary hypertension, unloading of the right ventricle with single lung transplantation has been adequate, and replacement of both lungs has not been necessary in most cases. Cystic fibrosis patients do well after lung transplantation, but double lung transplant is frequently necessary because of chronic infections. Secondary pulmonary hypertension is due to left ventricular failure with concomitant increases in pulmonary pressures secondary to increases in left ventricular end-diastolic pressures. Reactive secondary pulmonary hypertension is best treated with heart transplantation. Long-standing secondary pulmonary hypertension that is chiefly fixed is best treated with combined heart-lung transplantation.

206. The answer is a. *(Mulholland, p 601.)* Rejection after pancreas transplantation should be suspected in the presence of hyperamylasemia, hyperlipasemia, or hyperglycemia. However, these are not diagnostic. Percutaneous, open, or laparoscopic biopsy of the transplanted pancreas with histologic examination is necessary to confirm the diagnosis. Grading of the severity of rejection is dependent on the presence and extent of active septal inflammation, acinar inflammation, and arteritis. In pancreas transplant recipients with bladder drainage (connection of the donor duodenum to the bladder), a decreasing urinary amylase is suggestive of rejection.

207. The answer is a. *(Mulholland, pp 543-547.)* Specific exclusion criteria for liver transplantation are not formally established. Some of the more common contraindications to liver transplantation are ongoing or recent substance abuse, presence of active sepsis, current extrahepatic malignancy, poor cardiac or pulmonary function, and patients with hepatocellular carcinoma with metastatic disease, obvious vascular invasion, or significant tumor burden. Patients with hepatocellular carcinoma who would not tolerate resection because of portal hypertension and uncompensated liver disease can be successfully treated with liver transplantation. The best candidates are patients with a single lesion less than 5 cm in size or no more than 3 lesions, none of which are greater than 3 cm in size. The presence of hepatorenal syndrome is an indication, not a contraindication, to liver transplantation. Patients with hepatorenal syndrome requiring hemodialysis may require liver/kidney transplantation. Presence of an extrahepatic malignancy should defer transplantation for 2 years after curative therapy for their malignancy.

208. The answer is d. (*Brunicardi, pp 274-280.*) Muromonab-CD3 is the treatment of choice for severe acute rejection that does not respond to steroid treatment. It can be used as the primary treatment or second-line therapy for acute rejection, rejection prophylaxis, and induction therapy. It is a monoclonal antibody against the CD3 antigen complex on mature T cells. In addition to minor side effects such as fevers and headaches that result from cytokine release after administration, severe complications may occur such as noncardiogenic pulmonary edema, encephalopathy, aseptic meningitis, and nephrotoxicity. Cyclosporine, tacrolimus, and azathiorpine are all used for maintenance of immunosuppression, and sirolimus is used to to withdraw or avoid the use of steroids in immunosuppressive protocols.

209. The answer is b. (*Mulholland, pp 1954-1955.*) In following patients with nonseminomatous testicular tumors, elevated serum levels of the β subunit of human chorionic gonadotropin (hCG), alpha-fetoprotein (AFP), and lactate dehydrogenase have been found to be useful indicators of tumor activity or recurrence. PSA has been utilized in screening for prostate cancer, although its role is controversial. CA125 has been used to follow ovarian cancers; it is fairly nonspecific but can alert the physician to the need for a more aggressive search for persistent disease when relative increases are noted in a patient after therapy. The p53 oncogenes have been found in soft tissue sarcomas, osteogenic sarcomas, and colon cancers; they have no role in the detection of recurrence.

210. The answer is a. (*Brunicardi, p 503.*) Isolated enlarged cervical lymph nodes in adults are malignant nearly 80% of the time (excluding benign tumors of the thyroid gland). They are usually metastatic squamous cell carcinomas arising from primary sources above the clavicles in the aerodigestive tract. Fine-needle aspiration cytology is commonly used to obtain histologic confirmation of suspected cancer. Aspiration cytology can usually diagnose carcinoma accurately, but lymphoma may be difficult to identify by this method, and open biopsy is often necessary. Bone marrow biopsy is not indicated prior to lymph node biopsy. It is done as part of the staging process after a diagnosis of lymphoma has been made. Endoscopy and scanning of the oropharynx and nasopharynx are part of the diagnostic workup of a suspected malignant cervical lymph node, but do not provide histologic proof of cancer.

211. The answer is e. (*Brunicardi, pp 254-255, 1288-1289.*) The management of malignant tumors may be guided by knowledge obtained by grading and staging the tumors. Histologic grading reflects the degree of anaplasia of tumor cells. Tumors in which histologic grading seems to have prognostic value include soft tissue sarcoma, transitional cell cancers of the bladder, astrocytoma, and chondrosarcoma. Grading has been of little predictive value in melanoma, hepatocellular carcinoma, or osteosarcoma. Staging is based on the extent of spread rather than histologic appearance and is more relevant in predicting the course of lung and colorectal cancers.

212. The answer is e. (*Brunicardi, pp 1448-1449.*) The mass shown is a nephroblastoma (Wilms tumor) adherent to the left kidney. Wilms tumor is the most common abdominal malignancy of childhood, but represents only about 10% of childhood malignant tumors. The deletion of 2 contiguous genes, WT1 (Wilms tumor gene) and PAX6 on chromosome band 11p13, results in the WAGR syndrome—Wilms tumor, Aniridia, Genitourinary anomalies, and mental retardation. Wilms tumor is also associated with the Beckwith-Wiedemann syndrome—an overgrowth disorder that results in gigantism, macroglossia, and hypoglycemia—and hemihypertrophy. Most patients present with an asymptomatic mass found by a parent. Less than one-third of patients experience hematuria. As would be expected in over half such cases, this child is hypertensive, probably due to compression of the renal artery by the mass. CT scan is used to assess the tumor characteristics and evaluate for metastases. Ultrasonography is utilized to assess for vascular invasion into the renal vein or vena cava. Surgical treatment consists of resection of the kidney and ureter. Chemotherapy is indicated in patients with malignancy confined to 1 kidney, and chemoradiation is indicated after surgical excision for more advanced disease. Cure rates approaching 90% are achieved, even in patients with hematogenous metastases.

213. The answer is a. (*Brunicardi, pp 1367-1369.*) Most medullary thyroid carcinomas (MTC) occur sporadically. However, approximately 25% occur in inherited syndromes such as familial medullary thyroid cancer and MEN types 2A and 2B. These syndromes result secondary to germline mutations in the RET proto-oncogene. MEN2A consists of medullary thyroid cancer, pheochromocytomas or adrenal medullary hyperplasia, and primary hyperparathyroidism. MEN2B consists of MTC, pheochromocytoma, mucosal neuromas, gangliomas, and a Marfan-like habitus. These patients may develop medullary carcinoma at a very young age, and any patient with MEN2A or MEN2B should be assumed to have medullary cancer until proved otherwise. Patients are followed carefully for pheochromocytoma with urine VMA, for hyperparathyroidism with serum calcium, and for medullary carcinoma with serum calcitonin. However, as some patients have a normal basal calcitonin, a pentagastrin or provocative calcium infusion test should be performed in these high-risk patients. Patients thought to have MEN1 syndrome (pituitary, parathyroid, and pancreatic tumors) or Zollinger-Ellison syndrome should be assayed for serum gastrin, insulin, glucagon, and somatostatin. These assays may prove to be inappropriately high in MEN1 syndrome due to pancreatic islet cell tumors.

214. The answer is c. *(Brunicardi, pp 1289-1295.)* Benign soft tissue tumors far outnumber their malignant counterparts. Because of this, prolonged delays are common before definitive treatment of soft tissue sarcomas is instituted. Risk for malignancy is increased for tumors greater than 5 cm in largest diameter, as well as for those lesions that are symptomatic or that have enlarged rapidly over a short period of time. Properly performed biopsy is critical in the initial treatment of any soft tissue mass. Improperly performed biopsies can complicate the care of the sarcoma patient and, in rare circumstances, even eliminate certain surgical options. Excisional biopsies should be reserved for small masses for which complete excision would not jeopardize subsequent treatment should a sarcoma be found. For all other masses, incisional biopsy should be performed. The incision should be placed directly over the mass and should be oriented along the long axis of the extremity.

215. The answer is e. *(Mulholland, p 733; Brunicardi, pp 935-937.)* Gastric lymphomas can develop from B-cell proliferation in mucosa-associated lymphoid tissue (MALT) which is associated with chronic *Helicobacter pylori* infection. The initial therapy for low-grade MALT lymphomas is an antibiotic regimen to treat *H pylori*; eradication of *H pylori* has been associated with complete regression of low-grade MALT lymphomas. Chemotherapy and/or external beam radiation are used to treat persistent lymphoma after antibiotic therapy or advanced (stage III/IV or high-grade) MALT lymphomas. Surgery is rarely indicated.

216. The answer is d. *(Brunicardi, pp 507-508.)* Acinar, adenoid cystic, and low grades of mucoepidermoid carcinomas exhibit moderately malignant behavior. Undifferentiated, squamous, and high grades of mucoepidermoid carcinomas are considered highly malignant tumors. Facial nerve preservation should be attempted when the margins are adequate and the tumor is well localized. The minimal appropriate procedure for parotid carcinoma is a superficial parotidectomy with nerve preservation. The nerve must be partially or totally sacrificed if the tumor directly involves the nerve trunk or its branches. Invasion of the deep lobe of the parotid requires total parotidectomy with facial nerve preservation unless there is encasement or direct involvement of the nerve. Regional node dissection is indicated for malignant tumors because of the high (up to 50%) incidence of occult regional metastases.

217. The answer is b. (*Brunicardi, pp 260-262.*) A surgeon is frequently asked to evaluate patients who are receiving systemic chemotherapy. Most complications of chemotherapy do not require surgical therapy. Perirectal abscesses are more common in these immunosuppressed patients. GI bleeding occurs secondary to mucosal irritation and thrombocytopenia. Pancreatitis is uncommon, but is associated with L-asparaginase use. Up to 20% of patients treated with floxuridine by continuous hepatic artery infusion develop some degree of inflammation and obstruction of the bile duct. Systemic chemotherapy does not increase the likelihood of acute cholecystitis, appendicitis, incarcerated femoral hernia, or diverticulitis.

218. The answer is e. (*Brunicardi, p 1462.*) Early-stage seminomas should be treated with orchiectomy and external beam radiation. Seminoma is extremely radiosensitive; therefore retroperitoneal lymph node dissection is unnecessary. After radical orchiectomy, lymph node dissection is indicated in embryonal carcinoma, teratocarcinoma, and adult teratoma if there is no supradiaphragmatic spread. This dissection increases the 5-year survival and helps in staging. Choriocarcinoma are frequently associated with pulmonary metastases and are treated with chemotherapy. Orchiectomy for a testicular mass is approached via an inguinal incision in order to perform a high ligation of the cord and to eliminate spread of the tumor. Cryptorchidism (undescended testicle) is associated with decreased spermatogenesis and carries a lifelong risk of malignant degeneration even after being surgically corrected.

219. The answer is d. (*Brunicardi, pp 289-290.*) Kidney transplant is the treatment of choice for patients with end-stage renal disease. It offers the patients a chance to lead healthy, normal lives. Compared with dialysis, it is associated with better patient survival, improved quality of life, and decreased long-term costs. Dialysis is less expensive than renal transplantation if the graft functions for less than 2 years. Renal transplantation requires lifelong immunosuppression which has its associated risks.

220. The answer is e. *(Brunicardi, pp 1399-1400.)* Pheochromocytoma is associated with MEN2A, MEN2B, von Hippel-Lindau disease, and neurofibromatosis I. Hereditary pheochromocytomas are more likely to be multiple and bilateral.

221. The answer is e. *(Brunicardi, pp 1044-1045.)* The Amsterdam criteria are used to clinically diagnose hereditary nonpolyposis colorectal cancer (HNPCC) and consist of (a) at least 3 relatives with histologically confirmed colorectal cancer, one of whom is a first-degree relative of the other; (b) involvement of at least 2 successive generations; and (c) diagnosis of at least one of the cancers before age 50. Screening for patients with HNPCC should start either between the ages of 20 and 25 or 10 years earlier than the youngest family member with colorectal cancer, whichever comes earlier. This recommendation differs than that for the average-risk patient, for whom screening should begin at age 50.

222. The answer is b. *(Brunicardi, pp 1049-1052.)* The patient has clinical stage III rectal cancer (because of clinically positive regional lymph nodes). The best treatment option to preserve her sphincter and potentially achieve a cure is neoadjuvant chemoradiation followed by low anterior resection (resection of the rectum with a colorectal anastomosis). One advantage of preoperative or neoadjuvant chemoradiation is potential downstaging of shrinkage of the tumor which may allow for improved respectability and/or a sphincter-preserving operation. Studies suggest that neoadjuvant chemoradiation also improves local control and survival. Disadvantages include an increase in postoperative complications and may impair wound healing and functioning of the neorectum. Abdominoperineal resection (APR) involves resection of the rectum and anus with formation of a permanent colostomy, which is against the patient's preferences. Transanal excision is indicated for early-stage rectal tumors accessible transanally (within 10 cm of the anal verge). However, transanal excision does not evaluate the lymph nodes and has a high rate of local recurrence in the absence of adjuvant chemoradiation.

223. The answer is c. *(Brunicardi, pp 258-260, 458-450.)* The sentinel lymph node is the first node to receive drainage from a tumor in a regional lymph node basin. The sentinel lymph node can be identified using blue dye, technetium-labeled sulfur colloid, or both. Sentinel lymph node biopsy is used most frequently in patients with breast cancer and melanoma who do not have clinically positive lymph node disease (ie, palpable lymph nodes, biopsy-proven malignancy) or metastases. In breast cancer, sentinel lymph node biopsy is not recommended in patients with ductal carcinoma in situ (DCIS) not undergoing mastectomy. Patients with extensive DCIS requiring mastectomy may benefit from a sentinel lymph node biopsy in the event that there was an occult carcinoma present in the specimen, since sentinel lymph node biopsy cannot be performed after a mastectomy. Sentinel lymph node biopsy is also not indicated in patients who are pregnant or who have had prior surgery either in the axilla or in the breast (unrelated to cancer).

224. The answer is d. (*Mulholland, pp 532-534, 567.*) Cardiac allograft has become an accepted treatment for end-stage heart disease. One-year cardiac allograft survival exceeds 80%, which is comparable to renal allograft survival. Cardiac allografts have a cold ischemia preservation time of 4 to 5 hours, and therefore tissue typing is not practical. Cardiac donors are matched to recipients only by size and ABO blood type. Tissue typing remains an important component of cadaveric kidney allograft matching. The mainstay of immunosuppression for both cardiac and renal allografts continues to include calcineurin inhibitors (FK506, cyclosporine), steroids, and antimitotic agents (azathioprine, mycophenolate mofetil).

225. The answer is b. (*Mulholland, pp 1385-1389.*) Resection of metastases of lung, liver, and brain can result in occasional 5-year cures. In general, surgery should be undertaken only when the primary tumor is controlled, diffuse metastatic disease has been ruled out, and the affected patient's condition and the location of the metastasis permit safe resection. The best results have come from resection of pulmonary metastases, in which 5-year survival rates exceed those for resection for primary bronchogenic carcinoma. For example, resection of pulmonary metastases in patients with osteogenic sarcoma can have survival rates up to 25% to 35%.

226. The answer is c. (*Brunicardi, pp 262-263, 1297-1299.*) Greater understanding of cancer biology has led to the development of numerous targeted therapies. Gastrointestinal stromal tumors (GISTs) express the *c-kit* receptor; *c-kit* is a tyrosine kinase. Imatinib is a selective tyrosine kinase inhibitor that is used as neoadjuvant or palliative therapy for metastatic GIST. Ceutximab and bevacizumab are monoclonal antibodies directed against epidermal growth factor receptor (EGFR) and vascular endothelial growth factor A (VEGF-A), respectively. Both are used as adjuncts for treating various malignancies. Infliximab, which is a monoclonal antibody against tumor necrosis factor α (TNF α), is used for the treatment of autoimmune diseases including inflammatory bowel disease. Daclizumab, which is a monoclonal antibody against a subunit of the interleukin-2 (IL-2) receptor, is used in to treat rejection in organ transplantation. --

227. The answer is c. *(Brunicardi, pp 463-467.)* Trastuzumab is a monoclonal antibody against HER-2/neu and is indicated for patients with breast cancers that overexpress HER-2/neu. Antiestrogen therapies are used as adjuvant therapy for patients with hormone receptor–positive cancers and as chemoprevention in patients with a high risk of breast cancer. Tamoxifen is an estrogen receptor antagonist and raloxifene is a selective estrogen receptor modulator. Aromatase inhibitors block the synthesis of estrogen. 5-fluorouracil is used in some adjuvant chemotherapy regimens for breast cancer, but it does not confer additional benefit in patients with tumors overexpressing HER-2/neu.

228. The answer is c. *(Brunicardi, pp 246-247.)* Li-Fraumeni syndrome is associated most commonly with a mutation in the p53 tumor suppressor gene. Li-Fraumeni syndrome in an individual is based on (1) bone or soft tissue sarcoma in that person before the age of 45, (2) a first-degree relative with cancer before the age of 45, and (3) a first- or second-degree relative with sarcoma at any age or any cancer before the age of 45. The APC gene is associated with familial adenomatous polyposis (FAP). The RET proto-oncogene is associated with MEN2. The PTEN tumor suppressor gene is associated with Cowden disease, or multiple hamartoma syndrome. The p16 tumor suppressor gene is associated with hereditary malignant melanoma.

229. The answer is a. *(Brunicardi, pp 260-262, 1294.)* Doxorubicin, an antibiotic derived from *Streptomyces* species, has activity against sarcomas and carcinomas of the breast, liver, bladder, prostate, head and neck, esophagus, and lung. Its major side effect is production of a dilated cardiomyopathy. Patients receiving this agent should have an echocardiogram before and after treatment in order to monitor potential cardiac toxicity.

230. The answer is e. (*Brunicardi, pp 248-249, 439-440.*) Both BRCA1 and BRCA2 are associated with an increased cumulative risk of both breast and ovarian cancer. Prophylactic bilateral mastectomy and reconstruction is recommended for BRCA mutation carriers. If prophylactic mastectomy is not performed, intensive surveillance for breast cancer with biannual clinical examinations and annual mammograms starting at age 25 is recommended. Tamoxifen is not routinely indicated for al BRCA1 carriers since most breast cancers in BRCA1 mutation carriers are estrogen receptor-negative. BRCA2 breast cancers are more likely to be estrogen receptor-positive. Approximately 10% of women under the age of 40 who develop breast cancer have a mutation in BRCA1 or 2. BRCA1 is associated with an increased risk of colon cancer and prostate cancer in males. BRCA2 is associated with an increased risk of gallbladder, bile duct, and pancreatic cancers as well as gastric cancer, malignant melanoma, and in men, prostate cancer.

231. The answer is e. (*Brunicardi, pp 260-262.*) Cyclophosphamide is an alkylating agent used in the treatment of a variety of solid tumors. Its major side effect is hemorrhagic cystitis. Bleomycin can cause pulmonary fibrosis. Vincristine is an alkaloid that can cause peripheral and central neuropathies. Cisplatin is an alkylating agent that can lead to ototoxicity, neurotoxicity, and nephrotoxicity. 5-fluorouracil is an antimetabolite that can cause mucositis, dermatitis, and cerebellar dysfunction.

232. The answer is d. (*Townsend, pp 675-676.*) Posttransplant lymphoproliferative disorders (PTLD) are associated with the EBV. PTLD has a range of clinical presentations, and treatment can include multiple modalities including withdrawal of immunosuppression, antiviral therapy with ganciclovir, chemotherapy, or immunotherapy with monoclonal antibodies. Other common posttransplantation malignancies include hepatocellular carcinomas, which are associated with hepatitis B and C; Kaposi sarcoma, which is associated with human herpesvirus 8; and cervical cancers, which are associated with human papillomavirus. Although CMV infection can occur when CMV-seronegative recipients receive an organ from a CMV-seropositive donor, CMV does not predispose transplantation patients to malignancy.

233. The answer is d. (*Brunicardi, pp 1376-1377.*) The patient has tertiary hyperparathyroidism, which is manifested by persistent hypercalcemia secondary to autonomous parathyroid function after renal transplantation.

Treatment is total parathyroidectomy with autotransplantation or subtotal parathyroidectomy. The imaging modalities described would be more appropriate in the workup of primary hyperparathyroidism—24-hour urinary calcium levels are low in familial hypercalciuric hypercalcemia. Ultrasound, sestamibi scintigraphy, and CT scanning are all modalities that can be utilized to identify a parathyroid adenoma preoperatively.

234. The answer is e. *(Brunicardi, pp 255-256.)* CEA is a glycoprotein that is present in early embryonic and fetal cells (an oncofetal antigen) and in colon cancer. It is not found in normal colon mucosa. It is not tumor-specific and may be elevated in a variety of benign and malignant conditions, including cirrhosis, ulcerative colitis, renal failure, pancreatitis, pancreatic cancer, stomach cancer, breast cancer, and lung cancer. However, the CEA assay is a sensitive serologic tool for identifying recurrent disease. In about two-thirds of patients with recurrent disease, an increased CEA level is the first indicator of tumor reappearance. A rising CEA following colon cancer surgery, in the absence of other conditions associated with an elevated CEA, predicts the appearance of liver metastases within 1 year with an accuracy approaching 70%. Although an elevated CEA level preoperatively predicts a higher risk of recurrence, the use of preoperative CEA levels as an indication for postoperative adjuvant chemotherapy is controversial and currently not supported by clinical practice guidelines.

235 to 237. The answers are 235-a, 236-g, 237-e. *(Brunicardi, pp 1048-1051.)* In order to resect the tumor with an adequate margin (traditionally 5 cm) on its proximal and distal ends and remove the draining lymph node basin, a left hemicolectomy should be performed. Patients with lymph node involvement are at significant risk for both local and distant recurrence, and adjuvant chemotherapy is routinely recommended in these patients. The liver is the most common site of bloodborne metastases from primary colorectal cancers. If the liver is the only site of metastasis and the lesion is able to be resected with clear margins, then survival is improved with hepatic resection.

238 to 241. The answers are 238-f, 239-a, 240-d, 241-b *(Brunicardi, pp 274-280.)* Routine postoperative immunosuppression for a renal transplant recipient includes cyclosporine, azathioprine, and steroids. Cyclosporine is nephrotoxic and is frequently withheld in the postoperative period until the creatinine returns to normal following transplantation. Azathioprine has bone marrow toxicity as its major side effect, and both WBC and platelet counts need to be monitored in the immediate posttransplant period. The patient's decrease in WBCs is secondary to azathioprine toxicity, and the most appropriate step is to decrease the dose of azathioprine. Viral infections are a serious cause of morbidity following transplantation. A buffy coat is the supernatant of a centrifuged blood sample that contains the WBCs. Viral cultures from this supernatant as well as localization of inclusion bodies can identify transplant patients infected with CMV. This patient has CMV pneumonitis and needs to be treated with high-dose gancyclovir.

An elevation in creatinine at 3-month follow-up can be secondary to rejection, anastomotic problems, urologic complications, infection, or nephrotoxicity of various medications. With a normal ultrasound, no fever, and no graft tenderness, the most likely cause is cyclosporine-induced nephrotoxicity and the most appropriate step is a reduction in the cyclosporine dose. Finally, at 6 months with graft tenderness, fever, and an edematous kidney on ultrasound, rejection must be suspected. Negative cultures make infection unlikely, and a steroid boost is appropriate. Addition of monoclonal antibodies to CD3 (Muromonab-CD3) or pooled antibodies against lymphocytes (ALGs) is also appropriate in the treatment of a first rejection.

Endocrine Problems and the Breast

Questions

242. A 45-year-old woman complains to her primary care physician of nervousness, sweating, tremulousness, and weight loss. The thyroid scan shown here exhibits a pattern that is most consistent with which of the following disorders?

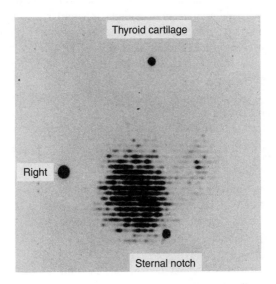

a. Hypersecreting adenoma
b. Graves disease
c. Lateral aberrant thyroid
d. Papillary carcinoma of thyroid
e. Medullary carcinoma of thyroid

243. A patient with mild skin pigmentation is admitted emergently to your service because of sudden abdominal pain, fever, and a rigid abdomen. Her blood work indicates a marked leukocytosis, a blood sugar of 55 mg/dL, a sodium value of 119 mEq/dL, and a potassium value of 6.2 mEq/dL. Her blood pressure is 88/58 mm Hg. She undergoes an exploratory laparotomy. Which of the following is the definitive treatment for her primary condition?

a. 10% dextrose infusion
b. Bicarbonate
c. Hypertonic saline
d. Corticosteroids
e. Vasopressors

244 A 35-year-old woman with a history of previous right thyroidectomy for a benign thyroid nodule now undergoes completion thyroidectomy for a suspicious thyroid mass. Several hours postoperatively, she develops progressive swelling under the incision, stridor, and difficulty breathing. Orotracheal intubation is successful. Which of the following is the most appropriate next step?

a. Fiberoptic laryngoscopy to rule out bilateral vocal cord paralysis
b. Administration of intravenous calcium
c. Administration of broad-spectrum antibiotics and debridement of the wound
d. Wound exploration
e. Administration of high-dose steroids and antihistamines

245. A 62-year-old woman presents with invasive ductal carcinoma of the right breast. Which of the following findings would still allow her to receive breast conservation surgery (partial mastectomy)?

a. Diffuse suspicious microcalcifications throughout the breast
b. Multifocal disease
c. Previous treatment of a breast cancer with lumpectomy and radiation
d. Large tumor relative to breast size
e. Persistently positive margins after multiple reexcisions of the breast cancer

246. A 29-year-old woman presents with a 6-month history of erythema and edema of the right breast with palpable axillary lymphadenopathy. A punch biopsy of the skin reveals neoplastic cells in the dermal lymphatics. Which of the following is the best next step in her management?

a. A course of nafcillin to treat the overlying cellulitis and then neoadjuvant chemotherapy for breast cancer
b. Modified radical mastectomy followed by adjuvant chemotherapy
c. Modified radical mastectomy followed by hormonal therapy
d. Combined modality chemotherapy and radiation therapy to the right breast with surgery reserved for residual disease
e. Combined modality therapy with chemotherapy, surgery, and radiation

247. A 15-year-old otherwise healthy female high school student begins to notice galactorrhea. A pregnancy test is negative. Which of the following is a frequently associated physical finding?

a. Gonadal atrophy
b. Bitemporal hemianopsia
c. Exophthalmos and lid lag
d. Episodic hypertension
e. Buffalo hump

248. A 52-year-old woman sees her physician with complaints of fatigue, headache, flank pain, hematuria, and abdominal pain. She undergoes a sestamibi scan that demonstrates persistent uptake in the right superior parathyroid gland at 2 hours. Which of the following laboratory values is most suggestive of her diagnosis?

a. Serum acid phosphatase above 120 IU/L
b. Serum alkaline phosphatase above 120 IU/L
c. Serum calcium above 11 mg/dL
d. Urinary calcium below 100 mg/day
e. Parathyroid hormone levels below 5 pmol/L

249. A 53-year-old woman presents with weight loss and a persistent rash to her lower abdomen and perineum. She is diagnosed with necrolytic migrating erythema and additional workup demonstrates diabetes mellitus, anemia and a large mass in the tail of the pancreas. Which of the following is the most likely diagnosis?

a. Verner-Morrison syndrome (VIPoma)
b. Glucagonoma
c. Somatostatinoma
d. Insulinoma
e. Gastrinoma

250. A 49-year-old obese man has become irritable, his face has changed to a round configuration, he has developed purplish lines on his flanks, and he is hypertensive. A 24-hour urine collection demonstrates elevated cortisol levels. This is confirmed with bedtime cortisol measurements of 700 ng/mL. Which of the following findings is most consistent with the diagnosis of Cushing disease?

a. Decreased ACTH levels
b. Glucocorticoid use for the treatment of inflammatory disorders
c. A 3-cm adrenal mass on computed tomography (CT) scan
d. Suppression with high-dose dexamethasone suppression testing
e. A 1-cm bronchogenic mass on magnetic resonance imaging (MRI)

251. A 35-year-old woman presents with a lump in the left breast. Her family history is negative for breast cancer. On examination the mass is rubbery, mobile, and nontender to palpation. There are no overlying skin changes and the axilla is negative for lymphadenopathy. An ultrasound demonstrates a simple 1-cm cyst in the area of the palpable mass in the left breast. Which of the following represents the most appropriate management of this patient?

a. Reassurance and reexamination
b. Immediate excisional biopsy
c. Aspiration of the cyst with cytologic analysis
d. Fluoroscopically guided needle localization biopsy
e. Mammography and reevaluation of options with new information

252. A 55-year-old woman presents with a slow-growing painless mass on the right side of the neck. A fine-needle aspiration of the nodule shows a well-differentiated papillary carcinoma. A complete neck ultrasound demonstrates a 1-cm nodule in the right thyroid without masses in the contralateral lobe or lymph node metastasis in the central and lateral neck compartments. With regards to this patient, which of the following is associated with a poor prognosis?

a. Age
b. Sex
c. Grade of tumor
d. Size of tumor
e. Lymph node status

253. A 55-year-old woman presents with a 6-cm right thyroid mass and palpable cervical lymphadenopathy. Fine-needle aspiration (FNA) of one of the lymph nodes demonstrates the presence of calcified clumps of sloughed cells. Which of the following best describes the management of this thyroid disorder?

a. The patient should be screened for pancreatic endocrine neoplasms and hypercalcemia.
b. The patient should undergo total thyroidectomy with modified radical neck dissection.
c. The patient should undergo total thyroidectomy with frozen section intraoperatively, with modified radical neck dissection reserved for patients with extracapsular invasion.
d. The patient should undergo right thyroid lobectomy followed by iodine 131 (^{131}I) therapy.
e. The patient should undergo right thyroid lobectomy.

254. A 45-year-old woman is found to have suspicious appearing calcifications in the right breast on a screening mammogram. Stereotactic biopsy of the calcifications shows lobular carcinoma in situ (LCIS). On examination both breasts are dense without palpable masses. The neck and bilateral axilla are negative for lymphadenopathy. Which of the following is the most appropriate management of this patient?

a. Frequent self breast examinations and yearly screening mammograms
b. Chemotherapy
c. Radiation
d. Right total mastectomy with sentinel lymph node biopsy
e. Bilateral modified radical mastectomy

255. A 14-year-old black girl has her right breast removed because of a large mass. The tumor weighs 1400 g and has a bulging, very firm, lobulated surface with a whorl-like pattern, as illustrated here. Which of the following is the most likely diagnosis?

a. Cystosarcoma phyllodes
b. Intraductal carcinoma
c. Malignant lymphoma
d. Fibroadenoma
e. Juvenile hypertrophy

256. A 53-year-old woman presents with complaints of weakness, anorexia, malaise, constipation, and back pain. While being evaluated, she becomes somewhat lethargic. Laboratory studies include a normal chest x-ray, serum albumin 3.2 mg/dL, serum calcium 14 mg/dL, serum phosphorus 2.6 mg/dL, serum chloride 108 mg/dL, blood urea nitrogen (BUN) 32 mg/dL, and creatinine 2.0 mg/dL. Which of the following is the most appropriate initial management?

a. Intravenous normal saline infusion
b. Administration of thiazide diuretics
c. Administration of intravenous phosphorus
d. Use of mithramycin
e. Neck exploration and parathyroidectomy

257. Which of the following patients with primary hyperparathyroidism should undergo parathyroidectomy?

a. A 62-year-old asymptomatic woman
b. A 54-year-old woman with fatigue and depression
c. A 42-year-old woman with a history of kidney stones
d. A 59-year-old woman with mildly elevated 24-hour urinary calcium excretion
e. A 60-year-old woman with mildly decreased bone mineral density measured at the hip of less than 2 standard deviations below peak bone density

258. A 45-year-old woman presents with hypertension, development of facial hair, and a 7-cm suprarenal mass. Which of the following is the most likely diagnosis?

a. Myelolipoma
b. Cushing disease
c. Adrenocortical carcinoma
d. Pheochromocytoma
e. Carcinoid

259. A 36-year-old woman presents with palpitations, anxiety, and hypertension. Workup reveals a pheochromocytoma. Which of the following is the best approach to optimizing the patient preoperatively?

a. Fluid restriction 24 hours preoperatively to prevent intraoperative congestive heart failure
b. Initiation of an α-blocker 24 hours prior to surgery
c. Initiation of an α-blocker at 1 to 3 weeks prior to surgery
d. Initiation of a β-blocker 1 to 3 weeks prior to surgery
e. Escalating antihypertensive drug therapy with β-blockade followed by α-blockade starting at least 1 week prior to surgery

260. A 33-year-old pregnant woman notices a persistent, painless lump in the left breast. On examination the left breast has a single mobile mass without evidence of skin changes or lymphadenopathy in the neck or axilla. An ultrasound demonstrates a solid, 1-cm mass in the upper outer quadrant of the breast. A core-needle biopsy shows invasive ductal carcinoma. The patient is in her first trimester of pregnancy. Which of the following is the most appropriate management of this patient?

a. Termination of the pregnancy followed by modified radical mastectomy
b. Immediate administration of chemotherapy followed by modified radical mastectomy after delivery of the baby
c. Administration of radiation in the third trimester followed by modified radical mastectomy after delivery of the baby
d. Total mastectomy with sentinel lymph node biopsy
e. Modified radical mastectomy

261. A 40-year-old woman presents with a rash involving the nipple-areola complex for the last month with associated itching. On physical examination there is crusting and ulceration of the nipple with surrounding erythema involving the areola and surrounding skin, no palpable breast masses, and no cervical or axillary lymphadenopathy. Which of the following is the most appropriate next step in the management of this patient?

a. Reexamine the patient in 1 month
b. Corticosteroid cream to the affected area
c. Administration of oral antibiotics
d. Mammogram and biopsy of the affected area
e. Modified radical mastectomy

262. A 50-year-old man presents with intractable peptic ulcer disease, severe esophagitis, and abdominal pain. Which of the following is most consistent with the diagnosis of Zollinger-Ellison syndrome?

a. Hypercalcemia
b. Fasting gastrin level of 10 pg/mL
c. Fasting gastrin level of 100 pg/mL
d. Increase in gastrin level (> 200 pg/mL) after administration of secretin
e. Decrease in gastrin level (> 200 pg/mL) after administration of secretin

263. A 29-year-old woman with a history of difficulty becoming pregnant presents to her primary care physician and is diagnosed with Grave disease on iodine uptake scan; her thyrotropin (TSH) level is markedly suppressed and her free thyroxine (T_4) level is elevated. She desires to conceive as soon as possible and elects to undergo thyroidectomy. After she is rendered euthyroid with medications preoperatively, which of the following management strategies should also be employed to reduce the risk of developing thyroid storm in the operating room?

a. Drops of Lugol iodine solution daily beginning 10 days preoperatively.
b. Preoperative treatment with phenoxybenzamine for 3 weeks.
c. Preoperative treatment with propranolol for 1 week.
d. Twenty-four hours of corticosteroids preoperatively.
e. No other preoperative medication is required.

264. A 30-year-old woman presents with hypertension, weakness, bone pain, and a serum calcium level of 15.2 mg/dL. Hand films below show osteitis fibrosa cystica. Which of the following is the most likely cause of these findings?

a. Sarcoidosis
b. Vitamin D intoxication
c. Paget disease
d. Metastatic carcinoma
e. Primary hyperparathyroidism

265. A 35-year-old woman presents with a serum calcium level of 15.2 mg/dL and an elevated parathyroid hormone level. Following correction of the patient's hypercalcemia with hydration and furosemide, which of the following is the best therapeutic approach?

a. Administration of steroids
b. Radiation treatment to the neck
c. Neck exploration and resection of all 4 parathyroid glands
d. Neck exploration and resection of a parathyroid adenoma
e. Avoidance of sunlight, vitamin D, and calcium-containing dairy products

266. A 58-year-old man presents with tachycardia, fever, confusion, and vomiting. Workup reveals markedly elevated (triiodothyronine) T_3 and (thyroxine) T_4 levels. He is diagnosed as having a thyroid storm. Which of the following is the most appropriate next step in the management of this patient?

a. Emergent subtotal thyroidectomy
b. Emergent total thyroidectomy
c. Emergent hemodialysis
d. Administration of fluid, antithyroid drugs, β-blockers, iodine solution, and steroids
e. Emergent radiation therapy to the neck

267. A 34-year-old woman presents with hypertension, generalized weakness, and polyuria. Her electrolyte panel is significant for hypokalemia. Which of the following is the best initial test given her presentation and laboratory findings?

a. Plasma renin activity and plasma aldosterone concentration
b. Urine electrolytes
c. Plasma cortisol level
d. Overnight low-dose dexamethasone suppression test
e. Twenty-four-hour urinary aldosterone level

268. Incisional biopsy of a breast mass in a 35-year-old woman demonstrates cystosarcoma phyllodes at the time of frozen section. Which of the following is the most appropriate management strategy for this lesion?

a. Wide local excision with a rim of normal tissue
b. Lumpectomy and axillary lymphadenectomy
c. Modified radical mastectomy
d. Excision and postoperative radiotherapy
e. Excision, postoperative radiotherapy, and systemic chemotherapy

269. A 36-year-old woman, 20 weeks pregnant, presents with a 1.5-cm right thyroid mass. FNA is consistent with a papillary neoplasm. The mass is cold on scan and solid on ultrasound. Which of the following methods of treatment is contraindicated in this patient?

a. Right thyroid lobectomy
b. Subtotal thyroidectomy
c. Total thyroidectomy
d. Total thyroidectomy with lymph node dissection
e. ^{131}I radioactive ablation of the thyroid gland

270. A 63-year-old woman notices lumps on both sides of her neck. A fine-needle aspirate is nondiagnostic, and she undergoes total thyroidectomy. Final pathology reveals a 2-cm Hürthle cell carcinoma. Which of the following is the most appropriate postsurgical management of this patient?

a. No further therapy is indicated.
b. Chemotherapy.
c. External beam radiotherapy.
d. Radioiodine ablation.
e. Chemotherapy, external beam radiotherapy, and radioiodine ablation.

271. A 51-year-old man presents with a 2-cm left thyroid nodule. Thyroid scan shows a cold lesion. FNA cytology demonstrates follicular cells. Which of the following is the most appropriate initial treatment of this patient?

a. External beam radiation to the neck.
b. Multidrug chemotherapy.
c. TSH suppression by thyroid hormone.
d. Prophylactic neck dissection is indicated along with a total thyroidectomy.
e. Thyroid lobectomy.

272. A 41-year-old woman has noted bilateral thin serous discharge from her breasts. There seems to be no mass associated with it. Which of the following statements would be appropriate to tell the patient?

a. Intermittent thin or milky discharge can be physiologic.
b. Expressible nipple discharge is an indication for open biopsy.
c. Absence of a mass on mammogram rules out malignancy.
d. Galactorrhea is indicative of an underlying malignancy.
e. Pathologic discharge is usually bilateral.

273. A 52-year-old woman presents with hypertension, obesity, and new skin striae. You are concerned about possible Cushing syndrome. Which of the following is the most common cause of Cushing syndrome?

a. Adrenocortical hyperplasia
b. Adrenocorticotropic hormone (ACTH)–producing pituitary tumor
c. Primary adrenal neoplasms
d. Ectopic adrenocorticotropic hormone (ACTH)–secreting carcinoid tumor
e. Pharmacologic glucocorticoid use

274. A 34-year-old woman has recurrent fainting spells induced by fasting. She also reports palpitations, trembling, diaphoresis, and confusion prior to the syncopal episodes. She has relief of symptoms with the administration of glucose. Which of the following findings is most consistent with the diagnosis of an insulinoma?

a. Serum glucose level > 50 mg/dL, elevated serum insulin levels, elevated C-peptide levels
b. Serum glucose level > 50 mg/dL, elevated serum insulin levels, decreased C-peptide levels
c. Serum glucose level < 50 mg/dL, elevated serum insulin levels, elevated C-peptide levels
d. Serum glucose level < 50 mg/dL, elevated serum insulin levels, decreased C-peptide levels
e. Serum glucose level < 50 mg/dL, decreased serum insulin levels, decreased C-peptide levels

275. A 36-year-old woman whose mother has just undergone treatment for breast cancer is asking about how this affects her and what can be done to lessen her chances of having the disease. Which of the following has the lowest risk factor for breast cancer?

a. Dietary fat intake
b. Paternal relative with breast cancer 1 (*BRCA1*) mutation
c. Excessive estrogen exposure—early menarche, late menopause, nulliparity
d. Previous biopsy with atypical hyperplasia
e. Exposure to ionizing radiation

Questions 276 to 280

For each clinical description, select the appropriate stage of breast cancer. Each lettered option may be used once, more than once, or not at all.

a. Stage 0
b. Stage I
c. Stage II
d. Stage III
e. Stage IV

276. Tumor not palpable, clinically positive ipsilateral axillary lymph nodes fixed to one another, no evidence of metastases.

277. Tumor 4.0 cm; clinically positive, movable axillary ipsilateral lymph nodes; no evidence of metastases.

278. Tumor 2.1 cm, clinically negative lymph nodes, no evidence of metastases. Final pathology shows only ductal carcinoma in situ.

279. Tumor not palpable, but breast diffusely enlarged and erythematous, clinically positive supraclavicular nodes; no evidence of metastases.

280. Tumor 0.5 cm, clinically negative lymph nodes, pathological lumbar fracture.

Questions 281 to 285

A 43-year-old man presents with signs and symptoms of peritonitis in the right lower quadrant. The clinical impression and supportive data suggest acute appendicitis. At exploration, however, a tumor is found; frozen section suggests carcinoid features. For each tumor described, choose the most appropriate surgical procedure. Each lettered option may be used once, more than once, or not at all.

a. Appendectomy
b. Segmental ileal resection
c. Cecectomy
d. Right hemicolectomy
e. Hepatic wedge resection and appropriate bowel resection

281. A 2.5-cm tumor at the base of the appendix.

282. A 1.0-cm tumor at the tip of the appendix.

283. A 0.5-cm tumor with serosal umbilication in the ileum.

284. A 1.0-cm tumor of the midappendix; a 1-cm firm, pale lesion at the periphery of the right lobe of the liver.

285. A 3.5-cm tumor encroaching onto the cecum and extensive liver metastases.

Questions 286 to 290

For each clinical problem outlined, select acceptable treatment options. Each lettered option may be used once, more than once, or not at all.

a. No further surgical intervention
b. Wide local excision
c. Wide local excision with adjuvant radiation therapy
d. Wide local excision with axillary lymph node dissection and radiation therapy
e. Simple mastectomy (without axillary lymph node dissection)
f. Modified radical mastectomy (simple mastectomy with in-continuity axillary lymph node dissection)
g. Radical mastectomy
h. Bilateral prophylactic simple mastectomies

286. A 49-year-old woman undergoes biopsy of a 5.0-cm left breast mass; she has no palpable axillary lymph nodes. Biopsy of the mass shows cystosarcoma phyllodes.

287. A 42-year-old woman has a mammogram that demonstrates diffuse suspicious mammographic calcifications suggestive of multicentric disease. Biopsy of one of the lesions reveals ductal carcinoma in situ (DCIS).

288. A 51-year-old (premenopausal) woman undergoes needle localization biopsy for microcalcifications. Pathology reveals sclerosing adenosis.

289. A 49-year-old woman has a 6-cm palpable mass that is biopsy-proven ductal adenocarcinoma. She undergoes neoadjuvant chemotherapy which reduces the tumor to 3 cm in size. However, she has palpable axillary lymph nodes; FNA demonstrates adenocarcinoma. She desires breast conservation therapy if possible.

290. A neglected 82-year-old woman presents with a locally advanced breast cancer that is invading the pectoralis major muscle over a broad base. She is otherwise in good health.

Endocrine Problems and the Breast

Answers

242. The answer is a. (*Brunicardi, pp 1353-1355.*) The thyroid scan shows a single focus of increased isotope uptake, often referred to as a hot nodule. Hyperfunctioning adenomas or hot nodules become independent of TSH control and secrete thyroid hormone autonomously, which results in clinical hyperthyroidism. The elevated thyroid hormone levels ultimately diminish TSH levels severely and thus depress function of the remaining normal thyroid gland. An isolated focus of increased uptake on a thyroid scan is virtually diagnostic of a hyperfunctioning adenoma. Graves disease demonstrates diffuse uptake of radioactive iodine by the thyroid gland. Carcinomas usually display diminished uptake and are called cold nodules. Multinodular goiter would display many nodules with varying activity.

243. The answer is d. (*Townsend, pp 1006-1007.*) This patient has adrenal insufficiency and needs treatment with corticosteroids. Chronic adrenal insufficiency (classic Addison disease) should be recognizable preoperatively by the constellation of skin pigmentation, weakness, weight loss, hypotension, nausea, vomiting, abdominal pain, hypoglycemia, hyponatremia, and hyperkalemia. Failure to recognize adrenal cortical insufficiency, particularly in the postoperative patient, may be a fatal error that is especially regrettable because therapy is effective and easy to administer. Adrenal insufficiency may occur in a host of settings including infections (eg, tuberculosis, [human immunodeficiency virus] HIV-associated infections), autoimmune states, adrenal hemorrhage (classically, during meningococcal septicemia), pituitary insufficiency, after burns, in the setting of coagulopathy, and after interruption of chronically administered exogenous steroids. Adrenal insufficiency may also develop insidiously in the postoperative period, progressing over a course of several days. This insidious course is seen when adrenal injury occurs in the perioperative period, as would be the case with adrenal damage from hemorrhage into the gland in a patient receiving postoperative anticoagulant therapy. The other answers all address individual components of the patient's condition but not the underlying disease.

244. The answer is d. (*Brunicardi, pp 1372-1374.*) The clinical presentation is consistent with a wound hematoma and necessitates exploration of the wound, drainage of the hematoma, and identification and control of any bleeding vessels. If airway control is unable to be obtained prior to the operating room, the wound should be opened at the bedside. Bilateral vocal cord dysfunction can be a cause of postoperative stridor and difficulty breathing, particularly after reoperative surgery; however, bilateral vocal cord dysfunction should manifest immediately after extubation. Hypocalcemia can occur in post-thyroidectomy due to ischemia or accidental removal of parathyroid tissue but is typically transient. Symptoms of hypocalcemia are usually neuromuscular and cardiac in nature.

245. The answer is b. (*Townsend, p 877.*) Multifocal disease refers to multiple tumors within 1 quadrant of the breast. If the lesions are small relative to the size of the breast, then the patient can still undergo breast conservation surgery with good results. Contraindications to breast conservation therapy include diffuse microcalcifications suspicious for malignancy, persistently positive margins in the face of multiple reexcisions, pregnancy (except in the third trimester with radiation therapy deferred until after delivery), multiple tumors in separate quadrants (multicentric disease), a previous history of therapeutic radiation to the breast, and expected poor cosmetic results (eg, large tumor, small breast).

246. The answer is e. (*Townsend, p 885.*) Currently, treatment of inflammatory breast cancer consists of multimodality therapy with neoadjuvant chemotherapy, surgery, and radiation, which results in a 50% 5-year survival rate. The clinical description of *peau d'orange* results from neoplastic invasion of dermal lymphatics with resultant edema of the breast; this clinical presentation and the skin biopsy findings are diagnostic for inflammatory breast cancer. Although the clinical picture may resemble that of a bacterial infection of the breast (mastitis), care must be taken to differentiate between the 2 pathologies.

247. The answer is b. (*Townsend, pp 2109-2110.*) Increased prolactin levels may be due to a variety of etiologies, including, but not limited to, medications, pregnancy, cirrhosis, or tumors. Prolactin-secreting tumors in the pituitary gland may cause bitemporal hemianopsia because of compression of the optic chiasm. They are typically associated with amenorrhea and galactorrhea in women. In both sexes, lack of libido and impotence or infertility may be noted. Sexual vigor is usually restored after removal of the adenomas. Observation alone is recommended for asymptomatic patients. Symptomatic relief can be afforded by dopaminergic agonists (eg, bromocriptine), which usually cause tumor shrinkage. Surgery is reserved for those individuals with persistent symptoms despite adequate therapy or who do not desire long-term medical therapy.

248. The answer is c. *(Brunicardi, pp 1376-1381.)* Elevated parathyroid hormone (PTH) levels in conjunction with elevated calcium levels are diagnostic for hyperparathyroidism. Primary hyperparathyroidism is a common disease, affecting 100,000 individuals each year in the United States. Essential to the diagnosis of hyperparathyroidism is the finding of hypercalcemia. Though there are many causes of hypercalcemia, hyperparathyroidism is by far the most prevalent. The majority of patients with primary hyperparathyroidism have a single parathyroid adenoma, which can be localized in 75% to 80% of patients with sestamibi scanning. Technetium 99m–labeled sestamibi is taken up by the parathyroid and thyroid glands. Hyperfunctioning parathyroid glands take up the sestamibi to a greater extent than normal glands, and therefore sestamibi scanning can be used to identify parathyroid adenomas. Patients with primary hyperparathyroidism have either normal or elevated urinary calcium. As the name suggests, patients with familial hypocalciuric hypercalcemia (FHH) have hypercalcemia. They also usually have elevated PTH, but urine calcium excretion is low (as opposed to normal to high as with a parathyroid adenoma). Surgery is not indicated in this relatively rare setting of hypercalcemia.

249. The answer is b. *(Townsend, p 992.)* A tumor in the tail of the pancreas with a rash called necrolytic migrating erythema is most consistent with a glucagonoma. Glucagonoma, a tumor of islet alpha cells, causes a syndrome of a characteristic rash, diabetes mellitus, anemia, weight loss, and elevated levels of circulating glucagon. Glucagonomas are usually present in the body or tail of the pancreas and easily identifiable on CT scanning of the abdomen. Treatment is surgical excision with a distal pancreatectomy. Metastases are common and should be resected whenever feasible. Medical management of symptoms involves administration of total parenteral nutrition containing amino acids and octreotide. The other islet cell tumors do not cause a characteristic rash.

250. The answer is d. (*Townsend, pp 1011-1013.*) Cushing disease is cortisol excess caused by an ACTH-hypersecreting pituitary adenoma. In these patients the ACTH level is normal or elevated and cortisol is suppressed with administration of high-dose dexamethasone. Cushing syndrome is an endocrine disorder caused by prolonged exposure of the body to elevated levels of cortisol, independent of the source. Clinical manifestations of glucocorticoid excess include hypertension, obesity, moon facies, buffalo hump, purple abdominal striae, and hirsutism. The most common cause of Cushing syndrome is pharmacologic glucocorticoid use for treatment of inflammatory disorders. Endogenous Cushing syndrome is rare, and the majority (75%) will have Cushing disease. The remainder will have primary adrenal Cushing syndrome or ectopic ACTH syndrome (most commonly arising from either neuroendocrine tumors or bronchogenic tumors).

251. The answer is a. (*Brunicardi, pp 435-436.*) Most clinicians would recommend reassurance and reexamination in this situation. Cysts are common lesions in the breasts of women in their thirties and forties and carry a very low risk for malignancy. A simple cyst is almost never associated with a malignancy. A complex cyst may be associated with an underlying malignancy and aspiration is usually recommended. If the cyst disappears with aspiration and the contents are not grossly bloody, the fluid does not need to be sent for cytologic analysis. If the lesion does not completely disappear or recurs multiple times after aspiration, then the fluid should be sent for cytology. Excision of a cyst is indicated if the cytologic findings are suspicious for malignancy. In young women, the breast parenchyma is dense, which limits the diagnostic value of mammography. A fluoroscopically guided needle localization biopsy is reserved for nonpalpable solid lesions of the breast.

252. The answer is a. (*Brunicardi, pp 1361-1363.*) Age is a very important prognostic indicator in papillary and follicular thyroid cancer. Age > 45 years is associated with a worse prognosis. Papillary carcinoma occurs more often in women, with a 2:1 female-to-male ratio. However, sex of the patient does not factor into the prognosis. Tumor grade is a measure of differentiation, the extent to which cancer cells are similar in appearance and function to healthy cells of the same tissue type. The degree of differentiation often relates to the clinical behavior of the particular tumor. Based on the microscopic appearance of cancer cells, pathologists commonly describe tumor grade by 4 degrees of severity: Grades 1, 2, 3, and 4. The cells of Grade 1 tumors are often well-differentiated or low-grade tumors, and are generally considered the least aggressive in behavior. Conversely, the cells of Grade 3 or Grade 4 tumors are usually poorly differentiated or undifferentiated high-grade tumors, and are generally the most aggressive in behavior. This patient's tumor is well-differentiated and is associated with a good prognosis. Larger tumors (> 4 cm) and metastasis to lymph nodes in the neck compartments are associated with a worse prognosis. The patient in this question has a small tumor and no evidence of LN involvement on ultrasound.

253. The answer is b. (*Brunicardi, pp 1361-1363.*) Treatment of high-risk papillary carcinomas consists of near-total (or total) thyroidectomy. If patients have lymph node metastases in the lateral neck, concomitant modified radical neck dissection should be performed with total thyroidectomy. Papillary carcinoma of the thyroid frequently metastasizes to cervical lymph nodes, but distant metastasis is uncommon. Overall, survival at 10 years is greater than 95%. Several scoring systems for determining prognosis have been developed; one of the more common systems takes into account age, grade, extrathyroidal invasion and metastases, and size (AGES). The surgical management of low-risk papillary thyroid cancers is controversial (lobectomy versus total thyroidectomy). Medullary, but not papillary, thyroid carcinoma is associated with multiple endocrine neoplasia syndrome.

254. The answer is a. (*Brunicardi, p 466.*) Lobular carcinoma in situ (LCIS) is considered to be a risk factor for invasive breast carcinoma, not an anatomic precursor. The risk for breast cancer is equivalent in both breasts, lasts indefinitely, and is not correlated to the amount of LCIS in the biopsy specimen. Patients are encouraged to perform monthly self-breast examinations and commit to yearly screening mammograms. Chemotherapy, radiation, and surgery are treatments reserved for DCIS and invasive carcinomas of the breast.

255. The answer is d. (*Brunicardi, p 436.*) Fibroadenomas occur infrequently before puberty but are the most common breast tumors between puberty and the early thirties. They usually are well-demarcated and firm. Although most fibroadenomas are no larger than 3 cm in diameter, giant or juvenile fibroadenomas are very large frequently. The bigger fibroadenomas (> 5 cm) occur predominantly in adolescent black girls. The average age at onset of juvenile mammary hypertrophy is 16 years. This disorder involves a diffuse change in the entire breast and does not usually manifest clinically as a discrete mass; it may be unilateral or bilateral and can cause an enormous and incapacitating increase in breast size. Regression may be spontaneous and sometimes coincides with puberty or pregnancy. Cystosarcoma phyllodes may also cause a large lesion. Together with intraductal carcinoma, it characteristically occurs in older women. Lymphomas are less firm than fibroadenomas and do not have a whorl-like pattern. They display a characteristic fish flesh texture.

256. The answer is a. (*Brunicardi, pp 1376-1380.*) The patient described is exhibiting classic signs and symptoms of hyperparathyroidism. In addition, if a history is obtainable, frequently the patient will relate a history of renal calculi and bone pain—the syndrome characterized as "groans, stones, and bones." Acute management of the hypercalcemic state includes vigorous hydration to restore intravascular volume, which is invariably diminished. This will establish renal perfusion and thus promote urinary calcium excretion. Thiazide diuretics are contraindicated because they frequently cause patients to become hypercalcemic. Instead, diuresis should be promoted with the use of loop diuretics such as furosemide (Lasix). The use of intravenous phosphorus infusion is no longer recommended because precipitation in the lungs, heart, or kidney can lead to serious morbidity. Mithramycin is an antineoplastic agent that in low doses inhibits bone resorption and thus diminishes serum calcium levels; it is used only when other maneuvers fail to decrease the calcium level. Calcitonin is useful at times. Bisphosphonates are used for lowering calcium levels in resistant cases, such as those associated with humoral malignancy. Emergency neck exploration is seldom warranted. In unprepared patients, the morbidity is unacceptably high.

257. The answer is c. (*Brunicardi, p 1380.*) Patients with symptomatic primary hyperparathyroidism as manifested by kidney stones, renal dysfunction, or osteoporosis should undergo parathyroidectomy. However, management of "asymptomatic" patients is controversial. Indications for surgical intervention for asymptomatic primary hyperparathyroidism include age less than 50 years, markedly elevated urine calcium excretion, kidney stones on radiography, decreased creatinine clearance, markedly elevated calcium or 1 episode of life-threatening hypercalcemia, and substantially decreased bone mass.

258. The answer is c. *(Brunicardi, pp 1397-1398.)* The constellation of symptoms in this patient is typical of a functional adrenocortical tumor (androgens). Approximately 50% of adrenocortical tumors are functional and can secrete cortisol, androgens, estrogens, aldosterone, or multiple hormones. The single most important determinant of malignancy is the size of the tumor. Treatment consists of en bloc resection of the tumor and involved adjacent organs, such as the kidney or the tail of the pancreas. Symptoms related to hormone production can be minimized by complete resection despite the inability to cure advanced disease. Mitotane has been utilized as adjuvant therapy for unresectable or metastatic disease, but has not been proven to decrease mortality. Cushing disease refers to hypercortisolism due to a pituitary tumor and subsequent bilateral adrenal hyperplasia. Pheochromocytomas are characterized by hypertension and symptoms of excessive catecholamine production. Myelolipomas are benign adrenal lesions.

259. The answer is c. *(Brunicardi, pp 1399-1400.)* Patients with pheochromocytomas should be treated preoperatively with α-blockade using phenoxybenzamine 1 to 3 weeks before surgery. β-Blockade may be necessary in addition to α-blockade for optimal blood pressure control, but should not be started in the absence of α-blockade because of the risk of cardiovascular collapse. With α-blockade, patients also require volume expansion.

260. The answer is e. *(Townsend, pp 2241-2243.)* The most appropriate treatment is immediate surgery. There is no evidence that general anesthesia and nonabdominal surgery increase premature labor and therefore surgery should not be delayed until after delivery of the baby. Sentinel lymph node biopsy is not routinely recommended during pregnancy because the radioactivity may harm the fetus. Radiation therapy is contraindicated in all trimesters of pregnancy. Patients in later stages of pregnancy, however, can start radiation therapy shortly after delivery, and some may be candidates for breast-conserving surgery and adjuvant radiotherapy. Administration of chemotherapy to a pregnant patient should be delayed until after the first trimester due to the increased risk of fetal abnormalities. Chemotherapy does not appear to increase the risk of congenital malformation when given in the second or third trimester of pregnancy. Elective termination of the pregnancy to receive appropriate therapy without the risk to the fetus is no longer routinely recommended because it has not been demonstrated to improve survival.

261. The answer is d. (*Townsend, p 885.*) This patient has Paget disease of the breast until proven otherwise with a thorough workup for breast cancer. She needs a mammogram and biopsy of the affected area. Paget disease of the breast represents a small percentage (1%) of all breast cancers and is thought to originate in the retroareolar lactiferous ducts. It progresses toward the nipple-areola complex in most patients, where it causes the typical clinical finding of nipple eczema and erosion. Up to 50% of patients with Paget disease have an associated breast mass. Nipple-areolar disease alone usually represents in situ cancer; these patients have a 10-year survival rate of over 80%. In contrast, if Paget disease presents with a mass, the mass is likely to be an infiltrating ductal carcinoma. The generally recommended surgical procedure for Paget disease is currently a modified radical mastectomy. Watchful waiting, steroid creams, and antibiotics are not appropriate forms of management in a woman who presents with a rash involving the nipple.

262. The answer is d. (*Townsend, pp 986-987.*) Zollinger-Ellison syndrome (ZES) refers to hypergastrinemia resulting from an endocrine tumor. ZES must be excluded in all patients with intractable peptic ulcers. The diagnosis depends on elevated levels of gastrin along with increased secretion of gastric acid. Patients with Zollinger-Ellison tumors have very high basal levels of gastric acid (> 35 mEq/h) and serum gastrin (usually > 1000 pg/mL). In equivocal cases, when the gastrin level is not markedly elevated, a secretin stimulation test is usually obtained. In this test, a fasting gastrin level is obtained before and after the administration of secretin (at 2, 5, 10, and 20 minutes). A paradoxical rise in serum gastrin after intravenous secretin is diagnostic of Zollinger-Ellison syndrome. Hypercalcemia is not a finding associated with ZES. However, the presence of hypercalcemia in a patient with ZES should prompt a workup for MEN1 (multiple endocrine neoplasia type 1). In MEN1 patients, the organ most involved is the parathyroid. The next most common syndrome is ZES, followed by insulinoma.

263. The answer is a. (*Brunicardi, p 1355.*) Drops of Lugol iodide solution daily beginning 10 days preoperatively should be prescribed to decrease the likelihood of postoperative thyroid storm, a manifestation of severe thyrotoxicosis. Propylthiouracil or methimazole can also be used preoperatively but are contraindicated in pregnant women. If thyroid storm occurs, treatment is β-blockade, for example, propranolol.

264. The answer is e. *(Brunicardi, pp 1377-1378.)* Osteitis fibrosa cystica is a condition associated with hyperparathyroidism that is characterized by severe demineralization with subperiosteal bone resorption (most prominent in the middle phalanx of the second and third fingers), bone cysts, and tufting of the distal phalanges on hand films. These specific bone findings would not be present in sarcoidosis, Paget disease, or metastatic carcinoma. Vitamin D deficiency can lead to osteitis fibrosa cystica, but it would also be associated with hypocalcemia, not hypercalcemia.

265. The answer is d. *(Brunicardi, pp 1381-1383.)* Treatment for primary hyperparathyroidism in this setting is resection of the diseased parathyroid glands after initial correction of the severe hypercalcemia. Parathyroidectomy without preoperative localization studies have a high success rate and low complication rate. Neck exploration will yield a single parathyroid adenoma in about 85% of cases. Two adenomas are found less often (approximately 5% of cases) and hyperplasia of all 4 glands occurs in about 10% to 15% of patients. If hyperplasia is found, treatment includes resection of 3½ glands. The remnant of the fourth gland can be identified with a metal clip in case reexploration becomes necessary. Alternatively, all 4 glands can be removed with autotransplantation of a small piece of parathyroid tissue into the forearm or sternocleidomastoid muscle. Subsequent hyperfunction, should it develop, can then be treated by removal of this tissue. Patients often need calcium supplementation postoperatively. Vitamin D supplementation may also be necessary if hypocalcemia develops and persists despite treatment with oral calcium. Steroids and radiation therapy have no role in the treatment of primary hyperparathyroidism.

266. The answer is d. *(Brunicardi, p 1355.)* Thyroid storm can be associated with high mortality rates if it is not appropriately managed in an intensive care unit setting. Treatment includes rapid fluid replacement, antithyroid medication such as propylthiouracil (PTU), β-blockers, iodine solutions, and steroids. β-Blockers are given to reduce peripheral conversion of T_4 to T_3 and decrease the hyperthyroid symptoms. Lugol iodine helps to decrease iodine uptake and thyroid hormone secretion. PTU therapy blocks formation of new thyroid hormone and reduces peripheral conversion of T_4 to T_3. Corticosteroids block hepatic thyroid hormone conversion. The thyroid storm needs to be treated before undergoing any surgery. Radiation therapy and hemodialysis have no role in the treatment of thyroid storm.

267. The answer is a. (*Brunicardi, p 1392.*) The biochemical diagnosis of hyperaldosteronism requires demonstration of elevated plasma aldosterone concentration (PAC) with suppressed plasma renin activity (PAR). A PAC: PAR ratio of 25 to 30:1 is strongly suggestive of the diagnosis. Hyperaldosteronism must be suspected in any hypertensive patient who presents with hypokalemia. Hypokalemia occurs spontaneously in up to 90% of patients with this disorder. Other individuals who should be evaluated for hyperaldosteronism include those with severe hypertension, hypertension refractory to medication, and young age at onset of hypertension. Plasma cortisol level and overnight low-dose dexamethasone suppression test are laboratory studies used in diagnosing Cushing syndrome. Neither urine electrolytes nor 24-hour urinary aldosterone level is beneficial in diagnosing hyperaldosteronism.

268. The answer is a. (*Brunicardi, p 468.*) Excision with adequate margins of normal breast tissue is curative. Cystosarcoma phyllodes is a tumor most often seen in younger women. It can grow to enormous size and at times ulcerate through the skin. Still, it is a lesion with low propensity toward metastasis. Local recurrence is common, especially if the initial resection was inadequate. Very large lesions may necessitate simple mastectomy to achieve clear margins. Axillary lymphadenectomy, however, is seldom indicated without biopsy-positive demonstration of tumor in the nodes. The low incidence of metastatic disease suggests that adjunctive therapy is indicated only for known metastatic disease, even when the tumors are quite large and ulcerated.

269. The answer is e. (*Brunicardi, pp 1361-1363.*) Radioactive ^{131}I is contraindicated in pregnancy and should be used with caution in women of childbearing age. This patient has cytologic evidence of a papillary lesion, possibly papillary carcinoma. Papillary carcinoma is a relatively nonaggressive lesion with 10-year survival of 95%. The lesion is frequently multicentric, which argues for more complete resection. Metastases, when they occur, are usually responsive to surgical resection or radioablation therapy. Removal of the involved lobe, and possibly the entire thyroid gland, is appropriate. Central and lateral lymph node dissection is performed for clinically suspect lymph nodes. Papillary carcinoma is frequently multifocal. Bilateral disease mandates total thyroidectomy.

270. The answer is d. *(Brunicardi, p 1367.)* The treatment of Hürthle cell carcinoma follows the same principles as follicular carcinoma. Primary treatment is surgical followed by radioiodine ablation. Hürthle cell cancer is a type of follicular cancer, but differs from follicular neoplasms in that it is more often multifocal and bilateral, and is more likely to spread to local nodes and distant sites. External beam radiotherapy is reserved for patients who need control of unresectable, locally invasive or recurrent disease. There is no role for routine chemotherapy in the treatment of Hürthle cell carcinoma. Chemotherapy has been used with little success in disseminated thyroid cancer.

271. The answer is e. *(Brunicardi, pp 1364-1367.)* For lesions less than 4 cm in size, thyroid lobectomy is adequate because at least 80% of follicular lesions are adenomas. For confirmed carcinomas or lesions greater than 4 cm in size, total thyroidectomy should be performed. Follicular carcinomas cannot be diagnosed by FNA; capsular or vascular invasion on histology confirms a diagnosis of malignancy. There is no role for prophylactic neck dissection for follicular carcinomas. Suppression with thyroid hormone (Synthroid) in the setting of abnormal cytology is not recommended. There is no role for external beam radiotherapy or chemotherapy in this patient.

272. The answer is a. *(Brunicardi, p 467.)* Nipple discharge from the breast may be classified as pathologic, physiologic, or galactorrhea. Galactorrhea may be caused by hormonal imbalance (hyperprolactinemia, hypothyroidism), drugs (oral contraceptives, phenothiazines, antihypertensives, tranquilizers), or trauma to the chest. Physiologic nipple discharge is intermittent, nonlactational (usually serous), and caused by stimulation of the nipple or to drugs (estrogens, tranquilizers). Both galactorrhea and physiologic discharge are frequently bilateral and arise from multiple ducts. Pathologic nipple discharge may be caused by benign lesions of the breast (duct ectasia, papilloma, fibrocystic disease) or by cancer. It may be bloody, serous, or gray-green. It is spontaneous and unilateral and can often be localized to a single nipple duct. When pathologic discharge is diagnosed, an effort should be made to identify the source. If an associated mass is present, it should be biopsied. If no mass is found, a terminal duct excision of the involved duct(s) should be performed.

273. The answer is e. (*Brunicardi, pp 1394-1395.*) The most common cause of Cushing syndrome is iatrogenic, via administration of synthetic corticosteroids. Cushing syndrome refers to the clinical manifestations of glucocorticoid excess due to any cause (Cushing disease, administration of exogenous glucocorticoids, adrenocortical hyperplasia, adrenal adenoma, adrenal carcinoma, ectopic ACTH-secreting tumors) and includes truncal obesity, hypertension, hirsutism, moon facies, proximal muscle wasting, ecchymoses, skin striae, osteoporosis, diabetes mellitus, amenorrhea, growth retardation, and immunosuppression. Cushing disease is caused by hypersecretion of ACTH by the pituitary gland. This hypersecretion, in turn, is caused by either a pituitary adenoma (90% of cases) or diffuse pituitary corticotrope hyperplasia (10% of cases) because of hypersecretion of corticotropin-releasing hormone (CRH) by the hypothalamus.

274. The answer is c. (*Brunicardi, pp 1217-1218.*) Laboratory studies in patients with insulinoma will uncover a low blood sugar (serum glucose < 50mg/dL), elevated serum insulin levels, and elevated levels of C-peptide. C-peptide levels are checked to rule out unauthorized administration of insulin and will only be elevated in cases of excess endogenous insulin production.

275. The answer is a. (*Brunicardi, pp 436-440.*) Studies have failed to demonstrate a correlation between diet and breast cancer risk. Age is the most common risk factor. Another important risk factor is family history in a first-degree relative or presence of a genetic mutation such as BRCA1 or 2, which can be inherited through either the maternal or the paternal side of the family. Other risk factors include excessive estrogen exposure, obesity, alcohol use, hormone replacement, ionizing radiation, and a history of a prior breast cancer or abnormal breast biopsy (LCIS or atypical hyperplasia).

276 to 280. The answers are 276-d, 277-c, 278-a, 279-d, 280-e. (*Brunicardi, pp 450-453.*) The TNM stage of breast cancer is assigned by measuring the greatest diameter of the tumor (T), assessing the axillary and clavicular lymph nodes for enlargement and fixation (N), and judging whether metastatic disease is present (M). T0 is indicated when there is no evidence of a primary tumor; Tis—carcinoma in situ; T1—tumors 2 cm or less; T2—tumors greater than 2 cm but not more than 5 cm; T3—tumors greater than 5 cm; and T4—tumors with extension into the chest wall or skin or inflammatory carcinomas. N0 is indicated when there is no evidence of regional lymph node metastasis; N1—positive, movable ipsilateral axillary nodes; N2—fixed ipsilateral axillary nodes or clinically apparent ipsilateral internal mammary nodes; N3—positive axillary nodes and ipsilateral internal mammary nodes or ipsilateral supra/infraclavicular nodes. Absence of evidence of metastatic disease is classified as M0 and distant metastatic disease as M1. The patient in question 277 has a T0N2M0 lesion. This is stage III (fixed or matted nodes are a poor prognostic sign). The patient in question 278 has a T2N1M0 lesion. This is stage II. The patient in question 279 has a TisN0M0 lesion. Carcinoma in situ lesions are by definition not invasive and therefore are classified as stage 0. The patient in question 280 has findings compatible with inflammatory breast cancer. A biopsy of the involved skin would confirm the diagnosis. Inflammatory breast cancer is a T4 lesion and would make this patient a stage III. The patient in question 281 has a T1N0M1 lesion. This is stage IV (stage IV is any T, any N, M1).

281 to 285. The answers are 281-d, 282-a, 283-b, 284-e, 285-c. (*Brunicardi, p 1088.*) Carcinoid tumors are most commonly found in the appendix and small bowel, where they may be multiple. They have a tendency to metastasize, which varies with the size of the tumor. Tumors less than 1 cm uncommonly metastasize and are adequately treated with an appendectomy. If the tumor is located at the base of the appendix, a right hemicolectomy is performed. Tumors greater than 2 cm are more often found to be metastatic. Metastasis to the liver and beyond may give rise to the carcinoid syndrome. The tumors cause an intense desmoplastic reaction. When metastatic lesions are found in the liver, they should be resected when technically feasible to limit the symptoms of the carcinoid syndrome. When extensive hepatic metastases are found, the disease is not curable. Resection of the appendix and cecum may be performed to prevent an early intestinal obstruction by locally encroaching tumor instead of a right hemicolectomy in patients with liver metastasis. Spread of the carcinoid tumor into the serosal lymphatics does not imply metastatic disease and local resection is potentially curative.

286 to 290. The answers are 286-b, 287-e, 288-a, 289-d, 290-g. (*Townsend, pp 871-896.*) Generally accepted treatment for stage I breast cancer in premenopausal women includes lumpectomy (wide excision, partial mastectomy, quadrantectomy), combined with axillary lymph node dissection (or sentinel lymph node biopsy) and adjuvant radiation therapy, or modified radical mastectomy. Both approaches offer equivalent chances of cure; there is a higher incidence of local recurrence with lumpectomy, axillary dissection, and radiation, but this observation has not been found to affect the overall cure rate in comparison with mastectomy. Patients with familial breast cancer (multiple first-degree relatives and penetrance of breast cancer through several familial generations) have extremely high risks of developing breast cancer in the course of their lifetimes. A subset of patients with familial breast cancer has been identified by a specific gene mutation (*BRCA1*); however, the genetic basis of most cases of familial breast cancer has yet to be elucidated. A patient with a history of familial breast cancer and multiple biopsies showing atypia may reasonably request bilateral prophylactic simple mastectomies. Alternatively, she may continue with routine surveillance. Lobular carcinoma in situ is a histologic marker that identifies patients at increased risk for the development of breast cancer. It is not a precancerous lesion in itself, and there is no benefit to widely excising it because the risk of subsequent cancer is equal for both breasts. As the risk for the future development of breast cancer is now estimated to be approximately 1% per year, prophylactic mastectomy is no longer recommended. Proper management consists of close surveillance for cancer by twice-yearly examinations and yearly mammography. Sclerosing adenosis is a benign lesion. DCIS is the precursor of invasive ductal carcinoma. It is described in 4 histologic variants (papillary, cribriform, solid, and comedo), of which the comedo subtype shows the greatest tendency to recur after wide excision alone. DCIS is treated with wide excision alone (for small noncomedo lesions) or wide excision plus radiation therapy. For multicentric DCIS, simple mastectomy is recommended. Cystosarcoma phyllodes is treated with wide local excision with at least 1-cm margins; axillary lymphadenectomy is not routinely recommended in the absence of clinically suspicious nodes. There are few indications for radical mastectomy, as it is both more traumatic and more disfiguring than any other method of local control of breast cancer and offers no greater survival benefit. However, one indication for radical mastectomy is locally advanced breast cancer with wide invasion of the pectoralis major in a patient who is physiologically able to tolerate general anesthesia.

Gastrointestinal Tract, Liver, and Pancreas

Questions

291. A 74-year-old woman is admitted with upper gastrointestinal (GI) bleeding. She is started on H_2 blockers, but experiences another bleeding episode. Endoscopy documents diffuse gastric ulcerations. Omeprazole is added to the H_2 antagonists as a therapeutic approach to the management of acute gastric and duodenal ulcers. Which of the following is the mechanism of action of omeprazole?

a. Blockage of the breakdown of mucosa-damaging metabolites of nonsteroidal anti-inflammatory drugs (NSAIDs)
b. Provision of a direct cytoprotective effect
c. Buffering of gastric acids
d. Inhibition of parietal cell hydrogen potassium ATPase (adenosine triphosphatase)
e. Inhibition of gastrin release and parietal cell acid production

292. A 35-year-old woman presents with frequent and multiple areas of cutaneous ecchymosis. Workup demonstrates a platelet count of 15,000/µL, evaluation of the bone marrow reveals a normal number of megakaryocytes, and ultrasound examination demonstrates a normal-sized spleen. Based on the exclusion of other causes of thrombocytopenia, she is given a diagnosis of immune (idiopathic) thrombocytopenic purpura (ITP). Which of the following is the most appropriate treatment upon diagnosis?

a. Expectant management with close follow-up of platelet counts
b. Immediate platelet transfusion to increase platelet counts to greater than 50,000/µL
c. Glucocorticoid therapy
d. Intravenous immunoglobulin (IVIG) therapy
e. Referral to surgery for laparoscopic splenectomy

293. A 59-year-old woman presents with right lower quadrant pain, nausea, and vomiting. She undergoes an uncomplicated laparoscopic appendectomy. Postoperatively, the pathology reveals a 2.5-cm mucinous adenocarcinoma with lymphatic invasion. Staging workup, including colonoscopy, chest x-ray, and computed tomography (CT) scan of the abdomen and pelvis, is negative. Which of the following is the most appropriate next step in her management?

a. No further intervention at this time; follow-up every 6 months for 2 years
b. Chemotherapy alone
c. Neoadjuvant chemotherapy followed by right hemicolectomy
d. Ileocecectomy
e. Right hemicolectomy

294. A 41-year-old man complains of regurgitation of saliva and of undigested food. An esophagram reveals a dilated esophagus and a bird's-beak deformity. Manometry shows a hypertensive lower esophageal sphincter with failure to relax with deglutition. Which of the following is the safest and most effective treatment of this condition?

a. Medical treatment with sublingual nitroglycerin, nitrates, or calcium-channel blockers
b. Repeated bougie dilations
c. Injections of botulinum toxin directly into the lower esophageal sphincter
d. Dilation with a Gruntzig-type (volume-limited, pressure-control) balloon
e. Surgical esophagomyotomy

295. A 32-year-old man with a 3-year history of ulcerative colitis (UC) presents for discussion for surgical intervention. The patient is otherwise healthy and does not have evidence of rectal dysplasia. Which of the following is the most appropriate elective operation for this patient?

a. Total proctocolectomy with end ileostomy
b. Total proctocolectomy with ileal pouch-anal anastomosis and diverting ileostomy
c. Total proctocolectomy with ileal pouch-anal anastomosis, anal mucosectomy, and diverting ileostomy
d. Total abdominal colectomy with ileal-rectal anastomosis
e. Total abdominal colectomy with end ileostomy and very low Hartmann

296. A 39-year-old previously healthy male is hospitalized for 2 weeks with epigastric pain radiating to his back, nausea, and vomiting. Initial laboratory values revealed an elevated amylase level consistent with acute pancreatitis. Five weeks following discharge, he complains of early satiety, epigastric pain, and fevers. On presentation, his temperature is 38.9°C (102°F) and his heart rate is 120 beats per minute; his white blood cell (WBC) count is 24,000/mm³ and his amylase level is normal. He undergoes a CT scan demonstrating a 6 cm by 6 cm rim-enhancing fluid collection in the body of the pancreas. Which of the following would be the most definitive management of the fluid collection?

a. Antibiotic therapy alone
b. CT-guided aspiration with repeat imaging in 2 to 3 days
c. Antibiotics and CT-guided aspiration with repeat imaging in 2 to 3 days
d. Antibiotics and percutaneous catheter drainage
e. Surgical internal drainage of the fluid collection with a cyst-gastrostomy or Roux-en-Y cyst-jejunostomy

297. A previously healthy 79-year-old woman presents with early satiety and abdominal fullness. CT scan of the abdomen, pictured here, reveals a cystic lesion in the body and tail of the pancreas. CT-guided aspiration demonstrates an elevated carcinoembryonic antigen (CEA) level. Which of the following is the most appropriate treatment option for this patient?

a. Distal pancreatectomy
b. Serial CT scans with resection if the lesion increases significantly in size
c. Internal drainage with Roux-en-Y cyst-jejunostomy
d. Percutaneous drainage of the fluid-filled lesion
e. Endoscopic retrograde cholangiopancreatography (ERCP) with pancreatic stent placement

298. A 56-year-old woman is referred to you about 3 months after a colostomy subsequent to a sigmoid resection for cancer. She complains that her stoma is not functioning properly. Which of the following is the most common serious complication of an end colostomy?

a. Bleeding
b. Skin breakdown
c. Parastomal hernia
d. Colonic perforation during irrigation
e. Stomal prolapse

299. A 56-year-old previously healthy physician notices that his eyes are yellow and he has been losing weight. On physical examination the patient has jaundice and scleral icterus with a benign abdomen. Transcutaneous ultrasound of the abdomen demonstrates biliary ductal dilation without gallstones. Which of the following is the most appropriate next step in the workup of this patient?

a. Esophagogastroduodenoscopy (EGD)
b. Endoscopic retrograde cholangiopancreatography (ERCP)
c. Acute abdominal series
d. Computed tomography (CT) scan
e. Positron emission tomography (PET) scan

300. A 45-year-old woman with history of heavy nonsteroidal anti-inflammatory drug ingestion presents with acute abdominal pain. She undergoes exploratory laparotomy 30 hours after onset of symptoms and is found to have a perforated duodenal ulcer. Which of the following is the procedure of choice to treat her perforation?

a. Simple closure with omental patch
b. Truncal vagotomy and pyloroplasty
c. Truncal vagotomy and antrectomy
d. Highly selective vagotomy with omental patch
e. Hemigastrectomy

301. A 45-year-old man with a history of chronic peptic ulcer disease undergoes a truncal vagotomy and antrectomy with a Billroth II reconstruction for gastric outlet obstruction. Six weeks after surgery, he returns, complaining of postprandial weakness, sweating, light-headedness, crampy abdominal pain, and diarrhea. Which of the following would be the best initial management strategy?

a. Treatment with a long-acting somatostatin analog
b. Dietary advice and counseling that symptoms will probably abate within 3 months of surgery
c. Dietary advice and counseling that symptoms will probably not abate but are not dangerous
d. Workup for neuroendocrine tumor (eg, carcinoid)
e. Preparation for revision to Roux-en-Y gastrojejunostomy

302. A 60-year-old male patient with hepatitis C with a previous history of variceal bleeding is admitted to the hospital with hematemesis. His blood pressure is 80/60 mm Hg, physical examination reveals splenomegaly and ascites, and initial hematocrit is 25%. Prior to endoscopy, which of the following is the best initial management of the patient?

a. Administration of intravenous octreotide
b. Administration of a β-blocker (eg, propranolol)
c. Measurement of prothrombin time and transfusion with cryoglobulin if elevated
d. Empiric transfusion of platelets given splenomegaly
e. Gastric and esophageal balloon tamponade (Sengstaken-Blakemore tube)

303. A 32-year-old alcoholic with end-stage liver disease has been admitted to the hospital 3 times for bleeding esophageal varices. He has undergone banding and sclerotherapy previously. He admits to currently drinking a 6 packs of beer per day. On his abdominal examination, he has a fluid wave. Which of the following is the best option for long-term management of this patient's esophageal varices?

a. Orthotopic liver transplantation
b. Transection and reanastomosis of the distal esophagus
c. Distal splenorenal shunt
d. End-to-side portocaval shunt
e. Transjugular intrahepatic portosystemic shunt (TIPS)

304. A 55-year-old man complains of chronic intermittent epigastric pain. A gastroscopy demonstrates a 2-cm prepyloric ulcer. Biopsy of the ulcer yields no malignant tissue. After a 6-week trial of medical therapy, the ulcer is unchanged. Which of the following is the best next step in his management?

a. Repeat trial of medical therapy
b. Local excision of the ulcer
c. Highly selective vagotomy
d. Partial gastrectomy with vagotomy and Billroth I reconstruction
e. Vagotomy and pyloroplasty

305. A 45-year-old man was discovered to have a hepatic flexure colon cancer during a colonoscopy for anemia requiring transfusions. Upon exploration of his abdomen in the operating room, an unexpected discontinuous 3-cm metastasis is discovered in the edge of the right lobe of the liver. Preoperatively, the patient was counseled of this possibility and the surgical options. Which of the following is the most appropriate management of this patient?

a. A diverting ileostomy should be performed and further imaging obtained
b. Right hemicolectomy
c. Right hemicolectomy with local resection of the liver metastasis
d. Closure of the abdomen followed by chemotherapy
e. Right hemicolectomy with postoperative radiation therapy to the liver

306. A 42-year-old man with no history of use of NSAIDs presents with recurrent gastritis. The patient was diagnosed and treated for *Helicobacter pylori* 6 months ago. Which of the following tests provides the least invasive method to document eradication of the infection?

a. Serology testing for *H pylori*
b. Carbon-labeled urea breath test
c. Rapid urease assay
d. Histologic evaluation of gastric mucosa
e. Culturing of gastric mucosa

307. A 22-year-old college student notices a bulge in his right groin. It is accentuated with coughing, but is easily reducible. Which of the following hernias follows the path of the spermatic cord within the cremaster muscle?

a. Femoral
b. Direct inguinal
c. Indirect inguinal
d. Spigelian
e. Interparietal

308. An 80-year-old man with history of symptomatic cholelithiasis presents with signs and symptoms of a small-bowel obstruction. Which of the following findings would provide the most help in ascertaining the diagnosis?

a. Coffee-grounds aspirate from the stomach
b. Pneumobilia
c. A leukocyte count of 40,000/mL
d. A pH of 7.5, P_{CO_2} of 50 kPa, and paradoxically acid urine
e. A palpable mass in the pelvis

309. A 42-year-old man has bouts of intermittent crampy abdominal pain and rectal bleeding. Colonoscopy is performed and demonstrates multiple hamartomatous polyps. The patient is successfully treated by removing as many polyps as possible with the aid of intraoperative endoscopy and polypectomy. Which of the following is the most likely diagnosis?

a. Ulcerative colitis
b. Villous adenomas
c. Familial polyposis
d. Peutz-Jeghers syndrome
e. Crohn colitis

310. A 70-year-old woman has nausea, vomiting, abdominal distention, and episodic crampy midabdominal pain. She has no history of previous surgery but has a long history of cholelithiasis for which she has refused surgery. Her abdominal radiograph reveals a spherical density in the right lower quadrant. Which of the following is the definitive treatment for this patient's bowel obstruction?

a. Ileocolectomy
b. Cholecystectomy
c. Ileotomy and extraction
d. Nasogastric (NG) tube decompression
e. Intravenous antibiotics

311. A 53-year-old man presents to the emergency room with left lower quadrant pain, fever, and vomiting. CT scan of the abdomen and pelvis reveals a thickened sigmoid colon with inflamed diverticula and a 7-cm by 8-cm rim-enhancing fluid collection in the pelvis. After percutaneous drainage and treatment with antibiotics, the pain and fluid collection resolve. He returns as an outpatient to clinic 1 month later. He undergoes a colonoscopy, which demonstrates only diverticula in the sigmoid colon. Which of the following is the most appropriate next step in this patient's management?

a. Expectant management with sigmoid resection if symptoms recur
b. Cystoscopy to evaluate for a fistula
c. Sigmoid resection with end colostomy and rectal pouch (Hartmann procedure)
d. Sigmoid resection with primary anastomosis
e. Long-term suppressive antibiotic therapy

312. A 29-year-old woman complains of postprandial right upper quadrant pain and fatty food intolerance. Ultrasound examination reveals no evidence of gallstones or sludge. Upper endoscopy is normal, and all of her liver function tests are within normal limits. Which of the following represents the best management option?

a. Avoidance of fatty foods and reexamination in 6 months.
b. Ultrasound examination should be repeated immediately, since the false-negative rate for ultrasound in detecting gallstones is 10% to 15%.
c. Treatment with ursodeoxycholic acid.
d. CCK-HIDA scan should be performed to evaluate for biliary dyskinesia.
e. Laparoscopic cholecystectomy for acalculous cholecystitis.

313. A 47-year-old asymptomatic woman is incidentally found to have a 5-mm polyp and no stones in her gallbladder on ultrasound examination. Which of the following is the best management option?

a. Aspiration of the gallbladder with cytologic examination of the bile
b. Observation with repeat ultrasound examinations to evaluate for increase in polyp size
c. Laparoscopic cholecystectomy
d. Open cholecystectomy with frozen section
e. En bloc resection of the gallbladder, wedge resection of the liver, and portal lymphadenectomy

314. A 48-year-old woman develops pain in the right lower quadrant while playing tennis. The pain progresses and the patient presents to the emergency room later that day with a low-grade fever, a WBC count of 13,000/mm^3 and complaints of anorexia and nausea as well as persistent, sharp pain of the right lower quadrant. On examination, she is tender in the right lower quadrant with muscular spasm, and there is a suggestion of a mass effect. An ultrasound is ordered and shows an apparent mass in the abdominal wall. Which of the following is the most likely diagnosis?

a. Acute appendicitis
b. Cecal carcinoma
c. Hematoma of the rectus sheath
d. Torsion of an ovarian cyst
e. Cholecystitis

315. A 32-year-old alcoholic man, recently emigrated from Mexico, presents with right upper quadrant pain and fevers for 2 weeks. CT scan of the abdomen demonstrates a non–rim-enhancing fluid collection in the periphery of the right lobe of the liver. The patient's serology is positive for antibodies to *Entamoeba histolytica*. Which of the following is the best initial management option for this patient?

a. Treatment with antiamebic drugs
b. Percutaneous drainage of the fluid collection
c. Marsupialization of the fluid collection
d. Surgical drainage of the fluid collection
e. Liver resection

316. A 45-year-old executive experiences increasingly painful retrosternal heartburn, especially at night. He has been chewing antacid tablets. An esophagogram shows a hiatal hernia. In determining the proper treatment for a sliding hiatal hernia, which of the following is the most useful modality?

a. Barium swallow with cinefluoroscopy during Valsalva maneuver
b. Flexible endoscopy
c. Twenty-four-hour monitoring of esophageal pH
d. Measurement of the size of the hernia on upper GI
e. Assessment of the patient's smoking and drinking history

317. A 22-year-old woman is seen in a surgery clinic for a bulge in the right groin. She denies pain and is able to make the bulge disappear by lying down and putting steady pressure on the bulge. She has never experienced nausea or vomiting. On examination she has a reducible hernia below the inguinal ligament. Which of the following is the most appropriate management of this patient?

a. Observation for now and follow-up in surgery clinic in 6 months
b. Observation for now and follow-up in surgery clinic if she develops further symptoms
c. Elective surgical repair of hernia
d. Emergent surgical repair of hernia
e. Emergent surgical repair of hernia with exploratory laparotomy to evaluate the small bowel

318. A 22-year-old woman presents with a painful fluctuant mass in the midline between the gluteal folds. She denies pain on rectal examination. Which of the following is the most likely diagnosis?

a. Pilonidal abscess
b. Perianal abscess
c. Perirectal abscess
d. Fistula-in-ano
e. Anal fissure

319. A 72-year-old man status post–coronary artery bypass graft (CABG) 5 years ago presents with hematochezia, abdominal pain, and fevers. Colonoscopy reveals patches of dusky-appearing mucosa at the splenic flexure without active bleeding. Which of the following is the most appropriate management of this patient?

a. Angiography with administration of intra-arterial papaverine
b. Emergent laparotomy with left hemicolectomy and transverse colostomy
c. Aortomesenteric bypass
d. Exploratory laparotomy with thrombectomy of the inferior mesenteric artery
e. Expectant management

320. A 62-year-old man has been diagnosed by endoscopic biopsy as having a sigmoid colon cancer. He is otherwise healthy and presents to your office for preoperative consultation. He asks a number of questions regarding removal of a portion of his colon. Which of the following is most likely to occur after a colon resection?

a. The majority (> 50%) of normally formed feces will comprise solid material.
b. Patients who undergo major colon resections suffer little long-term change in their bowel habits following operation.
c. Sodium, potassium, chloride, and bicarbonate will be absorbed by the colonic epithelium by an active transport process.
d. The remaining colon will absorb less water.
e. The remaining colon will absorb long-chain fatty acids that result from bacterial breakdown of lipids.

321. A 39-year-old woman with no significant past medical history and whose only medication is oral contraceptive pills (OCP) presents to the emergency room with right upper quadrant pain. CT scan demonstrates a 6-cm hepatic adenoma in the right lobe of the liver. Which of the following describes the definitive treatment of this lesion?

a. Cessation of oral contraceptives and serial CT scans
b. Intra-arterial embolization of the hepatic adenoma
c. Embolization of the right portal vein
d. Resection of the hepatic adenoma
e. Systemic chemotherapy

322. A 43-year-old man without symptoms is incidentally noted on CT scan to have a 4-cm lesion in the periphery of the left lobe of the liver. The lesion enhances on the arterial phase of the CT scan and has a central scar suggestive of focal nodular hyperplasia (FNH). Which of the following is the recommended treatment of this lesion?

a. No further treatment is necessary
b. Wedge resection of the lesion
c. Formal left hepatectomy
d. Intra-arterial embolization of the lesion
e. Radiofrequency ablation of the liver lesion

323. A 57-year-old previously alcoholic man with a history of chronic pancreatitis presents with hematemesis. Endoscopy reveals isolated gastric varices in the absence of esophageal varices. His liver function tests are normal and he has no stigmata of end-stage liver disease. Ultrasound examination demonstrates normal portal flow but a thrombosed splenic vein. He undergoes banding, which is initially successful, but he subsequently rebleeds during the same hospitalization. Attempts to control the bleeding endoscopically are unsuccessful. Which of the following is the most appropriate next step in management?

a. Transjugular intrahepatic portosystemic shunt
b. Surgical portocaval shunt
c. Surgical mesocaval shunt
d. Splenectomy
e. Placement of a Sengstaken-Blakemore tube

324. A previously healthy 15-year-old boy is brought to the emergency room with complaints of about 12 hours of progressive anorexia, nausea, and pain of the right lower quadrant. On physical examination, he is found to have a rectal temperature of 38.18°C (100.72°F) and direct and rebound abdominal tenderness localizing to McBurney point as well as involuntary guarding in the right lower quadrant. At operation through a McBurney-type incision, the appendix and cecum are found to be normal, but the surgeon is impressed by the marked edema of the terminal ileum, which also has an overlying fibrinopurulent exudate. Which of the following is the most appropriate next step?

a. Close the abdomen after culturing the exudate.
b. Perform a standard appendectomy.
c. Resect the involved terminal ileum.
d. Perform an ileocolic resection.
e. Perform an ileocolostomy to bypass the involved terminal ileum.

325. A 32-year-old woman undergoes a cholecystectomy for acute cholecystitis and is discharged home on the sixth postoperative day. She returns
to the clinic 8 months after the operation for a routine visit and is noted by
the surgeon to be jaundiced. Laboratory values on readmission show total
bilirubin 5.6 mg/dL, direct bilirubin 4.8 mg/dL, alkaline phosphatase 250
IU (normal 21-91 IU), serum glutamic oxaloacetic transaminase (SGOT) 52
kU (normal 10-40 kU), and serum glutamic pyruvic transaminase (SGPT)
51 kU (normal 10-40 kU). An ultrasonogram shows dilated intrahepatic
ducts. The patient undergoes the transhepatic cholangiogram seen here.
Which of the following is the most appropriate next management step?

a. Choledochoplasty with insertion of a T tube
b. End-to-end choledochocholedochal anastomosis
c. Roux-en-Y hepaticojejunostomy
d. Percutaneous transhepatic dilatation
e. Choledochoduodenostomy

326. After complete removal of a sessile polyp of 2.0 cm by 1.5 cm found 1 finger length above the anal mucocutaneous margin, the pathologist reports it to have been a villous adenoma that contained carcinoma in situ. Which of the following is the most appropriate next step in management?

a. Reexcision of the biopsy site with wider margins
b. Abdominoperineal rectosigmoid resection
c. Anterior resection of the rectum
d. External radiation therapy to the rectum
e. No further therapy

327. A 62-year-old man has been noticing progressive difficulty swallowing, first solid food and now liquids as well. A barium study shows a ragged narrowing just below the carinal level. Endoscopic biopsy confirms squamous cell carcinoma. Which of the following provides the most accurate information regarding the T stage of an esophageal carcinoma?

a. Computed tomography
b. Positron emission tomography
c. Magnetic resonance imaging
d. Endoscopic ultrasound
e. Bronchoscopy

328. A 53-year-old woman with a history of a vagotomy and antrectomy with Billroth II reconstruction for peptic ulcer disease presents with recurrent abdominal pain. An esophagogastroduodenoscopy (EGD) demonstrates that ulcer and serum gastrin levels are greater than 1000 pg/mL on three separate determinations (normal is 40-150). Which of the following is the best test for confirming a diagnosis of gastrinoma?

a. A 24-hour urine gastrin level
b. A secretin stimulation test
c. A serum glucagon level
d. A 24-hour urine secretin level
e. A serum glucose to insulin ratio

329. A 52-year-old man with a family history of multiple endocrine neoplasia type 1 (MEN1) has an elevated gastrin level and is suspected to have a gastrinoma. Which of the following is the most likely location for his tumor?

a. Fundus of the stomach
b. Antrum of the stomach
c. Within the triangle formed by the junction of the second and third portions of the duodenum, the junction of the neck and body of the pancreas, and the junction of the cystic and common bile duct
d. Tail of the pancreas
e. Within the triangle formed by the inferior edge of the liver, the cystic duct, and the common hepatic duct

330. A 73-year-old woman presents to the emergency room complaining of severe epigastric pain radiating to her back, nausea, and vomiting. CT scan of the abdomen demonstrates inflammation and edema of the pancreas. A right upper quadrant ultrasound demonstrates the presence of gallstones in the gallbladder. Which of the following is an important prognostic sign in acute pancreatitis according to Ranson's criteria?

a. Amylase level
b. Age
c. Total bilirubin level
d. Albumin level
e. Lipase level

331. A 55-year-old man who is extremely obese reports weakness, sweating, tachycardia, confusion, and headache whenever he fasts for more than a few hours. He has prompt relief of symptoms when he eats. Labarotory examination reveals an inappropriately high level of serum insulin during the episodes of fasting. Which of the following is the most appropriate treatment for this condition?

a. Diet modification to include frequent meals
b. Long-acting somatostatin analogue octreotide
c. Simple excision of the tumor
d. Total pancreatectomy
e. Chemotherapy and radiation

332. A 57-year-old woman sees blood on the toilet paper. Her doctor notes the presence of an excoriated bleeding 2.8-cm mass at the anus. Biopsy confirms the clinical suspicion of anal cancer. In planning the management of a 2.8-cm epidermoid carcinoma of the anus, which of the following is the best initial management strategy?

a. Abdominoperineal resection
b. Wide local resection with bilateral inguinal node dissection
c. Local radiation therapy
d. Systemic chemotherapy
e. Combined radiation therapy and chemotherapy

333. An 80-year-old man is admitted to the hospital complaining of nausea, abdominal pain, distention, and diarrhea. A cautiously performed transanal contrast study reveals an apple-core configuration in the rectosigmoid area. Which of the following is the most appropriate next step in his management?

a. Colonoscopic decompression and rectal tube placement
b. Saline enemas and digital disimpaction of fecal matter from the rectum
c. Colon resection and proximal colostomy
d. Oral administration of metronidazole and checking a *Clostridium difficile* titer
e. Evaluation of an electrocardiogram and obtaining an angiogram to evaluate for colonic mesenteric ischemia

334. A 46-year-old woman who was recently diagnosed with Crohn disease asks about the need for surgery. Which of the following findings would be an indication for an immediate exploratory laparotomy?

a. Intestinal obstruction
b. Enterovesical fistula
c. Ileum-ascending colon fistula
d. Enterovaginal fistula
e. Free perforation

335. A 50-year-old man presents to the emergency room with a 6-hour history of excruciating abdominal pain and distention. The abdominal film shown here is obtained. Which of the following is the most appropriate next diagnostic maneuver?

a. Emergency celiotomy
b. Upper GI series with small-bowel follow-through
c. CT scan of the abdomen
d. Barium enema
e. Sigmoidoscopy

336. A septuagenarian woman undergoes an uncomplicated resection of an abdominal aneurysm. Four days after surgery the patient presents with sudden onset of abdominal pain and distention. An abdominal radiograph demonstrates an air-filled, kidney-bean–shaped structure in the left upper quadrant. Which of the following is the most appropriate management at this time?

a. Decompression of the large bowel via colonoscopy
b. Placement of the NG tube and administration of low-dose cholinergic drugs
c. Administration of a gentle saline enema and encouragement of ambulation
d. Operative decompression with transverse colostomy
e. Right hemicolectomy

337. A 45-year-old man presents with right upper quadrant abdominal pain and fever. CT scan shows a large, calcified cystic mass in the right lobe of the liver. Echinococcus is suggested by the CT findings. Which of the following is the most appropriate management of echinococcal liver cysts?

a. Percutaneous catheter drainage.
b. Medical treatment with albendazole.
c. Medical treatment with steroids.
d. Medical treatment with metronidazole.
e. Total pericystectomy.

338. A 28-year-old woman who is 15 weeks pregnant has new onset of nausea, vomiting, and right-sided abdominal pain. She has been free of nausea since early in her first trimester. The pain has become worse over the past 6 hours. Which of the following is the most common nonobstetric surgical disease of the abdomen during pregnancy?

a. Appendicitis
b. Cholecystitis
c. Pancreatitis
d. Intestinal obstruction
e. Acute fatty liver of pregnancy

339. A 56-year-old woman has nonspecific complaints that include an abnormal sensation when swallowing. An esophagram is obtained. Which of the following is most likely to require surgical correction?

a. Large sliding esophageal hiatal hernia
b. Paraesophageal hiatal hernia
c. Traction diverticulum of esophagus
d. Schatzki ring of distal esophagus
e. Esophageal web

340. A 65-year-old man who is hospitalized with pancreatic carcinoma develops abdominal distention and obstipation. The following abdominal radiograph is obtained. Which of the following is the most appropriate initial management of this patient?

a. Urgent colostomy or cecostomy
b. Discontinuation of anticholinergic medications and narcotics and correction of metabolic disorders
c. Digital disimpaction of fecal mass in the rectum
d. Diagnostic and therapeutic colonoscopy
e. Detorsion of volvulus and colopexy or resection

341. A 48-year-old man presents with jaundice, melena, and right upper quadrant abdominal pain after undergoing a percutaneous liver biopsy. Endoscopy shows blood coming from the ampulla of Vater. Which of the following is the most appropriate first line of therapy for major hemobilia?

a. Correction of coagulopathy, adequate biliary drainage, and close monitoring
b. Transarterial embolization (TAE)
c. Percutaneous transhepatic biliary drainage (PTBD)
d. Ligation of bleeding vessels
e. Hepatic resection

342. A 30-year-old female patient who presents with diarrhea and abdominal discomfort is found at colonoscopy to have colitis confined to the transverse and descending colon. A biopsy is performed. Which of the following is a finding consistent with this patient's diagnosis?

a. The inflammatory process is confined to the mucosa and submucosa.
b. The inflammatory reaction is likely to be continuous.
c. Superficial as opposed to linear ulcerations can be expected.
d. Noncaseating granulomas can be expected in up to 50% of patients.
e. Microabscesses within crypts are common.

343. A 24-year-old man presents to the emergency room with abdominal pain and fever. CT scan of the abdomen reveals inflammation of the colon. He is referred to a gastroenterologist to be evaluated for inflammatory bowel disease (Crohn disease versus ulcerative colitis). Which of the following indications for surgery is more prevalent in patients with Crohn disease?

a. Toxic megacolon
b. Massive bleeding
c. Fistulas between the colon and segments of intestine, bladder, vagina, urethra, and skin
d. Intractable disease
e. Dysplasia or carcinoma

344. An upper GI series is performed on a 71-year-old woman who presented with several months of chest pain that occurs when she is eating. The film shown here is obtained. Investigation reveals a microcytic anemia and erosive gastritis on upper endoscopy. Which of the following is the most appropriate initial management of this patient?

a. Cessation of smoking, decreased caffeine intake, and avoidance of large meals before lying down
b. Antacids
c. Histamine-2 blocker
d. Proton-pump inhibitor
e. Surgical treatment

345. A 54-year-old man complains that his eyes are yellow. His bilirubin is elevated. His physical examination is unremarkable. A CT of the abdomen shows a small mass in the head of the pancreas encasing the superior mesenteric artery. Cytology from the ERCP is positive for cancer. Which of the following is the most appropriate treatment for this patient?

a. Pancreaticoduodenectomy
b. Pancreaticoduodenectomy with reconstruction of the superior mesenteric artery
c. Total pancreatectomy
d. Total pancreatectomy with reconstruction of the superior mesenteric artery
e. Chemoradiation therapy

346. A 28-year-old woman presents with hematochezia. She is admitted to the hospital and undergoes upper endoscopy that is negative for any lesions. Colonoscopy is performed and no bleeding sources are identified, although the gastroenterologist notes blood in the right colon and old blood coming from above the ileocecal valve. Which of the following is the test of choice in this patient?

a. Angiography
b. Small-bowel enteroclysis
c. CT scan of the abdomen
d. Technetium 99m (^{99m}Tc) pertechnetate scan
e. Small-bowel endoscopy

347. A 32-year-old woman undergoes an uncomplicated appendectomy for acute appendicitis. The pathology report notes the presence of a 1-cm carcinoid tumor in the tip of the appendix. Which of the following is the most appropriate management of this patient?

a. Right hemicolectomy
b. Right hemicolectomy and chemotherapy
c. Chemotherapy only
d. Radiation only
e. No further treatment

348. A 58-year-old man presents with a bulge in his right groin associated with mild discomfort. On examination the bulge is easily reducible and does not descend into the scrotum. Which of the following changes is most concerning for possible strangulation requiring emergent repair of the hernia?

a. Increase in size of the hernia
b. Descent of hernia into the scrotum
c. Development of a second hernia in the left groin
d. Inability to reduce hernia
e. Worsening pain over the hernia with walking

349. A 35-year-old woman presents with abdominal pain and jaundice. Subsequent ERCP reveals the congenital cystic anomaly of her biliary system illustrated in the film shown here. Which of the following is the most appropriate treatment?

a. Cholecystectomy with resection of the extrahepatic biliary tract and Roux-en-Y hepaticojejunostomy
b. Internal drainage via choledochoduodenostomy
c. Internal drainage via choledochocystojejunostomy
d. Percutaneous transhepatic biliary drainage
e. Liver transplantation

350. A 36-year-old man is in your intensive care unit on mechanical ventilation following thoracotomy for a 24-hour-old esophageal perforation. His WBC is markedly elevated, and he is febrile, hypotensive, and coagulopathic. His NG tube fills with blood and continues to bleed. Which of the following findings on upper endoscopy would be most suspicious for stress gastritis?

a. Multiple, shallow lesions with discrete areas of erythema along with focal hemorrhage in the antrum
b. Multiple, shallow lesions with discrete areas of erythema along with focal hemorrhage in the fundus
c. Multiple deep ulcerations extending into and through the muscularis mucosa in the antrum
d. Multiple deep ulcerations extending into and through the muscularis mucosa in the fundus
e. Single deep ulceration extending into and through the muscularis mucosa in the fundus

351. A 35-year-old man presents with right upper quadrant pain, fever, jaundice, and shaking chills. Ultrasound of the abdomen demonstrates gallstones, normal gallbladder wall thickness, and common bile duct of 1.0 cm. The patient is admitted to the hospital and given IV fluids and antibiotics. He continues to be febrile with increasing WBCs. Which of the following is the most appropriate next step in this patient's management?

a. Endoscopic retrograde cholangiopancreatography (ERCP)
b. Placement of a cholecystostomy tube
c. Laparoscopic cholecystectomy
d. Open cholecystectomy
e. Emergent operation and decompression of the common bile duct with a T tube

352. An 88-year-old man with a history of end-stage renal failure, severe coronary artery disease, and brain metastases from lung cancer presents with acute cholecystitis. His family wants "everything done." Which of the following is the best management option in this patient?

a. Tube cholecystostomy
b. Open cholecystectomy
c. Laparoscopic cholecystectomy
d. Intravenous antibiotics followed by elective cholecystectomy
e. Lithotripsy followed by long-term bile acid therapy

353. After a weekend drinking binge, a 45-year-old man presents to the hospital with abdominal pain, nausea, and vomiting. On physical examination, the patient is noted to have tenderness to palpation in the epigastrium. Laboratory tests reveal an amylase of 25,000 U/dL (normal < 180 U/dL). The patient is medically managed and sent home after 1 week. A CT scan done 4 weeks later is pictured here. Currently the patient is asymptomatic. Which of the following is the most appropriate initial management of this patient?

a. Distal pancreatectomy
b. Percutaneous catheter drainage
c. Endoscopic drainage
d. Surgical drainage
e. No intervention is warranted at this time

354. A 54-year-old man presents with sudden onset of massive, painless, recurrent hematemesis. Upper endoscopy is performed and reveals bleeding from a lesion in the proximal stomach that is characterized as an abnormally large artery surrounded by normal-appearing gastric mucosa. Endoscopic modalities fail to stop the bleeding. Which of the following is the most appropriate surgical management of this patient?

a. Wedge resection of the lesion
b. Wedge resection of the lesion with truncal vagotomy
c. Wedge resection of the lesion with highly selective vagotomy
d. Wedge resection of the lesion with truncal vagotomy and antrectomy
e. Subtotal gastrectomy

355. During an appendectomy for acute appendicitis, a 4-cm mass is found in the midportion of the appendix. Frozen section reveals this lesion to be a carcinoid tumor. Which of the following is the most appropriate management of this patient?

a. Appendectomy
b. Appendectomy followed by a colonoscopy
c. Appendectomy followed by a PET scan
d. Right hemicolectomy
e. Total proctocolectomy

356. A 45-year-old man is examined for a yearly executive physical. A mass is palpated in the rectum, and a biopsy suggests carcinoid. Which of the following findings is most likely to be associated with the carcinoid syndrome?

a. Tumor < 2 cm
b. Tumor < 2 cm with ulceration
c. Tumor > 2 cm
d. Involvement of regional lymph nodes
e. Hepatic metastases

357. An ultrasound is performed on a patient with right upper quadrant pain. It demonstrates a large gallstone in the cystic duct but also a polypoid mass in the fundus. Which of the following is an indication for cholecystectomy for a polypoid gallbladder lesion?

a. Size greater than 0.5 cm
b. Presence of clinical symptoms
c. Patient age of older than 25 years
d. Presence of multiple small lesions
e. Absence of shadowing on ultrasound

358. An alcoholic man has been suffering excruciating pain from chronic pancreatitis recalcitrant to analgesics and splanchnic block. A surgeon recommends total pancreatectomy. A patient who has a total pancreatectomy might be expected to develop which of the following complications?

a. Diabetes mellitus and steatorrhea
b. Diabetes mellitus and constipation
c. Hypoglycemia
d. Hypoglycemia and steatorrhea
e. Hypoglycemia and constipation

359. A 45-year-old woman has an incidental finding of a liver mass on a CT scan. Magnetic resonance imaging (MRI) is suggestive of a hemangioma. Which of the following is the most appropriate management strategy for this patient?

a. Observation
b. Discontinuation of oral contraceptive pills
c. Percutaneous biopsy of the lesion to confirm the diagnosis
d. Resection of the hemangioma
e. Liver transplantation

360. A 57-year-old woman presents with adenocarcinoma of the right colon. Laboratory evaluation demonstrates an elevation of carcinoembryonic antigen (CEA) to 123 ng/mL. Which of the following is the most appropriate use of CEA testing in patients with colorectal cancer?

a. As a screening test for colorectal cancer
b. To determine which patients should receive adjuvant therapy
c. To determine which patients should receive neoadjuvant therapy
d. To monitor for postoperative recurrence
e. To monitor for preoperative metastatic disease

361. A 61-year-old woman with a history of unstable angina complains of hematemesis after retching and vomiting following a night of binge drinking. Endoscopy reveals a longitudinal mucosal tear at the gastroesophageal junction, which is not actively bleeding. Which of the following is the next recommended step in the management of this patient?

a. Angiography with embolization
b. Balloon tamponade
c. Exploratory laparotomy, gastrotomy, and oversewing of the tear
d. Systemic vasopressin infusion
e. Expectant management

Questions 362 to 365

Select the most appropriate diagnosis for each patient. Each lettered option may be used once, more than once, or not at all.

a. Symptomatic cholelithiasis
b. Acute cholecystitis
c. Gallstone pancreatitis
d. Choledocholithiasis
e. Cholangitis

362. A 62-year-old man presents with right upper quadrant abdominal pain and jaundice. He is afebrile with normal vital signs. On laboratory findings he has elevated levels of bilirubin and alkaline phosphatase. Ultrasound demonstrates gallstones, normal gallbladder wall thickness, no pericholecystic fluid, and a common bile duct of 1.0 cm.

363. A 36-year-old woman presents with right upper quadrant abdominal pain and jaundice. She is febrile and tachycardic. On laboratory results she has leukocytosis and elevated levels of bilirubin and alkaline phosphatase. Ultrasound demonstrates gallstones, normal gallbladder wall thickness, no pericholecystic fluid, and a common bile duct of 1.0 cm.

364. A 55-year-old man presents with intermittent right upper quadrant abdominal pain. Each episode of pain lasts 1 to 2 hours. He is afebrile with normal vital signs. On laboratory results he has no leukocytosis and normal levels of bilirubin, alkaline phosphatase, amylase, and lipase. Ultrasound demonstrates gallstones, normal gallbladder wall thickness, no pericholecystic fluid, and a common bile duct of 3 mm.

365. A 23-year-old woman presents with epigastric abdominal pain and nausea. She is afebrile with normal vital signs. On laboratory results she has no leukocytosis with normal levels of bilirubin and alkaline phosphatase. The amylase and lipase are elevated. Ultrasound demonstrates gallstones, normal gallbladder wall thickness, no pericholecystic fluid, and a common bile duct of 3 mm.

Questions 366 to 369

Select the most appropriate surgical procedure for each patient. Each lettered option may be used once, more than once, or not at all.

a. Low anterior resection
b. Abdominoperineal resection
c. Subtotal colectomy with end ileostomy
d. Total proctocolectomy with ileoanal J-pouch
e. Sigmoid resection with end colostomy (Hartmann procedure)
f. Transanal excision
g. Diverting colostomy

366. A 37-year-old man with a 10-year history of ulcerative colitis who has a sessile polyp 10 cm from the anal verge with high-grade dysplasia.

367. A 60-year-old woman with recurrent squamous cell carcinoma of the anus after chemoradiation.

368. A 68-year-old woman with fecal incontinence who presents with a large fixed adenocarcinoma 3 cm from the anal verge.

369. A 33-year-old man with a history of Crohn disease presents with severe abdominal pain and fever. On examination, his heart rate is 130 beats per minute, blood pressure 105/62 mm Hg, and temperature 38.9°C (102°F). Workup reveals a leukocytosis of 32,000/mm³. Plain films reveal a markedly dilated large colon.

Gastrointestinal Tract, Liver, and Pancreas

Answers

291. The answer is d. *(Townsend, pp 1232-1233.)* Omeprazole (Prilosec) irreversibly inhibits the hydrogen-potassium-ATPase (proton pump) in the secretory canaliculus of the gastric parietal cell. This blocks the last step in the acid-secretory process. Omeprazole's duration of action exceeds 24 hours, and doses of 20 to 30 mg/day inhibit more than 90% of 24-hour acid secretion. Omeprazole provides excellent suppression of meal-stimulated and nocturnal acid secretion and seems very safe for short-term therapy. Prolonged administration in laboratory animals has been associated with significant hypergastrinemia, hyperplasia of enterochromaffin-like cells, and carcinoid tumors.

292. The answer is c. *(Townsend, pp 1628-1630.)* Patients with ITP who are asymptomatic and have a platelet count greater than 30,000/μL can be treated expectantly with follow-up. Of these patients, those with a platelet count between 30,000 and 50,000/μL have an increased risk for more severe thrombocytopenia. Patients with a platelet count lower than 30,000/μL or less than 50,000/μL with significant bleeding or risk factors for bleeding should be treated. Initial medical treatment with prednisone (1 mg/kg), and intravenous immunoglobulin is used in patients with severe bleeding or preoperatively prior to splenectomy. Platelet transfusions are reserved for patients with acute bleeding. Splenectomy is indicated in patients who have severe symptomatic thrombocytopenia, patients in whom remission is achieved only with toxic doses of steroids, patients with a relapse after initial steroid therapy, patients with persistent thrombocytopenia for more than 3 months and a platelet count less than 30,000/μL, and possibly in patients with a persistent platelet count of less than 10,000/μL after 6 weeks of therapy. The platelet count can be expected to rise shortly after splenectomy, and prolonged remissions are expected in approximately two-thirds of cases.

293. The answer is e. *(Townsend, p 1345.)* Patients with appendiceal adenocarcinoma, a rare neoplasm accounting for less than 0.5% of GI tumors, should undergo formal right hemicolectomy. Often affecting older patients, they may present with symptoms mimicking those of acute appendicitis. A thorough initial workup and follow-up are necessary because of the high rate of synchronous and metachronous tumors. Five-year survival is 55% but depends on the tumor stage.

294. The answer is e. *(Townsend, pp 1064-1069.)* This patient has achalasia, which is a functional disorder caused by failure of relaxation of the lower esophageal sphincter, typically present with dysphagia, chest pain, and regurgitation of saliva and undigested food. The safest and most effective treatment for this condition is surgical treatment with an esophagomyotomy. The operation of choice is a modified laparoscopic Heller myotomy. Initial management of achalasia may include medications (calcium-channel blockers or long-acting nitrates), and other management options such as endoscopic dilation or injection of botulinum toxin (Botox) into the LES. However, symptoms always recur and patients need to undergo repeated procedures with the associated risk of perforation. Surgery results in improvement in more than 90% of patients, compared with only 70% of patients treated by forceful dilatation.

295. The answer is b. *(Townsend, pp 1373-1384.)* Definitive surgical management options for UC include total proctocolectomy with end ileostomy (typically reserved for older or incontinent patients) and total proctocolectomy with ileoanal pouch anastomosis. In patients undergoing emergent colectomy for toxic megacolon, total abdominal colectomy without resection of the rectum can be performed initially. However, given that UC always involves the rectum, definitive management of UC requires resection of most of the rectal mucosa, although controversy exists regarding retention of the very distal rectal mucosa such as with a stapled ileoanal anastomosis. Avoiding the mucosectomy preserves the anal transition zone and provides superior postoperative continence. Therefore, a mucosectomy is not routinely performed for patients without rectal dysplasia.

296. The answer is d. *(Townsend, pp 1603-1606.)* The patient most likely has an infected pancreatic pseudocyst. Pseudocysts are nonepithelialized fluid collections that can present at earliest 4 to 6 weeks after an episode of acute pancreatitis. The treatment for infected pancreatic pseudocysts is similar to that for pancreatic abscesses—percutaneous catheter drainage with antibiotics. Aspiration of the fluid can be diagnostic but is not a definitive treatment, even with the addition of antibiotics. Internal drainage of pancreatic pseudocysts is contraindicated in the presence of infection but is the treatment of choice for mature, symptomatic, noninfected pseudocysts. Malignancy should be excluded if there is no preceding history of pancreatitis.

297. The answer is a. *(Townsend, pp 1610-1612.)* This woman has a cystadenocarcinoma arising from the pancreatic body and tail; the treatment is surgical resection. About 90% of primary malignant neoplasms of the exocrine pancreas are adenocarcinomas of duct cell origin. The remaining neoplasms include serous and mucinous cystadenomas/cystadenocarcinomas, solid pseudopapillary tumors, and intraductal mucinous papillary adenomas/tumors. Cystadenocarcinomas may be several times the size of typical ductal cancers and often arise in the body or tail of the pancreas. They may become very large without invading adjacent viscera and do not generally cause significant pain or weight loss. The clinical presentation is usually quite subtle, with symptoms related primarily to the enlarging mass. There are no diagnostic laboratory findings, and definitive preoperative diagnosis is rare. An elderly patient with no history of pancreatitis is unlikely to have a pseudocyst, and a benign neoplasm is also less likely in this age group. Endoscopic ultrasound and aspiration of the cyst fluid can assist with the diagnosis; a high CEA level and low amylase level in the cyst fluid can be suggestive of malignancy. Aggressive surgical resection is indicated for cystic neoplasms of the pancreas. Internal drainage is the treatment of choice for noninfected pancreatic pseudocysts (as opposed to external drainage which is the treatment of choice for infected pseudocysts) but is contraindicated if malignancy is suspected. ERCP with stent placement may be indicated in patients with pancreatic pseudocyst with fistula and proximal ductal stricture, but it has no role in the treatment of pancreatic malignancies. Percutaneous drainage is contraindicated in malignancies as well.

298. The answer is c. *(Townsend, pp 357-358.)* According to the United Ostomy Association Data Registry, the most frequent serious complication of end colostomies is parastomal herniation, which commonly occurs when the stoma is placed lateral to, rather than through, the rectus muscle. Symptomatic herniation requires operative relocation of the stoma or mesh herniorrhaphy. Minor problems are frequently encountered with colostomies. They include irregularity of function, irritation of the skin due to leakage of enteric contents, or bleeding from the exposed mucosa following trauma. Prolapse occurs most frequently with transverse loop colostomies and is likely due to the use of the transverse loop to decompress distal colon obstructions. As the intestine decompresses, it retracts from the edge of the surrounding fascia, which allows prolapse or herniation of the mobile transverse colon. Optimal treatment of stomal prolapse is restoration of intestinal continuity or conversion to an end colostomy. Perforation of a stoma is usually because of careless instrumentation with an irrigation catheter.

299. The answer is d. (*Townsend, pp 1614-1615.*) Painless jaundice with weight loss is suspicious for a pancreatic cancer involving the head or uncinate process of the pancreas. A helical contrast-enhanced CT scan is the most appropriate study to evaluate for a pancreatic mass. CT has a specificity of 95% or better with sensitivity exceeding 95% for tumors larger than 2 cm in diameter. PET scan may be of value in detecting small pancreatic tumors that are not seen on CT scan but the sensitivity and specificity remain to be established. An acute abdominal series is composed of three x-rays (upright chest, upright abdomen, supine abdomen) and is useful in evaluating patients for bowel perforation or bowel obstruction. An ERCP is helpful in evaluating patients with obstructive jaundice without a detectable mass on CT scan. An EGD is not useful in the evaluation of a patient with a pancreatic mass.

300. The answer is a. (*Townsend, pp 1245-1250.*) In patients with no prior history of peptic ulcer disease, simple closure with an omental patch is recommended. Patients with long-standing ulcer disease require a definitive acid-reducing procedure, except in high-risk situations and if the perforation is more than 24 hours old secondary to extensive peritoneal soilage. The choice of procedure is made by weighing the risk of recurrence against the incidence of undesirable side effects of the procedure, and considerable controversy persists about this issue. Antrectomy and truncal vagotomy offers a recurrence rate of 1%, but carries a 15% to 25% incidence of sequelae such as diarrhea, dumping syndrome, bloating, and gastric stasis. Highly selective vagotomy, if technically feasible, offers a 1% to 5% incidence of side effects but carries a recurrence rate of 10% to 13% in some series, although results are better when gastric and prepyloric ulcers are excluded. Pyloroplasty and truncal vagotomy carries intermediate rates of recurrence and side effects, but has the advantage of speed in the setting of very ill patients with acute perforation.

301. The answer is b. (*Townsend, pp 1252-1253.*) Though reminiscent of the carcinoid syndrome, this patient's complaints in the context of recent gastric surgery are highly suggestive of the dumping syndrome, which is characterized by intestinal symptoms (bloating, cramping, diarrhea) and vasomotor symptoms (weakness, flushing, palpitations, diaphoresis, and dizziness) after ingestion of a meal following surgical removal of part of the stomach or alteration of the pyloric sphincter. Early dumping occurs within 20 to 30 minutes of eating and is attributed to the rapid influx of fluid with a high osmotic gradient into the small intestine from the gastric remnant. Late dumping syndrome occurs 2 to 3 hours after a meal; symptoms resemble those of hypoglycemic shock. Medical management consists of reassurance and dietary measures (avoidance of large amounts of sugars, frequent small meals, and separation of fluids and solids). The majority of cases will resolve within 3 months of operation on this regimen. Octreotide, a long-acting somatostatin analogue, can be used as well, but cost is a limiting factor. Surgery for intractable dumping consists of creation of an antiperistaltic limb of jejunum distal to the gastrojejunostomy.

302. The answer is a. (*Townsend, pp 1210-1213.*) Restoration of circulating blood volume is the first priority in patients with an acute variceal bleed. Initial resuscitation should be with isotonic crystalloids followed by transfusion of blood. Elevated prothrombin times should be corrected with fresh-frozen plasma, and although mild hypersplenism and thrombocytopenia are associated with portal hypertension, platelet transfusion is indicated only for platelet counts less than 50,000/μL. Medical therapy consists of either octreotide or vasopressin to decrease splanchnic blood flow. Because of coronary vasoconstrictive effects, nitroglycerin is usually administered concomitantly with vasopressin. β-Blockade (eg, propranolol), with or without a long-acting nitrate, has been used to prevent recurrent variceal bleeding, but is not indicated in the acutely bleeding patients who are hemodynamically unstable. Balloon tamponade controls variceal hemorrhage immediately in more than 85% of patients. However, although balloon tamponade (Sengstaken-Blakemore tube) has reduced the mortality and morbidity from variceal hemorrhage in good-risk patients, an increased awareness of the associated complications (aspiration, asphyxiation, and ulceration at the tamponade site), as well as a rebleeding rate of 40%, have reduced its use. Balloon tamponade is indicated as a temporary measure when vasopressin or octreotide and sclerotherapy fail and other therapies are not immediately available (such as endoscopy with banding).

303. The answer is e. (*Townsend, pp 1210-1213.*) Patients with poorly compensated liver disease who develop recurrent variceal bleeds should undergo transjugular intrahepatic portosystemic shunting. β-Blockade and endoscopic therapy are typically used as initial therapeutic options for patients with variceal bleeds. In patients with well-compensated liver disease, portosystemic shunts can be used to prevent recurrent variceal bleeds. Portocaval, mesocaval, and splenorenal shunts are considered non-selective shunts and are associated with the development or worsening of encephalopathy postoperatively. The distal splenorenal shunt is a selective shunt procedure and is associated with a lower rate of encephalopathy. However, in patients with Child C cirrhosis (poorly compensated liver disease), surgical shunting should be avoided because of increased operative mortality. Hepatic transplantation is contraindicated in a patient who is actively drinking. Esophageal transection and reanastomosis, or the Sugiura procedure, are typically reserved for patients with splanchnic venous thrombosis who are not shunt candidates.

304. The answer is d. (*Townsend, pp 1236-1256.*) This patient has a persistent gastric ulcer and should undergo surgical resection via either a distal gastrectomy with gastroduodenostomy (Billroth I reconstruction) or with gastrojejunostomy (Billroth II reconstruction) to definitively rule out a malignancy. The initial management of a gastric ulcer consists of anti-microbial therapy directed against *H pylori*. Indications for surgical intervention are hemorrhage, perforation, disease refractory to medical therapy, and inability to rule out a malignancy. Only ulcers associated with acid hypersecretion require a vagotomy as well (type II—body of stomach, with concomitant duodenal ulcer, or type III—prepyloric). Type I (in the body and along the lesser curvature) and type IV (near the gastroesophageal junction) ulcers do not require vagotomy.

305. The answer is c. (*Townsend, pp 1406-1415.*) Five-year survival rates of 25% have been reported after synchronous resection of primary colorectal cancers and liver metastases. Because approximately 5% of colorectal cancers are associated with resectable hepatic metastases, appropriate preoperative discussion should include obtaining permission for removal of synchronous peripheral hepatic lesions if they are found. Adequate local resection, either by wedge or by limited partial hepatectomy, may be carried out whenever no extrahepatic disease is found and the hepatic lesion is technically removable. Any option that leaves the symptomatic colon cancer (bleeding) would be unacceptable. Radiation therapy has little to offer in colon cancer or its hepatic metastases.

306. The answer is b. (*Townsend, pp 1241-1242.*) The carbon-labeled urea breath test is the noninvasive method of choice to document eradication of a *H pylori* infection. This test samples the entire stomach and has sensitivity and specificity both greater than 95%. The test is performed by having the patient ingest a carbon-isotope labeled urea. After ingestion the urea will be metabolized to ammonia and labeled bicarbonate if a *H pylori* infection is present. The labeled bicarbonate is excreted in the breath as labeled carbon dioxide, which can then be quantified. Serology is another noninvasive test to establish the diagnosis of *H pylori* infection. However, it cannot be used to assess eradication after therapy because antibody titers can remain high for over a year. Endoscopy with biopsy is necessary to provide a specimen for the rapid urease test, histologic evaluation, and culturing of gastric mucosa.

307. The answer is c. (*Townsend, pp 1155-1157, 1175-1176.*) An indirect inguinal hernia leaves the abdominal cavity by entering the dilated internal inguinal ring and passing along the anteromedial aspect of the spermatic cord. The internal inguinal ring is an opening in the transversalis fascia for the passage of the spermatic cord; an indirect inguinal hernia, therefore, lies within the fibers of the cremaster muscle. A femoral hernia passes directly beneath the inguinal ligament at a point medial to the femoral vessels, and a direct inguinal hernia passes through a weakness in the floor of the inguinal canal medial to the inferior epigastric artery. Neither lies within the cremaster muscle fibers. Spigelian hernias, which are rare, protrude through an anatomic defect that can occur along the lateral border of the rectus muscle at its junction with the linea semilunaris. An interparietal hernia is one in which the hernia sac, instead of protruding in the usual fashion, makes its way between the fascial layers of the abdominal wall. These unusual hernias may be preperitoneal (between the peritoneum and transversalis fascia), interstitial (between muscle layers), or superficial (between the external oblique aponeurosis and the skin).

308. The answer is b. (*Townsend, p 1572.*) The finding of air in the biliary tract of a nonseptic patient is diagnostic of a biliary enteric fistula. When the clinical findings also include small-bowel obstruction in an elderly patient with history of gallstones and no prior abdominal surgery (a virgin abdomen), the diagnosis of gallstone ileus can be made with a high degree of certainty. In this condition, a large chronic gallstone mechanically erodes through the wall of the gallbladder into adjacent stomach or duodenum. A connection is formed between the biliary system and the GI tract which allows air into the biliary tract. When the gallstone arrives in the distal ileum, the caliber of the bowel no longer allows passage, and a small-bowel obstruction develops. Surgical removal of the gallstone is necessary. The diseases suggested by the other response items (bleeding ulcer, peritoneal infection, pyloric outlet obstruction, pelvic neoplasm) are common in elderly patients, but each would probably present with symptoms other than those of small-bowel obstruction.

309. The answer is d. (*Townsend, pp 1400-1414.*) Peutz-Jeghers syndrome is characterized by intestinal polyposis and melanin spots of the oral mucosa. Unlike the adenomatous polyps seen in familial polyposis, the lesions in this condition are hamartomas, which have no malignant potential. Surgery for symptomatic polyps involves polypectomy. Cancer of the colon in patients with chronic UC is 10 times more frequent than in the general population. Duration of disease is very important; the risk of developing cancer is low in the first 10 years but thereafter rises about 4% per year. The average age of cancer development in patients with chronic UC is 37 years; idiopathic carcinoma of the colon, however, develops at an average age of 65 years. Crohn colitis is currently felt to be a precancerous condition as well. The chance of development of carcinoma of the colon in patients with familial polyposis is essentially 100%. Treatment of the patient with familial polyposis generally consists of total proctocolectomy with ileoanal J-pouch. Villous adenomas have been demonstrated to contain malignant portions in about one-third of affected persons and invasive malignancy in another one-third of removed specimens. Anterior resection is performed for large lesions or those containing invasive carcinomas when the lesion is above the peritoneal reflection. Abdominalperineal resection (APR) is indicated for low-lying rectal villous adenomas when they have demonstrated invasive carcinomas. Transrectal excision with regular follow-up examinations is sufficient for lesions without invasive carcinomas.

310. The answer is c. (*Townsend, p 1572.*) Gallstone ileus is caused by erosion of a stone from the gallbladder into the GI tract (most commonly the duodenum). The stone becomes lodged in the small bowel (usually in the terminal ileum) and causes small-bowel obstruction. Plain films of the abdomen that demonstrate small-bowel obstruction and air in the biliary tract are diagnostic of the condition. Treatment consists of ileotomy, removal of the stone, and cholecystectomy if it is technically safe. If there is significant inflammation of the right upper quadrant, ileotomy for stone extraction followed by an interval cholecystectomy is often a safer alternative. Operating on the biliary fistula doubles the mortality rate compared with simple removal of the gallstone from the intestine.

311. The answer is d. (*Townsend, pp 1365-1369.*) The indications for surgical intervention for diverticular disease include hemorrhage secondary to diverticulosis, recurrent episodes of diverticulitis, intractability to medical therapy, and complicated diverticulitis. The latter includes perforated diverticulitis with or without abscess and fistulous disease. Diverticular abscesses are treated with percutaneous drainage initially followed by definitive resectional therapy. Initial percutaneous drainage allows for a 1-stage procedure that consists of resection of the affected colon with primary anastomosis. Perforated diverticulitis is typically treated with either the Hartmann procedure (sigmoid resection with end colostomy and rectal stump) or sigmoid resection, anastomosis, and diverting loop ileostomy.

312. The answer is d. (*Townsend, p 1562.*) This patient most likely has biliary dyskinesia. The diagnosis is confirmed by CCK-HIDA scan. Technetium-labeled hydroxy-iminodiacetic acid (HIDA) is injected intravenously, which is subsequently excreted into the biliary tract. After filling of the gallbladder, cholecystokinin (CCK), a hormone that is normally released by the duodenum after ingestion of a meal, is infused intravenously to stimulate gallbladder contraction. A gallbladder ejection fraction of less than 35% at 20 minutes is diagnostic of biliary dyskinesia. Cholecystectomy results in improvement in symptoms in 85% to 94% of patients with biliary dyskinesia. A laparoscopic cholecystectomy should not be performed without confirmation of the gallbladder as the etiology of the symptoms. There is no role for oral dissolutional therapy with ursodeoxycholic acid in the treatment of biliary colic, since no gallstones are present. Avoidance of fatty foods is a temporary measure to control the symptoms. It does not provide a long-term solution.

313. The answer is b. (*Townsend, pp 1578-1579.*) Gallbladder polyps can be observed with serial ultrasounds if they are less than 1 cm in size. Patients with suspected gallbladder carcinoma should undergo cholecystectomy with intraoperative frozen section, and if there is invasion of the serosa and no evidence of metastatic or extensive local disease, they should undergo a radical cholecystectomy (portal lymphadenectomy and either wedge or formal resection of the liver surrounding the gallbladder fossa in addition to the cholecystectomy). Bile aspiration does not have a role in the workup of gallbladder polyps or gallbladder carcinoma.

314. The answer is c. (*Townsend, p 1136.*) Hematomas of the rectus sheath are more common in the elderly, and a history of trauma, sudden muscular exertion, or anticoagulation can usually be elicited. The pain is of sudden onset and is sharp in nature. The hematoma typically presents as an abdominal mass that does not change with contraction of the rectus muscles. The diagnosis can be established preoperatively with an ultrasound or CT scan showing a mass within the rectus sheath. Management is conservative unless symptoms are severe and bleeding persists, in which case surgical evacuation of the hematoma and ligation of bleeding vessels may be required.

315. The answer is a. (*Townsend, p 1493.*) Amebic liver abscesses should be treated initially with metronidazole monotherapy, as opposed to pyogenic liver abscesses, which are treated initially with percutaneous catheter drainage and antibiotics against gram-negative and anaerobic organisms (eg, *Essherichia coli, Klebisella pneumoniae,* bacteroides, enterococcus, and anaerobic streptococci). If improvement fails to occur, then other antimicrobial agents can be added. Abscesses that are refractory to medical therapy may require laparotomy.

316. The answer is b. (*Townsend, pp 1111-1114.*) Endoscopy is an important step prior to undergoing operative intervention for GERD. It has the ability to exclude other diseases, such as tumors, and document the degree of peptic esophageal injury. Surgical treatment for sliding esophageal hernias (type I paraesophageal hernias) should be considered only in symptomatic patients with objectively documented esophagitis or stenosis. The overwhelming majority of sliding hiatal hernias are totally asymptomatic, even many of those with demonstrable reflux. Even in the presence of reflux, esophageal inflammation rarely develops because the esophagus is so efficient at clearing the refluxed acid. Symptomatic hernias should be treated vigorously by the variety of medical measures that have been found helpful. Patients who do have symptoms of episodic reflux and who remain untreated can expect their disease to progress to intolerable esophagitis or fibrosis and stenosis. Neither the presence of the hernia nor its size is important in deciding on surgical therapy. Once esophagitis has been documented to persist under adequate medical therapy, manometric or pH studies may help determine the optimum surgical treatment.

317. The answer is c. (*Townsend, pp 1167-1168.*) The patient has a bulge identified below the inguinal ligament which is consistent with a femoral hernia. A femoral hernia occurs through the femoral canal bounded superiorly by the iliopubic tract, inferiorly by Cooper ligament, laterally by the femoral vein, and medially by the junction of the iliopubic tract and Cooper ligament. The incidence of strangulation in femoral hernias is high. Therefore, all femoral hernias, even asymptomatic ones, should be repaired. This patient has no evidence of an acute incarceration and does not need emergent repair of her hernia at this time.

318. The answer is a. (*Townsend, pp 1449-1450.*) The patient has a pilonidal abscess which develops from an infected pilonidal cyst. It typically presents as a painful fluctuant mass extending from the midline and is located between the gluteal clefts. Perianal and perirectal abscesses are usually much closer to the anus and are very painful on rectal examination. A fistula-in-ano is a chronically draining tract in the perianal region. It may become plugged and develop a perianal or perirectal abscess. An anal fissure is a linear ulcer along the anal canal and is not associated with an abscess.

319. The answer is e. (*Townsend, pp 1389-1392.*) Ischemic colitis presents as hematochezia, fever, and abdominal pain. Unlike acute mesenteric ischemia, which affects the small intestine and requires emergent intervention, ischemic colitis rarely requires surgical intervention unless full-thickness necrosis, perforation, or refractory bleeding is present. Expectant management with intravenous fluids, bowel rest, and supportive care is the treatment of choice.

320. The answer is b. (*Townsend, pp 1360-1361.*) Patients may undergo resection of a large fraction of the colon and suffer little long-term change in bowel habits because the reserve capacity of the colon for water absorption greatly exceeds the normal requirements for maintaining stable bowel function. The colon absorbs electrolytes, water, short-chain fatty acids, and vitamins. The right colon absorbs more salt and water than the left colon. The majority of normal feces are composed of water. Sodium is absorbed by colonic epithelium by active transport, and potassium is excreted into the colonic lumen passively. Chloride and bicarbonate are exchanged across the epithelium–chloride is absorbed and bicarbonate is excreted.

321. The answer is d. *(Brunicardi, p 1120.)* Hepatic adenomas are associated with oral contraceptive use. Lesions greater than 4 cm in size have an increased risk of rupture with hemorrhage, which may in fact be the initial clinical presentation. Hepatic adenomas also have a risk of malignant transformation to a well-differentiated hepatocellular carcinoma.

322. The answer is a. *(Brunicardi, p 1120.)* Focal nodular hyperplasia is rarely symptomatic and unlike a hepatic adenoma does not carry an associated risk of malignant degeneration or rupture with hemorrhage. Therefore, surgical resection for FNH is indicated only if the lesion is symptomatic. If FNH cannot be distinguished from a hepatic adenoma on CT scan, a nuclear medicine scan can be obtained that may demonstrate a "hot" lesion in the setting of FNH and a "cold" lesion in the setting of hepatic adenoma.

323. The answer is d. *(Brunicardi, p 1205.)* Splenectomy is indicated for acute hemorrhage secondary to left-sided, or sinistral, portal hypertension, which is characterized by gastric varices in the setting of splenic or portal vein thrombosis in the absence of cirrhosis. Patients who have either had an episode of acute or have chronic pancreatitis can develop either splenic or portal venous thrombosis. In the absence of bleeding complications, surgery is indicated only if other surgical procedures are planned.

324. The answer is b. *(Brunicardi, pp 993-997, 1036-1038.)* This patient most likely has Crohn disease. In about 10% of patients, especially those who are young, the onset of the disease is abrupt and may be mistaken for acute appendicitis. Appendectomy is indicated in such patients as long as the cecum at the base of the appendix is not involved. Interestingly, about 90% of patients who present with the acute appendicitis-like form of regional enteritis will not progress to development of the full-blown chronic disease. Thus, resection or bypass of the involved areas is not indicated at this time. Patients with regional enteritis usually have a chronic and slowly progressive course with intermittent symptom-free periods. The usual symptoms are anorexia, abdominal pain, diarrhea, fever, and weight loss. Extraintestinal syndromes that may be seen include ankylosing spondylitis, polyarthritis, erythema nodosum, pyoderma gangrenosum, gallstones, hepatic fatty infiltration, and fibrosis of the biliary tract, pancreas, and retroperitoneum.

325. The answer is c. *(Brunicardi, pp 1159-1160.)* This scenario is typical for a patient with iatrogenic injury of the common bile duct. These injuries commonly occur in the proximal portion of the extrahepatic biliary system. The transhepatic cholangiogram documents a biliary stricture, which in this clinical setting is best dealt with surgically. Choledochoduodenostomy generally cannot be performed because of the proximal location of the stricture. The best results are achieved with end-to-side choledochojejunostomy (Roux-en-Y) performed over a stent. Percutaneous transhepatic dilatation has been attempted in select cases, but follow-up is too short to make an adequate assessment of this technique. Primary repair of the common bile duct may result in recurrent stricture.

326. The answer is e. *(Brunicardi, p 1048.)* The term *carcinoma in situ* refers to the presence of malignant cells in the mucosal layer only. Endoscopic polypectomy is adequate treatment when malignant cells are identified in a colonic polyp, even if an invasive component is identified, if: (1) no vascular or lymphatic invasion is present; (2) there is an adequate negative margin (2 mm), and the cancer is not poorly differentiated.

327. The answer is d. *(Townsend, pp 1092-1093.)* Endoscopic ultrasound (EUS) provides the most accurate T staging of an esophageal carcinoma. An experienced endoscopic ultrasonographer can identify the depth and length of the tumor, the degree of luminal compromise, the status of regional lymph nodes, and involvement of adjacent structures. In addition, biopsy samples can be obtained of the mass and the regional lymph nodes. The accuracy of EUS for T staging increases with the depth of invasion. For T1 lesions, EUS is 84% accurate, and increases to 95% accuracy for T_4 lesions. Computed tomography is helpful, but its accuracy is only 57% for T staging. An MRI can accurately detect T_4 lesions and metastatic lesions but overstages T and N status with only 74% accuracy. A PET scan is reliable for detecting metastatic disease but is equal to a CT scan for T staging. Bronchoscopy is useful in patients who present with a cough or cervical esophageal carcinoma to rule out a tracheoesophageal fistula or growth of tumor into the trachea.

328. The answer is b. (*Townsend, pp 986-987.*) A secretin stimulation test is highly useful to confirm the diagnosis of Zollinger-Ellison syndrome (ZES) (gastrinoma). In this test a fasting gastrin level is measured before administration of intravenous secretin and further samples of serum gastrin are obtained at 2, 5, 10, and 20 minutes after secretin administration. A rise in serum gastrin levels greater than 200 pg/mL above baseline after secretin administration is found in patients with ZES. The rest of the tests do not confirm the diagnosis of a gastrinoma.

329. The answer is c. (*Townsend, p 987.*) Ninety percent of gastrinomas are located within the gastrinoma triangle—the 3 corners of the triangle are defined by the junction of the second and third portions of the duodenum, the junction of the neck and body of the pancreas, and the junction of the cystic and common bile duct.

330. The answer is b. (*Townsend, p 1600.*) The patient has acute gallstone pancreatitis. Ranson criteria consist of 5 criteria on admission and 6 during the first 48 hours that predict mortality: less than 2 criteria are associated with 0% mortality, 3 to 5 criteria with 10% to 20% mortality, and 6 or more with greater than 50% mortality. The criteria are slightly different for gallstone pancreatitis and non–gallstone pancreatitis. The first five criteria assess age, WBC count, low-density hormone (LDH), aspartate aminotransferase (AST), and glucose. The second set of criteria assesses hematocrit fall, blood urea nitrogen (BUN) elevation, serum calcium, base deficit, and estimated fluid sequestration. Amylase, lipase, total bilirubin, and albumin are not part of the criteria and do not correlate with the severity of disease.

331. The answer is c. (*Townsend, pp 983-986.*) The patient's presentation is classic for an insulinoma. These tumors are treated surgically, and simple excision of an adenoma is curative in the majority of cases. Seventy-five percent of these tumors are benign adenomas, and in 15% of affected patients the adenomas are multiple. Tumors arising from the pancreatic β cells give rise to hyperinsulinism. Symptoms relate to a rapidly falling blood glucose level and are caused by epinephrine release triggered by hypoglycemia (sweating, weakness, tachycardia). Cerebral symptoms of headache, confusion, visual disturbances, convulsions, and coma are caused by glucose deprivation of the brain. Whipple triad summarizes the clinical findings in patients with insulinomas: (1) attacks precipitated by fasting or exertion, (2) fasting blood glucose concentrations below 50 mg/dL, and (3) symptoms relieved by oral or intravenous glucose administration.

332. The answer is e. *(Townsend, pp 1459-1460.)* Epidermoid cancers of the anal canal metastasize to inguinal nodes as well as to the perirectal and mesenteric nodes. The results of local radical surgery have been disappointing. Combined external radiation with synchronous chemotherapy (fluorouracil and mitomycin), also known as the Nigro protocol, has been used as the standard treatment of the disease, whereas radical surgical approaches are now generally reserved for treatment failures and recurrences.

333. The answer is c. *(Townsend, pp 1371-1372.)* A markedly distended colon could have many causes in this 80-year-old man. The contrast study, however, reveals a classic apple-core lesion appropriate prior to relief of this large-bowel obstruction. After medical preparation (eg, hydration, normalization of electrolytes), this patient should undergo prompt surgical management of his mechanical obstruction; conservative management by resection and proximal colostomy would generally be preferred in this elderly patient with an obstructed, unprepared bowel.

334. The answer is e. *(Townsend, pp 1385-1387.)* Perforation of bowel into the free abdominal cavity is obviously a surgical emergency. Surgical treatment of Crohn disease is aimed at correcting complications that are causing symptoms. Fistula formation in itself is not an indication for surgery. An ileum-ascending colon fistula is very common yet rarely symptomatic. Fistulas between the intestine and the bladder and the intestine and the vagina, however, generally cause significant symptoms and warrant surgical intervention. Intestinal obstruction is usually partial and secondary to a fixed stricture that is not responsive to anti-inflammatory agents. When the obstruction causes symptoms that compromise nutritional status, surgery is warranted.

335. The answer is e. *(Townsend, pp 1369-1370.)* The film shows a markedly distended colon. The differential diagnosis includes tumor, foreign body, and colitis, but far more likely is either cecal or sigmoid volvulus. Sigmoid volvulus may be ruled out quickly by proctosigmoidoscopy, which is preferable to barium enema, since sigmoid volvulus may be treated successfully by rectal tube decompression via the sigmoidoscope. If sigmoidoscopy is negative, the working diagnosis, based on this classic film, must be cecal volvulus; barium enema would clinch the diagnosis, but the colon might rupture in the intervening 1 to 2 hours. Emergency celiotomy should be done.

336. The answer is e. (*Townsend, pp 1370-1371.*) The patient has a cecal volvulus and the procedure of choice is a right hemicolectomy. A cecal volvulus involves axial rotation of the terminal ileum, cecum, and ascending colon with concomitant twisting of the associated mesentery. Immediate operation is required to correct the volvulus and prevent ischemia. Colonoscopic decompression is usually unsuccessful and does not prevent recurrence of a cecal volvulus. A transverse colostomy "decompression" would not decompress the cecum, nor would it provide detorsion of the cecal mesentery to allow restoration of adequate blood supply to the right colon.

337. The answer is e. (*Townsend, pp 1494-1496.*) Definitive treatment requires surgical resection, enucleation, or evacuation of the cysts. As long as there is no evidence of biliary communication with the cyst, agents such as 0.5% silver nitrate or hypertonic saline are introduced into the cyst at the time of surgery, and efforts are made to avoid spillage and contamination of the peritoneal cavity. Spontaneous rupture of the cyst or leakage of cyst fluid during diagnostic or therapeutic aspiration may cause anaphylactic reactions or peritoneal dissemination of the disease. Steroids and epinephrine are available during surgery should an anaphylactic reaction occur. Treatment of patients with mebendazole or albendazole is effective at shrinking the cysts. However, chemotherapy alone is not effective at eradicating the disease without definitive resection or drainage. Simple drainage of the cyst without injection of scolicidal agents or administration of chemotherapy is not recommended. Metronidazole is used to treat amebic abscesses of the liver.

338. The answer is a. (*Townsend, pp 2231-2233.*) Appendicitis complicates approximately 1 in 1700 pregnancies at an incidence comparable with that in nonpregnant women matched for age. It is the most prevalent extrauterine indication for laparotomy in pregnancy. The duration of gestation does not influence the severity of the disease, but the diagnosis does become more difficult as the pregnancy progresses. By the twentieth week of gestation, the appendix often lies at the level of the umbilicus and more lateral than usual. Pregnancy should not delay surgery if appendicitis is suspected; appendiceal perforation greatly increases the chance of premature labor and fetal mortality (approximately 20% for each). After appendicitis, biliary tract disease (biliary colic, cholecystitis) is the second most common nonobstetric surgical disease of the abdomen during pregnancy. Pancreatitis, intestinal obstruction, and acute fatty liver of pregnancy are all less common general surgical conditions encountered during pregnancy.

339. The answer is b. (*Brunicardi, pp 842-846.*) Normal respiration creates negative pressure in the thoracic cavity. As a result of the pressure gradient, blood enters the chest via the vena cava and air via the trachea; both are life-sustaining results of this pressure gradient. The pathophysiologic consequence of a hole in the diaphragm is that eventually abdominal viscera will be aspirated into the thorax. The sliding hernia, contained in the lower mediastinum by intact pleura, may rarely cause symptoms of reflux that would justify surgical attention, but such patients are in no danger of vascular compromise or of obstructive displacement of hollow viscera. The paraesophageal hernia, on the other hand, leaves the patient at substantial risk for both strangulation and obstruction. Either result would be a surgical catastrophe; with rare exceptions, paraesophageal hernias should be surgically repaired whenever diagnosed. A traction diverticulum is usually caused by inflammatory contraction around mediastinal nodes, is rarely of any symptomatic consequence, and need not be repaired. Neither the Schatzki ring nor the esophageal web justifies esophageal surgery. They can be ignored or dilated as symptoms demand.

340. The answer is b. (*Brunicardi, p 1056.*) This patient has Ogilvie syndrome which describes a condition in which massive cecal and colonic dilation is seen in the absence of mechanical obstruction. Other terms used to describe this condition are acute colonic pseudo-obstruction, colonic ileus, and functional colonic obstruction. Initial treatment consists of discontinuing anticholinergics, narcotics, or other medications that may contribute to the ileus. Strict bowel rest, with IV hydration, and correction of electrolytes are crucial. In patients with persistent distention or a dilated cecum greater than 10 cm, cautious endoscopic colonic decompression can be performed, or a sympatholytic agent such as neostigmine can be administered, with appropriate hemodynamic monitoring. Surgery is indicated in all patients in whom perforation or ischemic bowel is suspected.

341. The answer is b. (*Townsend, pp 1515-1517.*) The first line of therapy for major hemobilia is transarterial embolization (TAE). The classic Quincke triad of abdominal pain in the right upper quadrant, jaundice, and GI bleeding is present in 30% to 40% of patients with hemobilia. With more frequent use of percutaneous liver procedures (eg, transhepatic cholangiogram, transhepatic catheter drainage), iatrogenic injury has replaced other trauma as the most common cause of bloody bile. Other causes include spontaneous bleeding during anticoagulation, gallstones, parasitic infections/abscesses, and neoplastic lesions. Angiography and endoscopy are useful diagnostic studies, and intrahepatic bleeding can be controlled by angiographic embolization in up to 95% of cases. Most cases of minor hemobilia can be managed conservatively with correction of coagulopathy, adequate biliary drainage (if needed), and close monitoring. Surgical treatment is reserved for cases in which conservative therapy and TAE have failed. Percutaneous transhepatic biliary drainage (PTBD) is a cause of hemobilia with incidence of up to 10%.

342. The answer is d. (*Townsend, pp 1373-1385.*) The patient depicted in this question has Crohn disease of the colon (Crohn colitis). Crohn colitis is characterized by linear mucosal ulcerations, discontinuous (skip) lesions, a transmural inflammatory process, and noncaseating granulomas in up to 50% of patients. Because their clinical features and management differ, Crohn colitis must be distinguished from UC. UC is usually found in the rectum, although in rare cases the rectum is spared involvement. The entire colon, from cecum to rectum, may be involved (pancolitis). UC typically presents as a grossly continuous inflammatory process (without skip lesions) that microscopically is confined to the mucosa and submucosa of the colon. In addition, crypt abscesses and superficial ulcerations are common in UC.

343. The answer is c. (*Townsend, pp 1373-1385.*) Patients with Crohn disease can develop fistulas between the colon and other segments of intestine, the bladder, the urethra, the vagina, the skin, or the prostate. Toxic megacolon, massive bleeding, dysplasia/carcinoma, and intractability of symptoms are indications for surgery found in both Crohn disease and ulcerative colitis.

344. The answer is e. *(Townsend, pp 1121-1123.)* The condition demonstrated is a paraesophageal hernia. Surgical repair is indicated in patients with paraesophageal hernias as soon as the patient can be properly prepared for the procedure, as bleeding, ulceration, obstruction, necrosis of the stomach wall, and perforation can occur. The remaining answer choices are appropriate initial treatments for GERD, not paraesophageal hernias.

345. The answer is e. *(Townsend, pp 1612-1619.)* The patient has unresectable pancreatic cancer and needs chemotherapy and radiation. Tumors involving critical peripancreatic arteries are T_4 lesions and are deemed unresectable. Tumors involving the portal vein or superior mesenteric vein (T_3 lesions) are technically resectable with venous resection and reconstruction, but the long-term survival of these patients is poor. Other CT changes suggestive of unresectability include extension beyond the pancreatic capsule and into the retroperitoneum, involvement of neural or nodal structures surrounding the origin of the celiac axis or superior mesenteric artery, and extension of the tumor along the hepatoduodenal ligament.

346. The answer is d. *(Townsend, pp 1321-1323.)* The patient most likely has bleeding from the small bowel, given the findings on endoscopy, and the most common cause of small intestinal bleeding in patients under the age of 30 is a Meckel diverticulum. Because Meckel diverticula can contain ectopic gastric mucosa, acid secretion can cause small-bowel ulcerations. Small-bowel enteroclysis is a contrast study that can sometimes identify masses or lesions in the small bowel. While enteroclysis, small-bowel endoscopy, angiography, and CT scanning can all be useful adjuncts in the workup of GI bleeding, the patient in this scenario should have a ^{99m}Tc pertechnetate scan, which is diagnostic for a Meckel diverticulum.

347. The answer is e. *(Brunicardi, p 1088.)* The most appropriate treatment for a 1-cm carcinoid tumor at the tip of the appendix is an appendectomy. Therapy for a carcinoid tumor of the appendix is based on tumor size and location. Simple appendectomy is adequate treatment for appendiceal carcinoid tumors less than 1 cm. Tumors larger than 2 cm should be treated with a right hemicolectomy to decrease locoregional recurrence. Treatment for tumors between 1 and 2 cm is based on location. Tumors located at the base of the appendix or invading the mesentery are best treated with a right hemicolectomy. No further treatment is needed after an appendectomy for a 1- to 2-cm tumor located at the tip of the appendix.

348. The answer is d. (*Brunicardi, pp 1331-1332.*) Acute incarceration of a previously reducible inguinal hernia may lead to strangulation. Therefore, immediate surgical repairs of inguinal hernias are indicated in cases of acute incarceration. Chronically incarcerated hernias do not have an increased risk for strangulation. Descent of the hernia into the scrotum, worsening of the pain over the hernia with walking, and development of a contralateral hernia are not indications for urgent surgical repair.

349. The answer is a. (*Townsend, pp 1577-1578.*) The patient has congenital cystic dilations of the extrahepatic biliary ducts. Nonsurgical treatment of these cysts results in high morbidity and mortality, and therefore surgery is advised in all cases. The present recommendation is for complete resection of the cyst with cholecystectomy and Roux-en-Y hepaticojejunostomy. Since malignant changes in choledochal cysts have been frequently described, complete resection rather than the performance of a drainage procedure is preferred whenever the resection can be done safely. Liver transplantation offers a potential cure for patients with intrahepatic cystic dilation (Caroli disease).

350. The answer is b. (*Townsend, pp 1256-1258.*) Stress ulceration refers to acute gastric or duodenal erosive lesions that occur following shock, sepsis, major surgery, trauma, or burns. These lesions tend to be superficial and can involve multiple sites. Unlike chronic benign gastric ulcers, which are generally found along the lesser curvature and in the antrum, acute erosive lesions usually involve the body and fundus and spare the antrum. McClelland and associates showed that patients subjected to trauma and subsequent hemorrhagic shock do not have increased gastric secretion, but rather show decreased splanchnic blood flow. Ischemic damage to the mucosa may therefore play a role.

351. The answer is a. (*Townsend, pp 1574-1575.*) Cholangitis is suggested by the presence of the Charcot triad: fever, jaundice, and pain in the right upper quadrant. In patients with suppurative cholangitis who fail to respond to intravenous antibiotics and fluid resuscitation, the nonoperative approach is the preferred intervention via either percutaneous or endoscopic drainage of the obstructed common bile duct. If endoscopic retrograde cholangiopancreatography (ERCP) or percutaneous transhepatic biliary drainage (PTBD) fails, surgery is indicated. This is usually best accomplished by surgical placement of a T tube into the duct. Cholecystostomy will be effective only if there is free flow of bile into the gallbladder via the cystic duct and in general should not be depended on to secure drainage of the common bile duct. A cholecystectomy would not provide drainage of the obstructed common bile duct.

352. The answer is a. *(Townsend, p 1560.)* High-risk, critically ill patients with multisystem disease and cholecystitis experience a significant increase in morbidity and mortality following operative intervention. Tube chole-cystostomy can be performed under local anesthesia in the operating room or via a percutaneous approach in the radiology suite. Open or laparo-scopic procedures would carry the same general anesthetic risk whether done urgently or in a delayed (elective) fashion. Lithotripsy has no role in the treatment of acute cholecystitis.

353. The answer is e. *(Townsend, pp 1603-1605.)* The patient has a pancreatic pseudocyst after his episode of acute pancreatitis. Pancreatic pseudocysts are cystic collections that do not have an epithelial lining and therefore have no malignant potential. Most pseudocysts spontaneously resolve. Therapy should not be considered for at least 6 weeks to allow for the possibility of spontaneous resolution, as well as to allow for maturation of the cyst wall if the cyst persists. Complications of pseudocysts include gastric outlet and extrahepatic biliary obstructions as well as spontaneous rupture and hemorrhage. Symptomatic or enlarging pseudocysts can be excised, externally drained, or internally drained into the GI tract (most commonly the stomach or a Roux-en-Y limb of jejunum). Percutaneous catheter drainage is not recommended because it can lead to catheter-induced infection and the development of a persistent pancreatic fistula.

354. The answer is a. *(Townsend, pp 1272-1273.)* The patient has a Dieu-lafoy lesion. It is characteristically located within 6 cm distal to the gas-troesophageal junction. Dieulafoy lesion typically consists of an abnormally large submucosal artery that protrudes through a small, solitary mucosal defect. For unclear reasons, the lesions may bleed spontaneously and mas-sively, in which case they require emergency intervention. Upper endoscopy is usually successful in localizing the lesion, and permanent hemostasis can be obtained endoscopically in most cases with injection sclerotherapy, elec-trocoagulation, or heater probe. If surgery is required, a gastrotomy and simple ligation or wedge resection of the lesion may be adequate. No large series have yet established the optimal surgical treatment for Dieulafoy lesion; however, acid-reducing procedures have not been successful in preventing further bleeding.

355. The answer is d. (*Brunicardi, p 1088.*) Carcinoid tumors arise from enterochromaffin cells in the crypts of Lieberkühn. When the tumors are larger than 1 to 2 cm or involve the base of the appendix a right hemicolectomy should be performed. When they are encountered in the tip of the appendix and are less than 1 cm in size, simple appendectomy is the procedure of choice. A total proctocolectomy is not needed for treatment of carcinoid tumors found in the appendix.

356. The answer is c. (*Brunicardi, p 1052.*) Rectal carcinoids are slowly growing tumors, but they can be locally invasive and metastasize in up to 15% of patients. Patients manifest systemic signs of the carcinoid syndrome only in the rare circumstance where hepatic metastases have occurred. The malignant potential is low in carcinoid tumors when they are less than 2 cm in diameter, as is typically the case when diagnosed. The tumors are curable by wide local transanal resection that includes the muscle layer. Endoscopic treatment leaves tumor cells near the margin of resection and is felt to increase the risk of recurrence. Whether more aggressive resection (abdominoperineal or low anterior resection [LAR]) improves the prognosis in larger tumors remains controversial. The prognosis is excellent for patients with local disease.

357. The answer is b. (*Townsend, pp 1578-1579.*) Symptomatic lesions should be removed regardless of their size. Polypoid lesions of the gallbladder are found most often in the third through fifth decades of life and are increasingly being detected by ultrasonography. These are generally small lesions that typically do not show a shadow on ultrasound. Ninety percent are benign lesions, such as cholesterol polyps (pseudotumors). True adenomas, which constitute about 10% of these benign lesions, can undergo malignant transformation. The indications for operative intervention remain controversial. Recent reviews suggest that the vast majority of malignant polypoid lesions are solitary, larger than 1.0 cm, and much more common in patients older than 50 years of age. There is also an increased incidence of malignancy if the lesions are associated with gallstones. Asymptomatic small lesions can probably be safely followed by ultrasonography.

358. The answer is a. (*Townsend, p 1610.*) Patients who undergo total pancreatectomy will have brittle diabetes and severe steatorrhea. Total or near total pancreatectomy is usually reserved for patients with chronic pancreatitis who have failed drainage procedures or who have small ducts and have already undergone distal pancreatectomy.

359. The answer is a. (*Townsend, pp 1499-1500.*) An asymptomatic patient with a hepatic hemangioma can be safely observed. Hepatic hemangiomas are the most common of all liver tumors. The diagnostic incidence of incidental hemangiomas in adults has increased in this era of noninvasive imaging of organs with MRI, ultrasonography, and CT. The mean age of presentation in adults is about 45 years, and the vast majority of these lesions are asymptomatic. There is no evidence that they undergo malignant transformation. The risk of rupture and severe hemorrhage into or from hemangiomas is extremely low. Given the typically benign and static nature of these lesions, management by angiographic embolization or resection should be reserved for the rare patient with symptomatic or complicated hemangioma (rupture, change in size, or development of Kasabach-Merritt syndrome). Percutaneous biopsy of a suspected hemangioma is dangerous and unnecessary. Hemangiomas are not associated with oral contraceptive use.

360. The answer is d. (*Brunicardi, pp 256-257.*) A CEA level is most useful as a marker for postoperative recurrence in colorectal cancer. A level is obtained every 3 months during the first 2 years after surgery to detect early recurrence that is amenable to treatment. CEA is a nonspecific tumor marker that is elevated in only about one-half of patients with colorectal tumors and is often elevated in patients with lung, pancreatic, gastric, or gynecologic malignancies. Use of CEA level as a screening test for colorectal cancer is not recommended. Although preoperative elevation of CEA level is an indicator of poor prognosis, CEA levels are not used to determine whether to give a patient adjuvant (or neoadjuvant) therapy. CEA levels are not routinely used in the preoperative setting to evaluate for metastasis in colorectal cancer. Most surgeons obtain a CT scan of the abdomen and pelvis to evaluate for metastases.

361. The answer is e. (*Brunicardi, p 876.*) Most of the time (90%), the bleeding from Mallory-Weiss syndrome will stop without any intervention. In these cases further treatment is not necessary. Patients with Mallory-Weiss syndrome typically present with a massive, painless hematemesis after severe vomiting or retching. The majority of tears occur just below the gastroesophageal junction. These tears occur more commonly in cirrhotics than in the normal population. When bleeding persists, balloon tamponade, endoscopic control of the bleeding, and surgical intervention with gastrotomy and oversewing of the tear have all been successful. Both intravenous and intra-arterial infusions of vasopressin are also useful in controlling bleeding but are contraindicated in patients with coronary artery disease.

362 to 365. The answers are 362-d, 363-e, 364-a, 365-c. (*Townsend, pp 1556-1575.*) A patient with symptomatic cholelithiasis has pain from the gallbladder as it contracts against a gallstone lodged in the cystic duct. If the stone gets dislodged with the contractions, then the pain resolves until another stone gets lodged in the cystic duct. If the gallstone remains stuck in the cystic duct, then the abdominal pain worsens as the gallbladder becomes more and more inflamed. The gallstones harbor bacteria and, if the bile becomes static with an obstructed cystic duct, infection develops. At this point the patient has acute cholecystitis and needs antibiotics or urgent cholecystectomy. Eventually the pressure in the wall of the gallbladder exceeds the perfusion pressure of the vessels in the gallbladder and the gallbladder becomes ischemic. At this stage the gallbladder becomes necrotic and can perforate causing life-threatening peritonitis and sepsis. A gallstone remaining in the common bile duct is called choledocholithiasis. Dilation of the common bile duct occurs and a CBD size > 4 mm is suspicious for a CBD stone. These patients may be asymptomatic, have abdominal pain, or progress to develop cholangitis depending on the status of the gallstone in the common bile duct. Stones that are not lodged in the sphincter of Oddi allow bile to empty out of the bile duct. Stones that become stuck in the common bile duct cause stasis of bile in the biliary system which can lead to cholangitis. The symptoms of cholangitis are right upper quadrant abdominal pain, fever, and jaundice (Charcot triad). Cholangitis is a life-threatening condition requiring emergent ERCP with stone extraction and common bile duct decompression. Sometimes patients develop acute pancreatitis with passage of the gallstone past the ampulla of Vater as it exits the common bile duct into the duodenum.

366 to 369. The answers are 366-d, 367-b, 368-b, 369-c. (*Townsend, pp 1379-1388, 1454–1460.*) The definitive operation of choice for patients with UC is total proctocolectomy with either end ileostomy or ileoanal J-pouch anastomosis. Indications for operation in UC include high-grade dysplasia or carcinoma, toxic megacolon, massive colonic bleeding, and intractability to medical therapy. Patients with either UC or Crohn can develop toxic megacolon, which is manifested by fever, abdominal pain, and marked dilation of the large bowel. Treatment consists of a subtotal colectomy with end ileostomy. For patients with UC and toxic megacolon, completion proctectomy can be performed at a later date.

For squamous cell carcinoma of the anus, the mainstay of therapy is chemoradiation with the Nigro protocol. However, recurrent or persistent disease after chemoradiation requires surgery—abdominal-perineal resection involves removing the rectum and anus with formation of a permanent end colostomy. APR is also the procedure of choice for distal rectal cancers that involve the sphincters or are too close to obtain an adequate margin (2 cm) and in patients for whom sphincter-sparing surgery is contraindicated because of fecal incontinence. Preoperative or neoadjuvant chemoradiation can sometimes cause distal rectal tumors to shrink in size such that a sphincter-sparing operation can be performed. For proximal and midrectal cancers, low anterior resection (LAR) is the procedure of choice. LAR involves the removal of the rectum to below the peritoneal reflection through an abdominal approach.

Cardiothoracic Problems

Questions

370. A 75-year-old woman with history of angina is admitted to the hospital for syncope. Examination of the patient reveals a systolic murmur best heard at the base of the heart that radiates into the carotid arteries. Electrocardiogram (ECG) is notable for left ventricular hypertrophy with evidence of left atrial enlargement. ECG reveals an aortic valve area of 0.7 cm^2. What is the most appropriate next step in her management?

a. Medical management with a nitrate and an angiotensin-converting enzyme inhibitor
b. Bilateral carotid endarterectomies
c. Percutaneous coronary artery angioplasty and stenting
d. Coronary artery bypass surgery
e. Aortic valve replacement

371. A 68-year-old man is diagnosed with lung cancer. In preparation for pulmonary resection he undergoes pulmonary function tests. Which of the following results indicate a favorable prognosis?

a. Elevated P_{CO_2}
b. Forced expiratory volume in 1 second (FEV$_1$) more than 60% of predicted
c. Carbon monoxide diffusing capacity (DLCO) less than 40%
d. Low FEV$_1$/FVC (forced vital capacity)
e. Normal FEV$_1$/FVC

372. A 71-year-old woman with a 40-year smoking history is noted to have a peripheral nodule in her left upper lobe on chest x-ray. Workup is consistent with small cell lung cancer with ipsilateral mediastinal lymph node involvement but no extrathoracic disease. What is the best treatment option for this patient?

a. Thoracotomy with left upper lobectomy and mediastinal lymph node dissection
b. Thoracotomy with left upper lobectomy and mediastinal lymph node dissection followed by adjuvant chemotherapy
c. Neoadjuvant chemotherapy followed by thoracotomy with left upper lobectomy and mediastinal lymph node dissection
d. Neoadjuvant chemoradiation followed by thoracotomy with left upper lobectomy and mediastinal lymph node dissection
e. Chemoradiation

373. A 42-year-old homeless man presents with a 3-week history of shortness of breath, fevers, and pleuritic chest pain. Chest x-ray (CXR) reveals a large left pleural effusion. Thoracentesis reveals thick, purulent-appearing fluid, which is found to have glucose less than 40 mg/dL and a pH of 6.5. A chest tube is placed, but the pleural effusion persists. Which of the following is the most appropriate management of this patient?

a. Placement of a second chest tube at the bedside and antibiotic therapy
b. Infusion of antibiotics via the chest tube
c. Intravenous antibiotics for 6 weeks
d. Thoracotomy with instillation of antibiotics into the pleural space
e. Thoracotomy with decortication and antibiotic therapy

374. A 63-year-old man is seen because of facial swelling and cyanosis, especially when he bends over. There are large, dilated subcutaneous veins on his upper chest. His jugular veins are prominent even while he is upright. Which of the following conditions is the most likely cause of these findings?

a. Histoplasmosis (sclerosing mediastinitis)
b. Substernal thyroid
c. Thoracic aortic aneurysm
d. Constrictive pericarditis
e. Bronchogenic carcinoma

375. During endoscopic biopsy of a distal esophageal cancer, perforation of the esophagus is suspected when the patient complains of significant new substernal pain. An immediate chest film reveals air in the mediastinum. Which of the following is the most appropriate management of this patient?

a. Placement of a nasogastric tube to the level of perforation, antibiotics, and close observation
b. Spit fistula (cervical pharyngostomy) and gastrostomy
c. Left thoracotomy, pleural patch oversewing of the perforation, and drainage of the mediastinum
d. Left thoracotomy with esophagectomy
e. Thoracotomy with chest tube drainage and esophageal exclusion

376. A 63-year-old woman with chronic obstructive pulmonary disease (COPD) presents with a several-week history of fever, night sweats, weight loss, and cough. Her CXR is noted to have a density in the left upper lobe with a relatively thin-walled cavity. Bronchoscopy and computed tomographic (CT) scan are suggestive of a lung abscess rather than a malignant process. Which of the following is the most appropriate initial management of this patient?

a. Percutaneous drainage of the lung abscess
b. Systemic antibiotics directed against the causative agent
c. Tube thoracostomy
d. Left upper lobectomy
e. Surgical drainage of the abscess

377. A 45-year-old man with poorly controlled hypertension presents with severe chest pain radiating to his back. An ECG demonstrates no significant abnormalities. A CT scan of the chest and abdomen is obtained, which demonstrates a descending thoracic aortic dissection extending from distal to the left subclavian takeoff down to above the iliac bifurcation. A Foley catheter is placed, and urine output is 30 to 40 cc/h. His feet are warm, with less than 2-second capillary refill. Which of the following is the most appropriate initial management?

a. Emergent operation for repair of the aortic dissection
b. Angiography to confirm the diagnosis of aortic dissection
c. Echocardiography to rule out cardiac complications
d. Initiation of a β-blocker
e. Initiation of a vasodilator such as nitroprusside

378. A stockbroker in his mid-40s presents with complaints of episodes of severe, often incapacitating chest pain on swallowing. Diagnostic studies on the esophagus yield the following results: endoscopic examination and biopsy—mild inflammation distally; manometry—prolonged high-amplitude contractions from the arch of the aorta distally, lower esophageal sphincter (LES) pressure 20 mm Hg with relaxation on swallowing; barium swallow—2-cm epiphrenic diverticulum. Which of the following is the best management option for this patient?

a. Myotomy along the length of the manometric abnormality
b. Diverticulectomy, myotomy from the level of the aortic arch to the fundus, fundoplication
c. Diverticulectomy, cardiomyotomy of the distal 3 cm of esophagus and proximal 2 cm of stomach with antireflux fundoplication
d. A trial of calcium-channel blockers
e. Pneumatic dilatation of the LES

379. A 4-year-old boy is seen 1 hour after ingestion of a lye drain cleaner. No oropharyngeal burns are noted. The CXR is normal, but the patient continues to complain of significant chest pain. Which of the following is the most appropriate next step in his management?

a. Parenteral steroids and antibiotics
b. Esophagogram with water-soluble contrast
c. Administration of an oral neutralizing agent
d. Induction of vomiting
e. Rapid administration of a quart of water to clear remaining lye from the esophagus and dilute material in the stomach

380. A previously healthy 20-year-old man is admitted to the hospital with acute onset of left-sided chest pain. Electrocardiographic findings are normal, but CXR shows a 40% left pneumothorax. Appropriate treatment consists of which of the following procedures?

a. Observation
b. Barium swallow
c. Thoracotomy
d. Tube thoracostomy
e. Thoracostomy and intubation

381. A 50-year-old salesman is on a yacht with a client when he has a severe vomiting and retching spell punctuated by a sharp substernal pain. He arrives in your emergency room 4 hours later and has a chest film in which the left descending aorta is outlined by air density. Which of the following is the most appropriate next step in his workup?

a. Contrast esophagram
b. Echocardiogram
c. Flexible bronchoscopy
d. Flexible esophagogastroscopy
e. Aortography

382. A 26-year-old man is brought to the emergency room after being extricated from the driver's seat of a car involved in a head-on collision. He has a sternal fracture and is complaining of chest pain. He is hemodynamically stable and his electrocardiogram (ECG) is normal. Which of the following is the most appropriate management strategy for this patient?

a. Admit to telemetry for 24-hour monitoring
b. Admit to the regular ward with serial ECGs for 24 hours
c. Emergent cardiac catheterization
d. Immediate operative plating of the sternal fracture
e. Discharge to home with nonsteroidal anti-inflammatory agents for the sternal fracture

383. A 63-year-old man underwent a 3-vessel coronary artery bypass graft (CABG) 5 hours ago. Initially, his mediastinal chest tube output was 300 mL blood/h, but an hour ago, there was no further evidence of bleeding from the tube. His mean arterial pressure has fallen, and several fluid boluses were administered. His central venous pressure (CVP) is elevated to 20 mm Hg, and he has required the addition of inotropes. Which of the following is the best management strategy?

a. Addition of vasopressors along with the inotropes
b. Transfusion of packed red blood cells
c. Return to the operating room for exploration of the mediastinum
d. Placement of an intraaortic balloon pump
e. Infusion of streptokinase into the mediastinal chest tube

384. Several days following esophagectomy, a patient complains of dyspnea and chest tightness. A large pleural effusion is noted on chest radiograph, and thoracentesis yields milky fluid consistent with chyle. Which of the following is the most appropriate initial management of this patient?

a. Immediate operation to repair the thoracic duct
b. Immediate operation to ligate the thoracic duct
c. Tube thoracostomy and low-fat diet
d. Observation and low-fat diet
e. Observation and antibiotics

385. A 56-year-old woman presents for evaluation of a murmur suggestive of mitral stenosis and is noted on echocardiography to have a lesion attached to the fossa ovalis of the left atrial septum. The mass is causing obstruction of the mitral valve. Which of the following is the most likely diagnosis?

a. Endocarditis
b. Lymphoma
c. Cardiac sarcoma
d. Cardiac myxoma
e. Metastatic cancer to the heart

386. A 56-year-old woman has been treated for 3 years for wheezing on exertion, which was diagnosed as asthma. Chest radiograph, shown here, reveals a midline mass compressing the trachea. Which of the following is the most likely diagnosis?

a. Lymphoma
b. Neurogenic tumor
c. Lung carcinoma
d. Goiter
e. Pericardial cyst

387. A 59-year-old man is found to have a 6-cm thoracoabdominal aortic aneurysm which extends to above the renal arteries for which he desires repair, but he is concerned about the risk of paralysis postoperatively. Which of the following maneuvers should be employed to decrease the risk of paraplegia after repair?

a. Infusion of a bolus of steroids immediately postoperatively with a continuous infusion for 24 hours
b. Maintenance of intraoperative normothermia
c. Clamping of the aorta proximal to the left subclavian artery
d. Cerebrospinal fluid (CSF) drainage
e. Extracorporeal membrane oxygenation

388. An 89-year-old man has lost 30 lb over the past 2 years. He reports that food frequently sticks when he swallows. He also complains of a chronic cough. Barium swallow is shown here. What is the best treatment option for this patient?

a. Placement of an esophageal stent
b. Diverticuloplasty
c. Excision of the diverticulum
d. Excision of the diverticulum and administration of a promotility agent
e. Excision of the diverticulum and cricopharyngeal myotomy

389. A 70-year-old woman undergoes a cardiac catheterization for exertional chest pain. Her pain continues to worsen and she is interested in having either surgery or percutaneous coronary intervention (PCI). Which of the following would be an indication for her to undergo either coronary artery bypass grafting or PCI?

a. Two-vessel coronary disease with proximal left anterior descending artery stenosis and depressed left ventricular ejection fraction
b. Isolated left main stenosis, no diabetes, and normal left ventricular ejection fraction
c. Isolated left main stenosis and diabetes
d. Left main stenosis and additional coronary artery disease with depressed left ventricular ejection fraction.
e. Three-vessel coronary artery disease and diabetes

390. A 27-year-old woman seeks your advice regarding pain and numbness in the right arm and hand. She reports that it is exacerbated by raising her arm over her head. On examination, the right radial pulse disappears when the patient takes a deep breath and turns her head to the left. A provisional diagnosis is made. Which of the following is the most appropriate initial treatment for this patient?

a. Physical rehabilitation
b. Gabapentin to treat neuropathic pain
c. Right first rib resection
d. Thoracoscopic sympathectomy
e. Upper thoracic discectomy

391. A 35-year-old man with a history of melanoma status post wide local excision with negative margins and lymph node dissection presents with 2, peripherally-located pulmonary lesions seen on chest CT scan. Percutaneous biopsy of the lesion is consistent with metastatic melanoma. He has no evidence of recurrence or extrathoracic disease and is in good general health. Which of the following is the most appropriate management of this patient?

a. Chemotherapy
b. Radiation therapy
c. Pulmonary metastasectomy
d. Pulmonary metastasectomy followed by radiation therapy
e. Neoadjuvant radiation therapy followed by pulmonary metastasectomy

392. A 65-year-old woman has had pain in her right shoulder and has been treated with analgesics without relief. The CXR reveals a mass in the apex of the right chest. A transthoracic needle biopsy documents carcinoma. Superior pulmonary sulcus carcinomas (Pancoast tumors) are bronchogenic carcinomas that typically produce which of the following clinical features?

a. Atelectasis of the involved apical segment
b. Horner syndrome
c. Pain in the T4 and T5 dermatomes
d. Nonproductive cough
e. Hemoptysis

393. A 63-year-old man has a chylothorax that after 2 weeks of conservative therapy appears to be persistent. The chest tube output is approximately 600 mL/day. Appropriate management at this time includes which of the following procedures?

a. Neck exploration and ligation of the thoracic duct
b. Subdiaphragmatic ligation of the thoracic duct
c. Thoracotomy and repair of the thoracic duct
d. Thoracotomy and ligation of the thoracic duct
e. Thoracotomy and abrasion of the pleural space

394. A 32-year-old woman has a CXR screening, and a 1.5-cm mass is noted in the right lower lobe. She is a nonsmoker. Bronchoscopy shows a mass in the right lower lobe orifice, covered with mucosa. Biopsy indicates this is compatible with a carcinoid tumor. Imaging suggests ipsilateral mediastinal lymph node involvement but no extrathoracic disease. Which of the following is the most appropriate treatment plan?

a. Right lower lobectomy and mediastinal lymph node dissection
b. Right lower lobectomy and mediastinal lymph node dissection followed by adjuvant chemotherapy
c. Neoadjuvant chemotherapy followed by right lower lobectomy and mediastinal lymph node dissection
d. Neoadjuvant chemoradiation followed by right lower lobectomy and mediastinal lymph node dissection
e. Chemoradiation

395. Six months ago at the time of lumpectomy for breast cancer, a 60-year-old female attorney quit a 30-year smoking habit of 2 packs per day. She had the chest radiograph shown here as part of her routine follow-up examination. Based on her age and history of smoking, you are concerned for either a new primary lung or metastatic breast malignancy. Which of the following is the most appropriate next step in the management of this lesion?

a. Follow-up CT scan in 3 months
b. Magnetic resonance imaging of bilateral breasts to evaluate for recurrence of the breast cancer
c. Transthoracic fine-needle aspiration of the lesion
d. Mediastinoscopy
e. Thoracotomy with lobectomy

396. A 42-year-old man presents with a solitary lung lesion. At the time of operation on this patient, a firm, rubbery lesion in the periphery of the lung is discovered. It is sectioned in the operating room to reveal tissue that looks like cartilage and smooth muscle. Which of the following is the most likely diagnosis?

a. Fibroma
b. Chondroma
c. Osteochondroma
d. Hamartoma
e. Aspergilloma

397. A 45-year-old woman presents with dysphagia, regurgitation of undigested food, and weight loss. She had x-rays shown here as part of her workup. Upper endoscopy reveals no evidence of malignancy and esophageal motility studies show incomplete lower esophageal sphincter relaxation. Which of the following is the next best step in the treatment of this patient?

a. Laparoscopic myotomy of the lower esophageal sphincter (Heller)
b. Laparoscopic posterior 180° (Toupet) fundoplication
c. Laparoscopic anterior 180° (Dor) fundoplication
d. Laparoscopic 360° (Nissen) fundoplication
e. Transhiatal esophagectomy

Questions 398 to 402

For each physical finding or group of findings, select the cardiovascular disorder with which it is most likely to be associated. Each lettered option may be used once, more than once, or not at all.

a. Massive tricuspid regurgitation
b. Aortic regurgitation
c. Coarctation of the aorta
d. Thoracic aortic aneurysm
e. Myocarditis

398. An elderly man with abnormal pupillary responses (Argyll Robertson pupil).

399. A 24-year-old drug addict with jugular venous distention and exophthalmos.

400. A patient with flushing and paling of the nail beds (Quincke pulse) and a bounding radial pulse.

401. A patient with conjunctivitis, urethral discharge, and arthralgia.

402. A patient with short stature, webbed neck, low-set ears, and epicanthal folds.

Questions 403 to 407

For each clinical scenario, select the mediastinal tumor with which it is most likely to be associated. Each lettered option may be used once, more than once, or not at all.

a. Thymoma
b. Hodgkin disease
c. Pheochromocytoma
d. Parathyroid adenoma
e. Cystic teratoma

403. A 23-year-old patient with hypertension and increased urinary catecholamine levels.

404. A 21-year-old woman presents with generalized weakness and double vision. During her workup, she is noted to have a widened mediastinum on her CXR prompting a CT scan, which demonstrates an anterior mediastinal mass.

405. A 63-year-old woman with vague symptoms of fatigue and depression presents with hematuria. CT scan of the abdomen and pelvis reveals a stone at the ureteropelvic junction.

406. A 35-year-old woman with fever and weight loss. CT scan revealed a mediastinal mass, which was biopsied and revealed Reed-Sternberg cells.

407. A 33-year-old woman presents with cough and chest pain for 2 months. More recently, she complains of coughing up hair. The CXR reveals a mediastinal mass.

Questions 408 to 412

For each clinical scenario, select the most appropriate pharmacologic agent for the patient. Each lettered option may be used once, more than once, or not at all.

a. Epinephrine
b. Norepinephrine
c. Phenylephrine
d. Dopamine
e. Dobutamine
f. Nitroprusside
g. Nitroglycerin

408. A 56-year-old man presents with a blood pressure of 220/110 mm Hg, chest pain, and ST elevations on an ECG.

409. A 65-year-old man presents with cardiogenic shock following a myocardial infarction.

410. A 30-year-old man presents with perforated appendicitis and heart rate of 120 beats per minute, blood pressure of 80/40 mm Hg, and central venous pressure of 17 mm Hg. The patient remains hypotensive after a continuous infusion of dopamine.

411. A 21-year-old man undergoes major abdominal surgery after a motor vehicle collision. He has a cardiac arrest in the intensive care unit shortly after returning from surgery.

412. A 45-year-old woman presents with a blood pressure of 220/130 mm Hg and a headache. After several hours of an intravenous drip of medication to control her hypertension, she becomes acidotic.

Cardiothoracic Problems

Answers

370. The answer is e. *(Townsend, pp 1841-1844.)* The patient's history, physical examination, and findings on heart studies are classic for aortic stenosis. The only effective therapy with good long-term results is aortic valve replacement, with most patients achieving symptom relief after surgery. Percutaneous aortic balloon valvuloplasty is an option for patients who are not candidates for aortic valve replacement or whose long-term survival is poor. Valvuloplasty involves passing balloon catheters through the aortic orifice and inflating them in an effort to break the calcium that is retarding leaflet motion. The results are not as durable as those for valve replacement, with a third of the patients having recurrent symptoms by 6 months.

Aortic stenosis is most often thought to result from calcification of the aortic valve associated with advanced age. The process is mostly idiopathic, with only a small percentage associated with rheumatic fever. Patients may not develop symptoms until the aortic valve area is about 1 cm^2. Symptoms may include angina, congestive heart failure, or syncope. The combination of aortic stenosis and congestive heart failure, which is the presenting symptom in nearly one-third of patients, has a worse prognosis. Medical management, percutaneous coronary artery angioplasty and stenting, and coronary artery bypass surgery are options for angina due to coronary artery disease. Carotid endarterectomy is the treatment of choice for carotid artery stenosis.

371. The answer is b. *(Townsend, pp 1700-1703.)* The predicted postoperative forced expiratory volume in 1 second is the most commonly used predictor of postoperative pulmonary reserve. Usually FEV$_1$ may be expressed as an actual value of liter per second or as a percentage. The percent predicted value takes into account the body habitus. Most patients will tolerate a lobectomy with an FEV$_1$ greater than 60% of predicted. An elevated PCO$_2$ greater than 45 mm Hg suggests severe pulmonary disease with nearly 50% functional loss of the lung. Carbon monoxide diffusing capacity measures the rate at which carbon monoxide moves from the alveolar space to combine with hemoglobin in the red blood cells. It is determined by calculating the difference between inspired and expired samples of gas. DLCO levels less than 40% to 50% are associated with increased perioperative risk. FEV_1/FVC is useful in determining obstructive versus restrictive lung disease. The ratio is low (FEV_1 is reduced and FVC is high) in obstructive disease. In restrictive disease the ratio is normal because both FEV_1 and FVC are reduced.

372. The answer is e. (*Townsend, p 1711.*) Small cell lung cancers are treated primarily with chemotherapy and radiation; they are rarely amenable to surgical resection because of extensive disease at presentation. Small cell lung cancer accounts for about 20% of primary lung cancers. Most are centrally located and characterized by an aggressive tendency to metastasize. They spread early to mediastinal lymph nodes and distant sites, most commonly to the bone marrow and the brain.

373. The answer is e. (*Mulholland, p 1414.*) The patient has an empyema or the accumulation of pus in the pleural cavity. Based on the history (3 weeks of symptoms) and the fluid analysis demonstrating a glucose level less than 40 mg/dL and a pH less than 7.0 and its thick consistency, the patient's empyema is in the most advanced stage or the chronic organizing phase. In this phase, the fluid collection is loculated and depositions of fibrin create a thick pleural rind, which prevents apposition of the lung to the parietal pleura. Reexpansion of the lung requires thoracotomy with decortication to remove the purulent fluid and the pleural rind. Antibiotic therapy tailored to the organism(s) identified is necessary but not sufficient to treat an empyema.

374. The answer is e. (*Mulholland, p 1423.*) Superior vena cava obstruction (SVC syndrome) is almost always due to malignancy (90% of cases) and in 3 out of 4 cases, results from invasion of the vena cava by bronchogenic carcinoma. Lymphomas are the second most common cause of the SVC syndrome. Fibrosing mediastinitis as a complication of histoplasmosis or ingestion of methysergide may occur, but is rare. Rarely, a substernal thyroid or thoracic aortic aneurysm may be responsible for the obstruction. SVC syndrome can be caused iatrogenically secondary to indwelling catheters. Although constrictive pericarditis may decrease venous return to the heart, it does not produce obstruction of the superior vena cava. Whatever the cause of the superior vena cava syndrome, the resultant increased venous pressure produces edema of the upper body, cyanosis, dilated subcutaneous collateral vessels in the chest, and headache. Cervical lymphadenopathy may also be present as a result of either stasis or metastatic involvement. Initial management of superior vena cava syndrome consists of diuresis, and for malignancies, the treatment consists of radiation and chemotherapy if applicable. Occasionally, surgical intervention or thrombolysis may be indicated for severe life-threatening complications.

375. The answer is d. (*Mulholland, pp 667-668.*) Perforation of the esophagus in the chest is a surgical catastrophe that requires aggressive intervention in virtually all circumstances. Diagnosis is typically confirmed with a contrast esophagogram. A study using water-soluble contrast (such as a Gastrografin swallow) is typically ordered initially; if no leak is identified, the study is repeated using thin barium. A water-soluble contrast is used initially because of concerns for mediastinitis due to barium in the presence of an esophageal perforation. The management, in a patient with no underlying esophageal disorder, is primarily surgical—directed at primary repair of the perforation and drainage of the mediastinum. In patients with an underlying motility disorder, stricture, or malignancy, surgical intervention must address both the perforation and the esophageal abnormality. For patients with a distal esophageal carcinoma, treatment usually requires esophagectomy. Esophageal exclusion or proximal diversion (with a cervical esophagostomy or "spit fistula") are typically reserved for patients in whom a late diagnosis of esophageal perforation was made.

376. The answer is b. (*Brunicardi, pp 541-551.*) Initial treatment of a lung abscess, once the diagnosis has been made, is systemic antibiotics directed against the causative agent. The duration of therapy is dependent on the severity of the underlying pneumonia that resulted in the abscess and can last up to 12 weeks. Often, the abscess drains spontaneously via the tracheobronchial tree, but, if it fails to resolve with medical therapy, intervention may be required, ranging from percutaneous to surgical drainage of the abscess or resectional therapy.

377. The answer is d. (*Brunicardi, pp 689-695.*) The initial treatment for a descending aortic dissection is to reduce the rate of change in blood pressure and to reduce shear on the aortic wall, which is achieved with β-blockade. Nitroprusside may be added after β-blockade has been achieved. Indications for operative intervention for a descending aortic dissection are end-organ failure (renal failure, lower extremity ischemia, intestinal ischemia), inadequate pain relief despite optimal medical therapy, and rupture or signs of impending rupture (increasing diameter or periaortic fluid).

378. The answer is a. (*Brunicardi, pp 851-852.*) The finding of prolonged high-amplitude contractions in the body of the esophagus in a highly symptomatic patient is diagnostic of diffuse esophageal spasm (DES). None of the findings revealed by the diagnostic studies listed (minimal reflux esophagitis, normal LES relaxation and pressure, and an incidental small epiphrenic diverticulum) justifies treatment and none explains the patient's symptoms. The cause of the hypermotility disorder known as DES is unknown, but its symptoms can be disabling. The recommended treatment for this relatively rare disorder is a long myotomy guided by the manometric evidence. More than 90% of patients treated in this fashion will experience acceptable relief of symptoms if the myotomy is performed correctly.

379. The answer is b. (*Mulholland, pp 671-672.*) Corrosive injuries of the esophagus most frequently occur in young children because of accidental ingestion of strong alkaline cleaning agents. Signs of airway injury or imminent obstruction warrant close observation and possibly tracheostomy. An initial esophagogram with water-soluble contrast (Gastrografin) is performed if a perforation is suspected or for localization of a perforation prior to surgical intervention. Vomiting should be avoided, if possible, to prevent further corrosive injury and possible aspiration. Administration of oral antidotes is ineffective unless given within moments of ingestion; even then, the additional damage potentially caused by the chemical reactions of neutralization often makes use of them unwise. Attempted dilution of the caustic agent is not recommended, given that most of the damage has already occurred, and increasing the gastric volume may induce nausea and vomiting. Based on lack of evidence of efficacy in preventing strictures and potential deleterious side effects, steroids are not recommended. Parenteral antibiotics are indicated in cases with significant esophageal injury. It is probably wise to avoid all oral intake until the full extent of injury is ascertained.

380. The answer is d. (*Mulholland, p 1409.*) Spontaneous pneumothorax usually results from the rupture of subpleural blebs in young men (age 20-40 years), which is often signaled by a sudden onset of chest and shoulder pain. Large pneumothoraxes require placement of a chest tube; thoracotomy with bleb excision and pleural abrasion is generally recommended if spontaneous pneumothorax is recurrent. Small pneumothoraces in patients with minimal symptoms usually resolve and therefore can simply be observed. A spontaneous perforation of the esophagus (Boerhaave syndrome) can result in hydropneumothorax as well as the more usual pneumomediastinum, but would not present with an isolated 40% pneumothorax. Gastrografin swallow followed by a barium study is appropriate diagnostic test for evaluation of a suspected leaking esophagus.

381. The answer is a. *(Townsend, pp 1082-1086)* The presence of air in the mediastinum after an episode of vomiting and retching is virtually pathognomonic of spontaneous rupture of the esophagus (Boerhaave syndrome). A contrast esophagram is the initial test of choice and is indicated with barium for a suspected thoracic perforation and water-soluble contrast (Gastrografin) for an abdominal perforation. Barium is inert in the chest but causes peritonitis in the abdomen, whereas aspirated Gastrografin can cause severe pneumonitis. CT scanning may be useful if a small, contained leak is suspected. A surgical endoscopy needs to be performed if the imaging studies are negative with a high degree of suspicion for an esophageal injury. If the leak is contained and the patient does not have any evidence of sepsis, then the leak can be managed with antibiotics and expectant management. For leaks associated with systemic signs, patients should undergo prompt surgical therapy. The operation of choice is dependent on the time to diagnosis. Leaks that are less than 24 hours old in patients without an underlying esophageal disorder may be managed with thoracotomy, repair, and drainage. Leaks older than 24 hours typically require more extensive surgery.

382. The answer is a. *(Moore, pp 578-583; Mulholland, pp 378-382.)* There are no universally accepted criteria for the diagnosis of myocardial contusion. Therefore, if there is a significant clinical suspicion, then the patient should be monitored on telemetry or in the intensive care unit for 24 hours. An initial ECG may demonstrate ST- or T-wave changes (which are not specific for a myocardial contusion), arrhythmias, or bundle branch blocks. However, a normal ECG does not rule out a myocardial contusion. Similarly, cardiac enzymes may be elevated, including the CKMB fraction, but are neither sensitive nor specific for a myocardial contusion. Echocardiography may demonstrate wall motion abnormalities, valvular disruption, or a pericardial effusion with or without tamponade. Antiarrhythmics are not indicated prophylactically in a patient with a myocardial contusion, but should be used to treat any rhythm disturbances. Supportive therapy for myocardial contusion is directed at inotropic support of the ventricle; the coronary arteries are usually intact after the injury, so there is little role for coronary vasodilators and less for coronary artery bypass surgery.

383. The answer is c. (*Townsend, pp 1819-1820.*) Cardiac tamponade is a life-threatening complication that can occur after CABG. If the patient has bleeding postoperatively, the patient's coagulopathy should be corrected. Clotting of the mediastinal chest tube followed by hemodynamic decompensation with decreased mean arterial pressures (MAPs) and cardiac output with increasing filling pressures is suggestive of tamponade. Equalization of pressures across the 4 chambers on Swan-Ganz catheter monitoring or collapse of the right atrium on echocardiography is diagnostic of tamponade. The patient should return to the operating room for exploration and drainage of the mediastinal hematoma.

384. The answer is c. (*Mulholland, pp 1879-1881.*) A low-fat, medium-chain triglyceride diet often reduces the flow of chyle. Chylothorax may occur after intrathoracic surgery, or it may follow malignant invasion or compression of the thoracic duct. Intraoperative recognition of a thoracic duct injury is managed by ligation of the duct. Direct repair is impractical owing to the extreme friability of the thoracic duct. Injuries not recognized until several days after intrathoracic surgery frequently heal following the institution of a low-fat diet and either repeated thoracentesis or tube thoracostomy drainage.

385. The answer is d. (*Brunicardi, pp 660-661.*) The most common benign cardiac tumor is a myxoma. Symptoms can include valvular obstruction (mitral or tricuspid valve) or embolization systemically. Histologic examination of a peripheral embolus can confirm the diagnosis. In the heart, they are often attached by a pedicle to the fossa ovalis of the left atrial septum. Treatment is resection.

386. The answer is d. (*Mulholland, pp 1860-1861.*) The boundaries of the mediastinum are the thoracic inlet, the diaphragm, the sternum, the vertebral column, and the pleura bilaterally. The mediastinum itself is divided into 3 portions delineated by the pericardial sac: the anterosuperior and posterosuperior regions are in front of and behind the sac, respectively, while the middle region designates the contents of the pericardium. In adults, mediastinal masses occur most frequently in the anterosuperior region and less often in the posterosuperior and middle regions. Cysts (pericardial, bronchogenic, or enteric) are the most common tumors of the middle region; neurogenic tumors are the most common of the primary tumors of the posterior mediastinum. The primary neoplasms of the mediastinum in the anteroposterior region (in order of descending frequency) are thymomas, lymphomas, and germ cell tumors. More commonly, though, a mass in this area represents the substernal extension of a benign substernal goiter. Diagnosis may be made by visualization of an enhancing structure on CT; radioactive iodine scanning is useful in management because it may make the diagnosis if the mediastinal tissue is functional and will also document the presence of functioning cervical thyroid tissue to prevent removal of all functional thyroid tissue during mediastinal excision.

387. The answer is a. *(Brunicardi, pp 678-679.)* Operative intervention is usually recommended for thoracic aortic aneurysms greater than 5 or 6 cm in diameter or those that are increasing in size. Spinal cord ischemia can result in paraplegia with a risk of 5% to 15%, depending on the extent of the repair. Various strategies that have been employed to prevent spinal cord ischemia include aggressive reattachment of segmental intercostal and lumbar arteries, minimizing cross-clamp time (moving the clamp sequentially more and more distally as branches are reattached), hypothermia, moderate systemic heparinization, left heart bypass, and cerebrospinal fluid drainage (using a lumbar drain). The rationale for cerebrospinal fluid drainage is that it decreases the pressure on the blood supply to the spinal cord and therefore improves perfusion. Postoperative steroids do not reduce the risk of paraplegia.

388. The answer is e. *(Brunicardi, pp 848-850.)* The barium swallow shows a pharyngoesophageal (Zenker) diverticulum, which is an outpouching of mucosa between the lower pharyngeal constrictor and the cricopharyngeus muscles. Surgical treatment is excision of the diverticulum (or diverticulopexy which inverts the diverticulum) and division of the cricopharyngeus muscle (cricopharyngeal myotomy), which can be done under local anesthesia in a cooperative patient. A Zenker diverticulum is thought to result from an incoordination of cricopharyngeal relaxation with swallowing. These diverticula occur in elderly patients and more commonly on the left. The typical patient presents with complaints of dysphagia, weight loss, and choking. Other patients present symptoms such as repeated aspiration, pneumonia, or chronic cough. A mass is sometimes palpable, and a gurgle may be heard. Diagnosis is made with a barium swallow; endoscopy is indicated if there is concern for malignancy (which is rarely associated with Zenker diverticulum). Esophagoscopy should be performed cautiously because the blind pouch is easily perforated. Even though the pouch may extend down into the mediastinum, the origin of the diverticulum is at the cricopharyngeus muscle near the level of the bifurcation of the carotid artery.

389. The answer is a. (*Townsend, pp 1802-1812; Mulholland, p 1472.*) Coronary artery bypass grafting (CABG) is indicated in patients with angina (chronic, unstable, or postinfarction) and in asymptomatic patients with ischemia on cardiac stress tests. CABG offers a long-term survival benefit in patients with multivessel disease, left main coronary artery disease, and 1-vessel and 2-vessel disease with proximal left anterior descending (LAD) coronary artery obstruction. CABG is the treatment of choice in diabetic patients. CABG and percutaneous coronary intervention (PCI) are both appropriate in patients with 2-vessel disease and proximal LAD obstruction. For all of the other choices, it is either uncertain or inappropriate to choose PCI over CABG.

390. The answer is a. (*Mulholland, pp 1401-1403.*) The patient has thoracic outlet syndrome. The initial treatment should be conservative management with an exercise program to strengthen shoulder girdle muscles and decrease shoulder droop. Operative treatment includes division of the scalenus anticus and medius muscles, first rib resection, cervical rib resection, or a combination of all three. Gabapentin may be prescribed to treat neuropathic pain, but is not the primary treatment of thoracic outlet syndrome. Thoracoscopic sympathectomy is a surgical treatment for hyperhidrosis. Carpal tunnel syndrome and cervical disk disease can be commonly confused with thoracic outlet syndrome. Since the innervation of the brachial plexus is derived from the nerve roots C5-T1, upper thoracic discectomy is unlikely to be helpful.

Thoracic outlet syndrome is felt to result from compression of the brachial plexus or subclavian vessels, or both, in the anatomic space bounded by the first rib, the clavicle, and the scalene muscles. Symptoms and signs include pain, paresthesias, edema, venous congestion, and digital vasospastic changes.

Positional dampening or obliteration of the radial pulse is an unreliable finding, since it is present in up to 70% of the normal population. Plain films may diagnose bony abnormalities, and MRI can be useful in detecting cervical disease. Neurologic abnormalities may be documented by nerve conduction studies. Angiographic studies are often negative.

391. The answer is c. *(Mulholland, pp 1381-1385; Brunicardi, p 549.)* The appropriate treatment for this patient is pulmonary metastasectomy. He meets all criteria for resection, including (a) control of the primary lesion, (b) no evidence of extrathoracic disease, (c) ability to tolerate pulmonary resection including possible single-lung ventilation, (d) predicted ability to achieve a complete resection, and (e) lack of a more effective systemic therapy. Pulmonary metastasectomy has been performed for sarcomas, melanomas, germ cell tumors, and carcinomas including colon, renal cell, endometrial, and head and neck. There is no role for radiation therapy pre- or postoperatively for melanoma.

392. The answer is b. *(Brunicardi, pp 544-546.)* Pancoast tumors are peripheral bronchogenic carcinomas that produce symptoms by involvement of extrapulmonary structures adjacent to the cupula. These structures include the nerve roots of C8 and T1, as well as the sympathetic trunk. Interruption of the cervical sympathetic trunk leads to miosis, ptosis, and anhidrosis, the triad of signs that constitutes Horner syndrome. Involvement of the nerve roots causes pain along the corresponding dermatomes. The peripheral location of the neoplasm makes pulmonary signs, such as atelectasis, cough, and hemoptysis, unlikely.

393. The answer is d. *(Mulholland, pp 1879-1881.)* The initial treatment for a chylothorax consists of nonoperative therapy: drainage of the chest cavity, bowel rest, and total parenteral nutrition. However, if chyle drainage continues to be greater than 500 mL/day, then operative ligation of the thoracic duct should be performed. The best approach if the site of the leak cannot be identified is from a right thoracotomy—the thoracic duct is ligated from the diaphragm to T6. The thoracic duct enters the chest from the abdomen through the aortic hiatus of the diaphragm, courses on the right side of the chest, and then curves to the left at the level of the fifth thoracic vertebra.

394. The answer is a. *(Mulholland, pp 1377-1378.)* The primary therapy for a bronchial carcinoid is operative resection, which may include a lobectomy or lesser resection as long as the tumor is completely excised as well as mediastinal lymph node sampling or dissection. Chemotherapy and radiation therapy do not have a role in the treatment of bronchial carcinoids. These are slow-growing, infrequently metastatic tumors that histologically resemble carcinoid tumors of the small intestine. More than 80% arise in the major proximal bronchi, and their intraluminal growth is responsible for the frequent presentation of bronchial obstruction. The low malignant potential for this lesion is reflected by a long-term survival rate that approaches 90%.

395. The answer is c. (*Brunicardi, pp 526-528.*) Coin lesions have been defined as densities within the lung field of up to 3 cm, usually round, and free of signs of infections such as cavitation or surrounding infiltrates. Coin lesions should be biopsied to rule out malignancy. The differential diagnosis for coin lesions includes primary pulmonary carcinomas, metastatic carcinomas to the lung, benign lung neoplasms such as chondromas, other benign lung processes such as granulomas, or vascular abnormalities such as arteriovenous malformations. Malignant solitary lesions may contain flecks of calcification, but heavy calcification or concentric rings of calcium generally suggest a benign etiology. Transthoracic fine-needle aspiration (FNA) can be used for diagnosis, with an accuracy of 95% for peripheral pulmonary lesions, but is associated with a high rate of complications. Thoracoscopic resection can be used for peripheral nodules not amenable to FNA. Bronchoscopy can be performed for lesions if an air-bronchogram is present or if the operator is experienced at endoscopic ultrasound and transbronchial biopsy. Observation with high-resolution CT scans at regular intervals should be reserved for lesions with a low suspicion of malignancy based on patient history and lesion characteristics. Workup for recurrence of breast cancer may be reasonable, but magnetic resonance imaging of the breasts will not rule out a new primary or metastatic malignancy of the lung.

396. The answer is d. (*Mulholland, pp 1385-1386.*) The term *hamartoma* denotes a tumor that arises from the disorganized arrangement of tissues normally found in an organ. Pulmonary hamartomas are solitary lesions of the pulmonary parenchyma and generally appear as asymptomatic peripheral nodules; they represent the most common benign epithelial and mesodermal elements. Pulmonary chondromas consist of mesodermal elements alone and arise centrally in major bronchi, where they produce signs and symptoms of bronchial obstruction. Fibromas are the most common benign mesodermal tumors found in the lung; they may occur either within the lung parenchyma or, more commonly, within the tracheobronchial tree. Osteochondromas are lesions of bone and are not found in the lung. Aspergillomas are caused by infection with the fungus *Aspergillus* and most commonly appear in the upper lobes as oval, friable, necrotic gray, or yellow masses often surrounded by evidence of preexisting parenchymal lung disease.

397. The answer is b. *(Brunicardi, pp 857-862.)* The studies are consistent with a diagnosis of achalasia, a motility disorder of the esophagus that usually affects persons between 30 and 50 years of age. Treatment options include botulinum toxin injection into the lower esophageal sphincter, balloon dilation, or surgical myotomy of the lower esophageal sphincter (Heller myotomy) with or without an accompanying antireflux procedure. Surgical myotomy can be performed open or laparoscopically and approached either through the chest or through the abdomen. Anterior 180° (Dor), posterior 180° (Toupet), and 360° fundoplications are all options for treating gastroesophageal reflux. Whether an antireflux procedure is necessary in addition to a Heller myotomy for achalasia is controversial, but these procedures are never used alone in the absence of a Heller myotomy. Esophagectomy is indicated for achalasia only in the presence of end-stage disease with loss of esophageal contractions or in the setting of esophageal cancer.

The diagnosis of achalasia is generally suspected on the basis of barium studies. The x-rays for this question show a classic beak-like narrowing of the distal esophagus and a large, dilated esophagus proximal to the narrowing. However, because other esophageal disorders may mimic achalasia, an esophageal motility study is usually required to confirm the diagnosis. The characteristic findings on a motility study are small-amplitude, repetitive, simultaneous postdeglutition contractions in the body of the esophagus, incomplete relaxation of the lower esophageal sphincter, and a higher-than-normal pressure in the body of the esophagus. Carcinoma of the esophagus is approximately 7 times more frequent in persons who have achalasia than in the general population.

398 to 402. The answers are 398-d, 399-a, 400-b, 401-e, 402-c. *(Mulholland, pp 1439-1440, 1453-1458, 1706-1710.)* The Argyll Robertson pupil (a pupil that constricts with accommodation but not in response to light) is characteristic of central nervous system syphilis and is associated with vascular system manifestations of that disease. *Treponema pallidum* invades the vasa vasorum and causes an obliterative endarteritis and necrosis. The resulting aortitis gradually weakens the aortic wall and predisposes it to aneurysm formation. Once an aneurysm has formed, the prognosis is grave. Massive isolated tricuspid regurgitation produces a markedly elevated venous pressure, usually manifested by a severely engorged (often pulsating) liver. If the venous pressure is sufficiently elevated, exophthalmos may result. Tricuspid regurgitation of rheumatic origin is almost never an isolated lesion, and the major symptoms of patients who have rheumatic heart disease are usually attributable to concurrent left heart lesions. Bacterial endocarditis from intravenous drug abuse is becoming an increasingly important cause of isolated tricuspid regurgitation. A Quincke pulse, which consists of alternate flushing and paling of the skin or nail beds, is associated with aortic regurgitation. Other characteristic features of the peripheral pulse in aortic regurgitation include the waterhammer pulse (Corrigan pulse, caused by a rapid systolic upstroke) and pulsus bisferiens, which describes a double systolic hump in the pulse contour. The finding of a wide pulse pressure provides an additional diagnostic clue to aortic regurgitation. Myocarditis, aortitis, and pericarditis have all been described in association with Reiter syndrome; the original description included conjunctivitis, urethritis, and arthralgias. Although its cause is unknown, Reiter syndrome is associated with HLA-B27 antigen, as are aortic regurgitation, pericarditis, and ankylosing spondylitis. Short stature, webbed neck, low-set ears, and epicanthal folds are the classic features of patients who have Turner syndrome. Persons affected by the syndrome, which is commonly linked with aortic coarctation, are genotypically XO. However, females and males have been described with normal sex chromosome constitutions (XX, XY) but with the phenotypic abnormalities of Turner syndrome. Additional cardiac lesions associated with Turner syndrome include septal defects, valvular stenosis, and anomalies of the great vessels.

403 to 407. The answers are 403-c, 404-a, 405-d, 406-b, 407e. (*Mulholland, pp 1862-1864.*) Mediastinal pheochromocytomas comprise less than 2% of all pheochromocytomas. Their presentation is consistent with overproduction of catecholamines, resulting in paroxysmal or sustained hypertension. Diagnosis is by measurement of urinary catecholamines and their metabolites. Thymomas are associated with myasthenia gravis, agammaglobulinemia, and red blood cell aplasia. These tumors are typically cystic and occur in the anterior mediastinum. Most thymic lesions associated with myasthenia gravis are hyperplastic rather than neoplastic. Renal stones occur in about half the cases of hyperparathyroidism. Other disorders sometimes associated with hyperparathyroidism include peptic ulcers, pancreatitis, and bone disease; central nervous system symptoms may also arise in connection with hyperparathyroidism. Occasionally, parathyroid adenomas occur in conjunction with neoplasms of other endocrine organs, a condition known as multiple endocrine adenomatosis. Persons afflicted with Hodgkin disease have impaired cell-mediated immunity and are particularly susceptible to mycotic infections and tuberculosis. The severity of the immune deficiency correlates with the extent of the disease. The nodular sclerosing variant of primary mediastinal Hodgkin disease is the most common type. Histology reveals Reed-Sternberg cells. Cystic teratomas, or dermoid cysts, include endodermal, ectodermal, and mesodermal elements. They are characteristically cystic and contain poorly pigmented hair, sebaceous material, and, occasionally, teeth. If there is a connection between the teratoma and the tracheobronchial tree, the patient may present with symptoms of coughing up hair or sebaceous material. Dermoid cysts occur in the gonads and central nervous system, as well as in the mediastinum. With rare exceptions, these lesions are benign.

408 to 412. The answers are 408-g, 409-e, 410-b, 411-a, 412-f. *(Mulholland, pp 163-164.)* Norepinephrine and dopamine are the first-line agents used for septic shock. Phenylephrine is often used as a first-line agent in the treatment of neurogenic shock (where there is a loss of sympathetic tone) or as a secondary agent for refractory hypotension in the setting of tachycardia which limits increases in other medications such as dopamine. Dobutamine is primarily used in patients with cardiogenic shock. Epinephrine is used as a short-term agent given in intravenous boluses during cardiac arrests and in patients with cardiac dysfunction refractory to other agents such as dobutamine. Nitroprusside can be used in severe cardiogenic shock to reduce afterload or to treat severe hypertension. Nitroglycerin is used to treat acute myocardial ischemia.

Epinephrine is a circulating endogenous catecholamine, released mainly from the adrenal medulla, whose effects are mediated by binding of free circulating hormone to β_1 and β_2 receptors, with lesser effects on α adrenoreceptors. At low infusion rates the β_1-adrenergic effects predominate causing increased heart rate, stroke volume, and contractility. At higher infusion rates, α-adrenergic receptors are stimulated, resulting in an increase in blood pressure and systemic vascular resistance. Prolonged use of high-dose epinephrine is limited by renal and splanchnic vasoconstriction, cardiac dysrhythmias, and increased myocardial oxygen demand. Norepinephrine is also endogenously produced, but acts locally through release at nerve synapses. It acts on α-adrenergic and β-adrenergic receptors, resulting in an increase in afterload and glomerular perfusion pressure with preservation of cardiac output. Norepinephrine is associated with increase in urine output in hypotensive, septic patients. Dopamine is an endogenous catecholamine that is released into the circulation and acts by binding to α_1 receptors as well as to specific dopamine receptors in the renal, mesenteric, coronary, and intracerebral vascular beds, causing vasodilation. It has effects that change with increasing doses by binding to different receptors. At low serum concentrations, dopamine binds to dopaminergic receptors in the renal and splanchnic beds leading to increased urine output and natriuresis. At modest concentrations, dopamine binds to cardiac β_1-adrenergic receptors leading to increased myocardial contractility and increased heart rate. At high doses, dopamine binds to α-adrenergic receptors and causes an increase in blood pressure and peripheral vascular resistance. Dopamine is an effective agent in increasing blood pressure in hypotensive patients with adequate fluid resuscitation. Dobutamine is a synthetic catecholamine that predominately binds to β-adrenergic receptors and enhances myocardial contractility with minimal changes in heart rate. It is often used in treatment of cardiogenic shock following myocardial infarction to support myocardial contractility while reducing peripheral resistance. Phenylephrine is a pure α-agonist and its use results in increased peripheral vascular resistance and blood pressure. The increase in afterload increases left ventricular work and oxygen demand, and may cause a decrease in stroke volume and cardiac output. Nitroprusside is an arterial and venous smooth muscle vasodilator. Continuous infusions of nitroprusside require monitoring of serum thiocyanate levels and arterial pH for cyanide toxicity. Nitroglycerin is primarily a venous smooth muscle vasodilator. It is an effective treatment for myocardial ischemia because it diminishes myocardial oxygen demand by reducing excessive preload and ventricular end-diastolic pressure.

Peripheral Vascular Problems

Questions

413. A 64-year-old woman complains of right calf pain and swelling. She recently underwent an uncomplicated left hemicolectomy for diverticular disease. A duplex ultrasound confirms the presence of deep vein thrombosis (DVT) of the calf. Which of the following is the most appropriate initial management of this patient?

a. Pneumatic compression stockings
b. Warfarin
c. Heparin
d. Thrombolysis
e. Inferior vena cava filter

414. For the first 6 hours following a long and difficult surgical repair of a 7-cm abdominal aortic aneurysm, a 70-year-old man has a total urinary output of 25 mL since the operation. Which of the following is the most appropriate diagnostic test to evaluate the cause of his oliguria?

a. Renal scan
b. Aortogram
c. Left heart preload pressures
d. Urinary sodium concentration
e. Creatinine clearance

415. A 72-year-old man undergoes an aortobifemoral graft for symptomatic aortoiliac occlusive disease. The inferior mesenteric artery (IMA) is ligated at its aortic attachment. Twenty-four hours after surgery the patient has abdominal distention, fever, and bloody diarrhea. Which of the following is the most appropriate diagnostic study for this patient?

a. Aortogram
b. Magnetic resonance imaging (MRI)
c. Computed tomographic (CT) scan
d. Sigmoidoscopy
e. Barium enema

416. A 25-year-old woman presents to the emergency room complaining of redness and pain in her right foot up to the level of the midcalf. She reports that her right lower extremity has been swollen for at least 15 years, but her left leg has been normal. On physical examination, she has a temperature of 39°C (102.2°F) and the right lower extremity is nontender with nonpitting edema from the groin down to the foot. There is cellulitis of the right foot without ulcers or skin discoloration. The left leg is normal. Which of the following is the most likely underlying problem?

a. Congenital lymphedema
b. Lymphedema praecox
c. Venous insufficiency
d. Deep venous thrombosis
e. Acute arterial insufficiency

417. A 76-year-old woman presents with acute onset of persistent back pain and hypotension. A CT scan is obtained (shown below), and the patient is taken emergently to the operating room. Three days after surgery she complains of abdominal pain and bloody mucus per rectum. Which of the following is the most likely diagnosis?

a. Staphylococcal enterocolitis
b. Diverticulitis
c. Bleeding arteriovenous (AV) malformation
d. Ischemia of the left colon
e. Bleeding colonic carcinoma

418. An 80-year-old man is found to have an asymptomatic pulsatile abdominal mass. An arteriogram is obtained (shown below). Which of the following is the most frequent and lethal complication of this condition?

a. Rupture
b. Acute thromboembolism
c. Dissection
d. High-output congestive heart failure
e. Myocardial infarction

419. A 75-year-old man is found by his internist to have an asymptomatic carotid bruit. Which of the following is the most appropriate next test?

a. Transcranial Doppler studies
b. Doppler ultrasonography (duplex)
c. Spiral CT angiography
d. Arch aortogram with selective carotid artery injections
e. Magnetic resonance arteriogram (MRA)

420. A 69-year-old man with mild hypertension and chronic obstructive pulmonary disease (COPD) presents with transient ischemic attacks and the angiogram shown here. Which of the following is the most appropriate treatment recommendation?

a. Medical therapy with aspirin 325 mg/day and medical risk factor management
b. Medical therapy with warfarin
c. Angioplasty of the carotid lesion followed by carotid endarterectomy if the angioplasty is unsuccessful
d. Carotid endarterectomy
e. Medical risk factor management and carotid endarterectomy if neurologic symptoms develop

421. A 55-year-old man with recent onset of atrial fibrillation presents with a cold, numb, pulseless left lower extremity. He is immediately taken to the operating room for an embolectomy of the left popliteal artery. Which additional procedure should be performed along with the embolectomy?

a. Electromyography (EMG) of the leg
b. Measurement of anterior compartment pressure in the leg
c. Fasciotomy of the anterior compartment in the leg
d. Fasciotomy of all the compartments in the leg
e. Application of a posterior splint to the leg

422. A 58-year-old man presents with pain in the left leg after walking more than one block that is relieved with rest. On physical examination, distal pulses are not palpable in the left foot and there is dry gangrene on the tip of his left fifth toe. An ankle-brachial index on the same side is 0.5. Which of the patient's symptoms or signs of arterial insufficiency qualifies him for reconstructive arterial surgery of the left lower extremity?

a. Ankle-brachial index less than 0.7
b. Rest pain
c. Claudication
d. Absent palpable pulses
e. Toe gangrene

423. A 64-year-old man with a history of a triple coronary artery bypass 2 years ago presents with peripheral arterial occlusive disease. His only medication is a thiazide diuretic. Which of the following medications would be most appropriate in the medical management of his atherosclerosis?

a. Aspirin
b. Warfarin
c. Low-dose heparin
d. High-dose heparin
e. Low-molecular-weight heparin

424. A patient who has had angina as well as claudication reports feeling light-headed on exertion, especially when lifting and working with his arms. The subclavian steal syndrome is associated with which of the following hemodynamic abnormalities?

a. Antegrade flow through a vertebral artery
b. Venous congestion of the upper extremities
c. Occlusion of the carotid artery
d. Occlusion of the vertebral artery
e. Occlusion of the subclavian artery

425. A 66-year-old woman presents with severe right lower extremity claudication. Surgery is considered, but her hypertension, smoking, and diabetes puts her at risk for associated coronary heart disease. What test is most predictive of postoperative ischemic cardiac events following surgery?

a. Exercise stress testing
b. Electrocardiography (ECG)
c. Coronary angiography
d. Dipyridamole-thallium imaging
e. Transesophageal echocardiography

426. A 60-year-old man is admitted to the coronary care unit with a large anterior wall myocardial infarction. On his second hospital day, he begins to complain of the sudden onset of numbness in his right foot and an inability to move his right foot. On physical examination, the right femoral, popliteal, and pedal pulses are no longer palpable. The left lower extremity is normal. Which of the following is the most appropriate management of this patient?

a. Duplex imaging of the right lower extremity arteries
b. CT angiogram of the right lower extremity
c. CT angiogram of bilateral lower extremities
d. Embolectomy of the right femoral artery
e. Embolectomy of the right femoral artery with exploration of the contralateral femoral artery

427. A 60-year-old man is found on a routine physical examination to have a 3-cm pulsatile mass in the right popliteal fossa. X-ray of the right of the right lower extremity is shown below. Which of the following is the most appropriate management of this patient?

a. Antiplatelet therapy
b. Anticoagulation
c. Thrombolytic therapy
d. Surgery
e. Reassurance and reexamination if the patient develops symptoms

428. A 65-year-old male cigarette smoker reports onset of claudication of his right lower extremity approximately 3 weeks previously. He can walk 3 blocks before the onset of claudication. Physical examination reveals palpable pulses in the entire left lower extremity, but no pulses are palpable below the right groin level. Noninvasive flow studies are obtained and are pictured here. What is the level of the occlusive process in this patient?

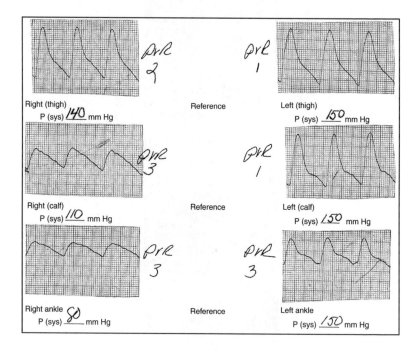

Right (thigh) P (sys) _140_ mm Hg — Reference — Left (thigh) P (sys) _150_ mm Hg

Right (calf) P (sys) _110_ mm Hg — Reference — Left (calf) P (sys) _150_ mm Hg

Right ankle P (sys) _80_ mm Hg — Reference — Left ankle P (sys) _150_ mm Hg

a. Right anterior tibial artery
b. Right superficial femoral artery
c. Right profunda femoris artery
d. Right external iliac artery
e. Right internal iliac artery

429. A 56-year-old woman presents to her primary care physician for a routine checkup. She states that she was recently hospitalized for surgery and was told she had some metal placed in a large blood vessel to prevent blood clots from moving to her lungs. An abdominal x-ray is shown here. Which of the following is the most appropriate indication for placement of this device?

a. Recurrent pulmonary embolus despite adequate anticoagulation therapy
b. Axillary vein thrombosis
c. Pulmonary embolus due to DVT of the lower extremity that occurs 2 weeks postoperatively
d. DVT in a patient with patient with metastatic carcinoma
e. Pulmonary embolus in a patient with metastatic carcinoma

430. Two days after admission to the hospital for a myocardial infarction, a 65-year-old man complains of severe, unremitting midabdominal pain. His cardiac index is 1.6. Physical examination is remarkable for an absence of peritoneal irritation or distention despite the patient's persistent complaint of severe pain. Serum lactate is 9 mmol/L (normal is < 3 mmol/L). Which of the following is the most appropriate next step in this patient's management?

a. Perform computed tomography.
b. Perform mesenteric angiography.
c. Perform laparoscopy.
d. Perform flexible sigmoidoscopy to assess the distal colon and rectum.
e. Defer decision to explore the abdomen until the arterial lactate is greater than 10 mmol/L.

431. A postoperative patient with swelling and pain in his right calf is suspected of having a deep venous thrombosis. Prior to initiating treatment with anticoagulants, he requires a confirmatory examination. Which of the following is a limitation of the duplex ultrasound in evaluating a DVT?

a. It is not very sensitive for detecting calf thrombi in symptomatic patients.
b. It is invasive.
c. It cannot differentiate between acute and chronic venous thrombi.
d. It is expensive.
e. It cannot image the proximal veins (iliac veins, IVC).

432. A 72-year-old woman with severe COPD who requires home oxygen is unable to ambulate inside her home without experiencing severe left hip pain. She was hospitalized 1 year ago for a viral pneumonia and was ventilator-dependent at that time for 6 weeks. On examination, her blood pressure is 165/80 mm Hg. She has weakly palpable bilateral femoral pulses. An angiogram demonstrates severe aortoiliac disease involving bilateral iliac vessels. Which of the following is the most appropriate vascular procedure for this patient?

a. Femorofemoral bypass
b. Axillofemoral bypass
c. Femoropopliteal bypass
d. Aortobifemoral bypass
e. Common femoral and profunda femoral endarterectomies

Peripheral Vascular Problems

Answers

413. The answer is c. *(Townsend, pp 2013-2016)* The initial treatment for DVT is therapeutic heparinization with either with intravenous heparin or low-molecular-weight heparin administered subcutaneously. Even following prompt, aggressive treatment of DVT of the calf, as many as half of affected patients will develop symptoms of chronic venous hypertension, and a larger number will have abnormal venous hemodynamic findings. Long-term anticoagulation for patients with DVT is achieved with warfarin; the appropriate duration of therapy is based on the risk factors (reversible or time-limited versus ongoing), the number of previous episodes, and the location (isolated calf versus femoral). Pneumatic compression stockings are an acceptable prophylactic measures in patients at moderate risk for DVT; however, they are not effective against established thrombosis. A small percentage of patients undergoing appropriate treatment of DVT can still develop a pulmonary embolus. These patients would then be candidates for an inferior vena cava filter. Thrombolytic therapy is not recommended for treatment of a routine DVT. It is reserved for patients with phlegmasia for relief of significant venous obstruction.

414. The answer is c. *(Townsend, pp 348-349.)* By far the most likely cause of the oliguria observed in this patient is hypovolemia. Volume status would be best assessed by placing a Swan-Ganz catheter to measure the preload pressures in the left atrium (by inference from the pulmonary capillary wedge pressures). Patients who undergo long, difficult operations in large surgical fields collect third-space fluids and become intravascularly depleted despite large volumes of intravenous fluid and blood replacement. The proper management usually involves titrating the cardiac output by providing as much fluid as necessary to keep the wedge pressures near 15 mm Hg. The other studies listed might become useful if urinary flow remains depressed after optimal cardiac output has been achieved, but in view of the probability of hypovolemia, they are not indicated as first diagnostic studies.

415. The answer is d. (*Townsend, pp 1923-1924.*) The patient has ischemia of the left colon and rectum. Intestinal ischemia develops when a patent inferior mesenteric artery is ligated in the setting of superior mesenteric artery (SMA) or bilateral hypogastric artery occlusion. Ligation of the IMA too far from the aorta can also interfere with the collateral blood supply to the rectosigmoid and lead to ischemia. Abdominal distention, fever, elevation of white blood cell count, and/or bloody diarrhea in the postoperative period should raise suspicion for colon ischemia. The best study to evaluate the sigmoid and rectum is sigmoidoscopy. Barium enema is not as accurate as sigmoidoscopy in determining depth of injury and carries grave risks of contamination by barium and feces if perforation occurs. CT, MRI, and aortography are not useful in evaluating the colon for early ischemia.

416. The answer is b. (*Townsend, pp 2022-2023.*) This patient's underlying problem is unilateral primary lymphedema. Lymphedema is classified as primary when the etiology is unknown. Hypoplasia of the lymphatic system of the lower extremity accounts for more than 90% of cases of primary lymphedema. If edema is present at birth, it is referred to as congenital; if it starts early in life (as in this woman), it is called praecox; if it appears after the age of 35 years, it is tarda. The inadequacy of the lymphatic system accounts for the repeated episodes of cellulitis that these patients experience. Swelling is not seen with acute arterial insufficiency. Deep venous thrombophlebitis will result in tenderness and is generally not a predisposing factor for cellulitis of the foot. Venous insufficiency is usually accompanied by varicose veins, brawny skin discoloration in the distal leg and ankle, and skin ulcers.

417. The answer is d. (*Townsend, pp 1923-1924.*) The patient's presentation of acute-onset, persistent back pain and hypotension is classic for ruptured abdominal aortic aneurysm. The CT scan reveals a fractured ring of calcification in the abdominal aorta with significant density (blood) in the para-aortic area. The incidence of ischemic colitis following abdominal aortic repair is about 2%. The incidence dramatically increases following a ruptured aneurysm repair. The sigmoid colon is affected most frequently. Blood flow to the left colon is normally derived from the IMA with collateral flow from the middle and inferior hemorrhoidal vessels. The SMA may also contribute via the marginal artery of Drummond. If the SMA is stenotic or occluded, flow to the left colon will be primarily dependent on an intact IMA. The IMA is usually ligated at the time of aneurysm repair. Patients at highest risk for diminished flow through collateral vessels are those with a history of visceral angina, those found to have a patent IMA at the time of operation, those who have suffered an episode of hypotension following rupture of an aneurysm, those in whom preoperative angiograms reveal occlusion of the SMA, and those in whom Doppler flow signals along the mesenteric border cease following occlusion of the IMA. Bowel ischemia recognized at the time of operation should be treated by reimplantation of the IMA into the graft to restore flow.

418. The answer is a. *(Townsend, pp 1912-1913.)* The patient has an asymptomatic abdominal aortic aneurysm (AAA). An aneurysm is defined as a focal dilation of an artery exceeding 1.5 times the normal diameter. The diameter of a normal abdominal aorta in a man is approximately 2 cm. This patient's arteriogram demonstrates an aneurysm diameter close to 3 times the size of his normal aorta. This would make the patient's aneurysm 5 to 6 cm in diameter. The most frequent and lethal complication of an AAA is rupture. All symptomatic AAAs should be repaired, regardless of size. In asymptomatic patients, the minimum size for repair is controversial. For good surgical candidates (young, low operative risks), repair is advocated for aneurysms larger than 4 cm in diameter. Smaller AAAs may warrant repair only if rapidly enlarging owing to the increased risk for rupture. Occasionally AAAs can lead to life-threatening conditions because of acute thromboembolism. Aortic dissection, high-output congestive heart failure, and myocardial infarction are not complications of an AAA.

419. The answer is b. *(Townsend, pp 1887-1890.)* Doppler ultrasonography (duplex) is the best initial test for screening patients with carotid disease. It has become a highly accurate test, often obviating the need for carotid arteriography prior to carotid endarterectomy. Carotid arteriography is seldom used solely for the diagnosis of carotid disease. It is invasive and reserved for cases in which other tests cannot be performed or fail to provide enough information to make an accurate diagnosis. MRA is also a modality that has enjoyed success in the investigation of carotid disease. Although not quite as accurate as standard arteriography, it has been used in conjunction with the duplex as a complementary study. Once again, because of its cost, MRA would not be used as the primary screening modality. CT angiograms are rapidly becoming almost as accurate as MRAs. It can be used in patients with metallic implants, but the need for iodinated contrast carries some risk for renal failure in patients with compromised renal function. Transcranial Doppler studies are used to assess the intracranial vasculature.

420. The answer is d. (*Townsend, pp 1890-1891.*) Although the patient has chronic COPD, surgery with a carotid endarterectomy is indicated because the risk for a future stroke is significantly increased with his history of TIAs. Randomized trials have led to some generally accepted criteria for carotid endarterectomy: (1) for symptomatic carotid arteries, more than 50% diameter reduction, and (2) for asymptomatic carotid arteries, more than 80% reduction. Warfarin has not been shown to be effective in the management of patients with carotid disease. Angioplasty of carotid stenoses is being performed in some institutions but to date has not replaced surgery as the treatment for high-grade carotid stenoses.

421. The answer is d. (*Townsend, pp 545-547.*) This patient should undergo four compartment fasciotomy (anterior, lateral, superficial posterior, and deep posterior) since he satisfies 2 conditions that lead to a compartment syndrome of the leg: acute arterial occlusion without collateral inflow and rapid reperfusion of ischemic muscle. Another common cause of compartment syndrome is orthopedic trauma to the leg. The need for fasciotomy is based on clinical judgment. If a fasciotomy is indicated, all 4 compartments should always be opened. Electromyographic studies and compartment pressure measurements would probably be abnormal, but are unnecessary in view of the known findings and would delay treatment. Application of a splint has no role in the acute management of this problem.

422. The answer is e. (*Brunicardi, pp 756-759.*) The major threat to patients with arterial occlusive disease is limb loss. Rest pain and gangrene represent advanced stages of arterial insufficiency and warrant arterial reconstructive surgery whenever clinically feasible. This patient does not have rest pain which is defined as persistent pain in the extremity. Claudication, in most cases, reflects mild ischemia; the majority of affected patients are successfully managed without surgery. Most will stabilize or improve with development of increased collateral blood flow following institution of a program of daily exercise, cessation of smoking, and weight loss. Ankle-brachial index is a useful preoperative tool but does not by itself determine whether someone is a candidate for revascularization. Palpable pulses are usually absent in patients with claudication. Vasodilator drugs have been shown to have little benefit in the conservative management of intermittent claudication.

423. The answer is a. *(Townsend, pp 122, 1949.)* Antiplatelet agents are generally used to prevent thrombotic and embolic events in the arterial circulation. Aspirin exerts an antiplatelet effect that will last for the life of the platelet (approximately 7-10 days). Aspirin interferes with platelet function by inhibiting the synthesis of thromboxane A2 and the subsequent production of prostaglandins. Other medical management options include lipid-lowering therapy and smoking cessation. Anticoagulation is not recommended in the medical management of atherosclerosis.

424. The answer is e. *(Townsend, pp 1902-1904.)* Atherosclerotic occlusion of the subclavian artery proximal to the vertebral artery is the anatomic situation that results in the subclavian steal syndrome. On being subjected to exercise, the involved extremity (usually the left, which is more prone to atherosclerosis because of anatomic differences) develops relative ischemia, which gives rise to reversal of flow through the vertebral artery with consequent diminished flow to the brain. The upper extremity symptom is intermittent claudication. Venous occlusive disease is not a feature of the syndrome. The operative procedure for treating the subclavian steal syndrome consists of delivering blood to the extremity by creating either a carotid-subclavian bypass or a subclavian-carotid transposition. Dilatation and stenting of the artery by endovascular techniques is effective as well.

425. The answer is d. *(Townsend, p 252)* Reversible perfusion defects on dipyridamole-thallium imaging are predictive of perioperative ischemic cardiac events among patients undergoing noncardiac surgery. Ischemic rest pain or early onset of claudication after minimal exercise limits the effectiveness of stress testing as a screening procedure for occult coronary artery disease in this group of patients. Coronary angiography is invasive and therefore not used as a screening tool to assess the cardiac status of patients undergoing noncardiac surgery. Angiography is used to exactly define the anatomic abnormalities contributing the ischemia in patients who have already been evaluated with noninvasive testing. Transesophageal echocardiography is invasive and has no role in the preoperative screening of peripheral vascular patients. An electrocardiogram is useful in detecting perioperative ischemia and infarction, not in predicting them.

426. The answer is d. *(Townsend, pp 1957-1958.)* Immediate surgical intervention is the appropriate management for patients presenting with acute arterial insufficiency with neurologic compromise of the lower extremities from thromboembolic disease. The heart is the most common source of arterial emboli and accounts for 90% of cases. Sources include diseased valves, endocarditis, the left atrium in patients with unstable atrial arrhythmias, and mural thrombus on the wall of the left ventricle in patients with myocardial infarction. The diagnosis in this patient is clear, and therefore neither noninvasive testing nor arteriography is indicated. These studies would only delay treatment and lead to limb loss. Embolectomy of the femoral artery can be performed under local anesthesia with minimal risk to the patient. Emboli typically lodge in 1 femoral artery; contralateral exploration is not indicated in the absence of signs or symptoms. The contralateral groin should always be prepared in case flow is not restored via simple thrombectomy, and femoral-femoral bypass is needed to provide inflow to the affected limb.

427. The answer is d. *(Townsend, pp 1934-1935.)* The patient has a popliteal artery aneurysm. Popliteal artery aneurysms are the most common peripheral arterial aneurysms and are bilateral in 53% of patients. Many patients are asymptomatic when diagnosed, but they can present with chronic limb ischemia or acute thromboembolism. Unlike abdominal aortic aneurysms, popliteal artery aneurysms rarely rupture. All symptomatic popliteal aneurysms should undergo surgical repair with exclusion of the aneurysm (which is ligated and left in situ) combined with a surgical bypass. Because of the risk of complications, asymptomatic popliteal aneurysms greater than 2 cm should be repaired as well. Thrombolytic therapy is reserved for patients who present with acute limb ischemia to improve runoff for revascularization and decrease limb loss. Neither antiplatelet therapy nor anticoagulation therapy are useful in the management of popliteal artery aneurysms.

428. The answer is b. *(Townsend, pp 1945-1946.)* This patient has occlusion of the right superficial femoral artery caused by atherosclerosis. This is confirmed by both the physical examination and the flow study findings which indicate a sharp decrease in the blood pressure below the level of the common femoral artery. Physical examination and flow studies indicate disease distal to the aortoiliac distribution.

429. The answer is a. *(Townsend, p 342.)* The Greenfield filter pictured on the x-ray is used to interrupt migration of emboli to the lungs from the veins below the level of the filter. It is indicated in patients who sustain a recurrent pulmonary embolus despite adequate anticoagulant therapy or in patients with pulmonary emboli who cannot receive anticoagulants because of a contraindication (eg, bleeding ulcer, intracranial hemorrhage). The filter is not used in patients who sustain a single pulmonary embolus. It is placed in the inferior vena cava just below the renal veins and therefore would not be effective for emboli that arise cephalad to its position. Despite the hypercoagulable state seen in some patients with metastatic pancreatic cancer, anticoagulation can still be used as a first-line defense.

430. The answer is b. (*Townsend, pp 1973-1976.*) Abdominal pain out of proportion to findings on physical examination is characteristic of intestinal ischemia. The etiology of ischemia may be embolic or thrombotic occlusion of the mesenteric vessels or nonocclusive ischemia due to a low cardiac index or mesenteric vasospasm. Differentiation among these etiologies is best made by mesenteric angiography. While not without serious risks, angiography also offers the possibility of direct infusion of vasodilators into the mesenteric vasculature in the setting of nonocclusive ischemia. This patient, with a recent myocardial infarction and a low cardiac index, is at risk for embolism of clot from a left ventricle mural thrombus as well as low-flow mesenteric ischemia. If embolism or thrombosis is found angiographically (usually involving the superior mesenteric artery), thrombolytic therapy can be attempted in the absence of suspicion of ischemic bowel. Otherwise, operative embolectomy or vascular bypass is indicated to restore flow. If occlusive disease cannot be demonstrated, efforts should be made to simultaneously increase cardiac output with inotropic agents and dilate the mesenteric vascular bed by angiographic instillation of papaverine, nitrates, or calcium-channel blockers. Computed tomography is not helpful in delineating the cause of intestinal ischemia because it does not provide a sufficiently detailed image of the mesenteric vessels. Laparoscopy and/or laparotomy would be useful if ischemic bowel were suspected, although laparoscopy would not allow for adequate assessment of the visceral vessels. Flexible sigmoidoscopy, while useful in patients with ischemic colitis, has no role in the workup of mesenteric ischemia, which involves primarily the small intestine and right colon. Serum lactate is helpful in raising the suspicion of intestinal ischemia, but no absolute level should be used to decide whether or not to explore a patient.

431. The answer is e. (*Townsend, p 2014.*) Duplex ultrasonography depends on the compressibility of the vein to evaluate for a venous thrombus. The proximal veins are not accessible due to their location and therefore cannot be adequately evaluated using the duplex ultrasound. Magnetic resonance venography is a useful test for evaluating the iliac veins and the IVC for DVTs. The sensitivity, specificity, and positive and negative predictive values of duplex scanning (Doppler analysis and B-mode ultrasonography) are more than 95% in *symptomatic* patients with acute DVT. Duplex scanning can differentiate between acute and chronic venous thromboses. Acute DVTs are characterized by an enlarged noncompressable vein without collateral vessels whereas chronic DVTs have normal-sized veins with significant collaterals. The duplex scanning device is portable, and therefore the study is easily performed at the bedside, in a vascular laboratory, or in a radiology suite. It is noninvasive, inexpensive, and safe.

432. The answer is b. (*Townsend, pp 1963-1964.*) Given her comorbidities, the patient should undergo axillofemoral bypass grafting. In a patient with severe symptoms of claudication that are interfering with his or her lifestyle, intervention is indicated. Axillofemoral bypass grafts are an alternative to aortofemoral procedures, but have a lower 5-year patency rate and should be reserved for high-risk patients with bilateral iliac disease or an infected aortic aneurysm or graft. In a young, healthy patient with unilateral iliac artery occlusive disease, when angioplasty is not a treatment option, an aortofemoral bypass offers excellent long-term relief. Aortobifemoral bypass, while clearly the most risky of the treatment options offered, provides the best long-term patency. In elderly patients with severe comorbidities who are considered at high risk for complications, extra-anatomic bypasses (femorofemoral or axillofemoral bypasses) offer fair long-term patencies while not subjecting the patient to the risks of general anesthesia. Femorofemoral bypass offers the additional benefit of not disturbing sexual function; however, femorofemoral bypass is not an option in a patient with bilateral iliac artery disease. Neither common femoral and profunda femoral endarterectomies nor femoropopliteal bypass is beneficial in this patient who has aortoiliac disease.

Urology

Questions

433. A 60-year-old man sees a urologist for what he describes as bloody urine. A urine sample is positive for cytologic evidence of malignancy. Cystoscopy confirms the presence of superficial transitional cell carcinoma. Which of the following is the recommended treatment for stage A (superficial and submucosal) transitional cell carcinoma of the bladder?

a. Topical (intravesicular) chemotherapy
b. Radical cystectomy
c. Radiation therapy
d. Local excision and topical (intravesicular) chemotherapy
e. Systemic chemotherapy

434. A 36-year-old man presents to the emergency room with renal colic. His vital signs are normal and a urinalysis shows microscopic hematuria. A radiograph reveals a 1.5-cm stone. Which of the following is the most appropriate management of this patient?

a. Hydration and analgesics
b. α-Adrenergic blocker
c. Extracorporeal lithotripsy
d. Percutaneous nephrostomy tube
e. Open surgery to remove the stone

435. An 8-month-old boy is seen by a pediatrician for the first time. The physician notes that there are no testes in the scrotum. Which of the following is the optimal management of bilateral undescended testicles in an infant?

a. Immediate surgical placement into the scrotum
b. Chorionic gonadotropin therapy for 1 month; operative placement into the scrotum before age 2 if descent has not occurred
c. Observation until age 2; operative placement into the scrotum if descent has not occurred
d. Observation until age 5; if no descent by then, plastic surgical scrotal prostheses before the child enters school
e. No therapy; reassurance of the parent that full masculinization and normal spermatogenesis are likely even if the testicle does not fully descend

436. A 32-year-old man presents with an asymptomatic mass in his right testicle. On examination, the mass cannot be transilluminated. Ultrasound shows a solid mass in the right testicle. Which of the following is the most accurate method in obtaining a diagnosis of testicular cancer?

a. Serum levels of alpha-fetoprotein and beta human chorionic gonadotrophin
b. Percutaneous biopsy of the testicular mass
c. Incisional biopsy of the testicular mass through a scrotal incision
d. Excisional biopsy of the testicular mass through a scrotal incision
e. Radical inguinal orchiectomy

437. A 10-year-old boy presents to the emergency room with pain in the left testicle. The pain was acute in onset and began 1 hour ago. On physical examination, he is noted to have a high-riding, firm, and markedly tender left testis. The right testicle is normal. Urinalysis is unremarkable. Which of the following is the most appropriate management of this patient?

a. Manual detorsion of the left testicle with external rotation toward the thigh; orchiopexy if the condition recurs
b. Manual detorsion of the left testicle with internal rotation toward the thigh; orchiopexy if the condition recurs
c. Orchiopexy of the left testicle
d. Orchiopexy of bilateral testicles
e. Orchiectomy of the left testicle

438. A 45-year-old woman presents with a 7-cm renal cell carcinoma with radiologic evidence of abdominal lymph node involvement with no distant metastases. Which of the following is the most appropriate management of this patient?

a. Radical nephrectomy
b. Radiation
c. Chemotherapy
d. Radiation followed by nephrectomy
e. Chemotherapy followed by nephrectomy

439. A 58-year-old man is found to have high serum prostate–specific antigen (PSA) concentration with a normal prostate examination. A biopsy of the prostate confirms low-grade carcinoma. The patient wishes to avoid therapy involving any risk for impotence. Which of the following is the most appropriate management of this patient?

a. Observation
b. Chemotherapy
c. Prostatectomy
d. Radiation therapy
e. Hormonal therapy

440. A 60-year-old man seeks medical attention because of recurrent urinary tract infections. The patient also reports a history of increasing difficulty in urination (decreased flow, straining, and hesitancy) over the last several months. A prostate-specific antigen (PSA) level is mildly elevated and a prostate biopsy proves benign. Which of the following is the most appropriate initial management of this patient with benign prostatic hyperplasia (BPH)?

a. α-Adrenergic blocker
b. 5-alpha reductase inhibitor
c. α-Adrenergic blocker and 5-alpha reductase inhibitor
d. Transurethral resection of the prostate (TURP)
e. Open prostatectomy

441. The left ureter is partially transected (50% of circumference) during the course of a difficult operation on an unstable, critically ill patient. Which of the following would be the most appropriate management of this injury given the patient's unstable condition?

a. Placement of an external stent through the proximal ureteral stump with delayed reconstruction
b. Ipsilateral nephrectomy
c. Placement of a catheter from the distal ureter through an abdominal wall stab wound
d. Placement of a closed-suction drain adjacent to the injury
e. Bringing the proximal ureter up to the skin as a ureterostomy

442. A pedestrian is hit by a speeding car. Radiologic studies obtained in the emergency room, including a retrograde urethrogram (RUG), are consistent with a pelvic fracture with a rupture of the urethra superior to the urogenital diaphragm. Which of the following is the most appropriate next step in this patient's management?

a. Immediate percutaneous nephrostomy
b. Immediate placement of a Foley catheter through the urethra into the bladder to align and stent the injured portions
c. Immediate reconstruction of the ruptured urethra after initial stabilization of the patient
d. Immediate exploration of the pelvis for control of hemorrhage from pelvic fracture and drainage of pelvic hematoma
e. Immediate placement of a suprapubic cystostomy tube

443. A 55-year-old man presents with fever and pain in the perineal region. Upon further questioning he also complains of frequency, urgency, dysuria, and a decreased urinary stream. On physical examination his abdomen is soft, nondistended, and nontender. Digital rectal examination demonstrates exquisite tenderness on the anterior aspect. Laboratory examination reveals leukocytosis and findings on urinalysis are consistent with a bacterial infection. Which of the following is the most likely diagnosis?

a. Urinary tract infection
b. Benign prostatic hyperplasia
c. Prostatitis
d. Pyelonephritis
e. Nephrolithiasis

Urology

Answers

433. The answer is d. *(Townsend, pp 2275-2277.)* Ninety percent of bladder cancers are of transitional cell origin. It is most prevalent among men with a history of heavy smoking and is usually multifocal and superficial, even when recurrent. When the disease is still superficial, transurethral resection of visible lesions and intravesicular chemotherapy are most often recommended. More radical surgical resection, systemic chemotherapy, and radiation are reserved for advanced stages of the disease.

434. The answer is c. *(Townsend, pp 2267-2269; Brunicardi, pp 1472-1473.)* The most appropriate treatment for this patient is extracorporeal shockwave lithotripsy given the size of his renal stone (1.5 cm). This procedure is completely noninvasive and uses a device that delivers convergent shockwave energy to the stone under fluoroscopic guidance. Many patients with renal stones smaller than 1 cm can be managed with hydration and analgesics until the stone passes spontaneously. α-Adrenergic blockers, which are usually used in the treatment of men with bladder outlet obstruction, have recently been shown to potentiate the likelihood of stone expulsion for small stones. Percutaneous nephrostomy tubes are reserved for unstable patients who present with a urinary infection coexisting with an obstructing stone. Open surgery for nephrolithiasis is rarely performed secondary to the successful management of this condition with minimally invasive techniques.

435. The answer is b. *(Brunicardi, p 1446.)* Chorionic gonadotropin is occasionally effective in patients with bilateral undescended testes. If there is no testicular descent after 1 month of endocrine therapy, surgical intervention consisting of inguinal orchidopexy should be performed before the age of 2. After 2 years of age, a testicle not in the cooler environment of the scrotal sac will begin to undergo histologic changes characterized by reduced spermatogonia. Testicles left longer in the undescended state not only have a higher incidence of malignant degeneration, but are inaccessible for examination. If a malignancy should occur, diagnosis will be delayed. There is also a substantial psychological burden when children reach school age or are otherwise subjected to exposure of their deformed genitalia. Gel-filled prostheses are generally inserted when a testicle cannot be placed in the scrotum. Close follow-up by a physician until the late teens is indicated in all patients who have had an undescended testicle. Since these patients may be at increased risk for malignancy throughout life, careful training should be given in self-examination.

436. The answer is e. (*Townsend, pp 2280-2284.*) The most accurate method to obtaining a diagnosis of any cancer is with histologic confirmation. In the case of testicular cancer, a radical inguinal orchiectomy with high ligation of the spermatic cord near the internal inguinal ring is the procedure of choice to provide histologic evaluation of the tumor. Violation of the scrotum must be avoided because it may alter the lymphatic drainage of the testis and lead to a poorer outcome. Serum levels of alpha-fetoprotein and beta human chorionic gonadotrophin are elevated in up to 85% of men with nonseminomatous germ cell tumors. However, these tests are not sensitive or specific enough to establish the diagnosis of testicular cancer in the absence of histologic confirmation.

437. The answer is d. (*Townsend, p 2266.*) The patient's presentation is consistent with testicular torsion and he needs to be taken to surgery immediately. During surgery, the affected testicle is rotated to its normal position. If it is viable, orchiopexy is performed on both the affected and the unaffected testes because the unaffected testes has a greater-than-normal chance of torsion in the future. If the affected testicle is nonviable, orchiectomy is performed with orchiopexy of the nonaffected testicle. Manual detorsion can be attempted by external rotation of the testicle toward the thigh, but the patient still needs to be taken to surgery following the initial presentation of testicular torsion. If left untreated, testicular torsion leads to strangulation of the blood supply to the testicle. Testicular torsion usually occurs in adolescent boys 12 to 18 years of age. The underlying pathology is secondary to an abnormally narrowed testicular mesentery with tunica vaginalis surrounding the testis and epididymis in a bell clapper deformity. As the testis twists, it comes to lie in a higher position within the scrotum. Presentation is acute onset of testicular pain and/or swelling. Diagnosis of testicular torsion is mainly made with clinical presentation and examination. A technetium 99m (^{99m}Tc) pertechnetate scan or Doppler ultrasound may be helpful in making the diagnosis if clinical suspicion of torsion is low; however, operation should not be delayed in order to maximize testicular salvage. This patient's presentation warrants immediate operation. If treated within the first 4 to 6 hours of onset of symptoms, the chance of saving the testicle is high.

438. The answer is a. *(Townsend, pp 2273-2274.)* Renal cell cancer is not responsive to radiation and chemotherapy; therefore, radical nephrectomy remains the main treatment for localized renal cancer. A radical nephrectomy should be offered as a possible curative procedure in this patient because many nodes initially suspected of having metastatic disease on imaging are enlarged due to reactive inflammation.

439. The answer is a. *(Townsend, pp 2277-2280.)* Observation, or active surveillance, is an appropriate management option in a patient with early prostate cancer who wishes to avoid the risk of impotence involved with radiation, surgery, and hormonal therapy. Most early prostate cancers are slow-growing tumors and will remain confined to the prostate gland for a significant length of time. Active surveillance involves frequent visits to the doctor (every 3-6 months) with questions about new or worsening symptoms and digital rectal examinations for any change in the prostate gland. In addition, blood tests are done to watch for a rising PSA, and imaging studies can be conducted to detect the spread of the cancer. Chemotherapy is not indicated in the treatment of early-stage prostate cancer and is most often given to patients with metastatic disease who no longer respond to hormonal therapy.

440. The answer is d. *(Townsend, pp 2269-2272.)* Recurrent urinary tract infection is an absolute indication for surgery in patients with benign prostatic hyperplasia (BPH). Other indications for surgery in patients with BPH include urinary retention refractory to medical therapy, upper tract dilation, renal insufficiency secondary to outflow obstruction, and bladder stones. Transurethral resection of the prostate (TURP) is the surgery of choice with proven long-term efficacy and safety. Open prostatectomy is more invasive than TURP and is reserved for patients with very large prostates (>100 g) and patients with orthopedic conditions preventing proper positioning (dorsal lithotomy for a TURP). Medical treatment is the first-line therapy for patients with symptomatic uncomplicated BPH. Medical management consists of α-Adrenergic antagonists and/or 5-alpha reductase inhibitor.

441. The answer is a. (*Moore, pp 811-814.*) If the patient is too unstable to perform a definitive repair, placement of a catheter into the proximal ureter is an acceptable alternative that will allow reconstruction to be performed later. Suction drainage adjacent to the injured segment alone is inadequate. If time and the patient's condition permit, primary ureteral reconstruction should be carried out. In the middle third of the ureter, this will usually consist of ureteroureterostomy (primary anastamosis) using absorbable sutures over a stent. If the injury involves the upper third, ureteropyeloplasty may be necessary. In the lower third, ureteral implantation into the bladder using a tunneling technique is preferred. The creation of a watertight seal is difficult and nephrectomy may be required if the injury occurs during a procedure in which a vascular prosthesis is being implanted (eg, an aortic reconstructive procedure) and contamination of the foreign body by urine must be avoided.

442. The answer is e. (*Townsend, p 2265.*) If a rupture of the urethra is suspected, a retrograde urethrogram should be obtained before any attempts are made to place a Foley catheter, as efforts to do so may result in the creation of multiple false passages or conversion of a partial laceration into complete rupture. If there is incomplete disruption of the urethra, a transurethral Foley catheter can be cautiously placed across the injury. However, if there is complete disruption, a suprapubic catheter is placed temporarily and definitive repair is delayed 4 to 6 months, at which time the hematoma will have resolved and the prostate will have descended into the proximity of the urogenital diaphragm. Percutaneous nephrostomy has no role in the management of this problem.

443. The answer is c. (*Brunicardi, p 1471.*) The patient has signs and symptoms classic for acute prostatitis. Occasionally, patients may present in shock with hypotension and tachycardia. On rectal examination, the prostate is extremely tender to palpation and it should be performed gently to prevent releasing bacteria into the blood stream. The treatment is broad-spectrum IV antibiotics until the patient is afebrile and hemodynamically normal. Then the treatment is continued for a total of 3 weeks with oral antibiotics. A urinary tract infection also presents with the same complaints of frequency, urgency, dysuria, and decreased urinary stream, but it is not associated with perineal pain or pain on rectal examination. Benign prostatic hyperplasia does not present with pain or fever. Pyelonephritis and nephrolithiasis are not associated with pain in the perineum.

Orthopedics

Questions

444. An 18-year-old football player is seen in the emergency ward with severe knee pain incurred after being hit by a tackler while running. Which of the following findings on physical examination is most sensitive for an anterior cruciate ligament injury?
a. Excessive valgus laxity of the knee
b. Excessive varus laxity of the knee
c. Locked knee
d. Positive Lachman test
e. Positive posterior drawer test

445. A 34-year-old man is extricated from an automobile after a motor vehicle collision. The patient has an obvious deformity of his right thigh consistent with a femur fracture. Upon closer examination of the right thigh, there is bone visible through an open wound. Which of the following is the most appropriate management of his open femur fracture?
a. Intravenous (IV) antibiotics and cast or splint placement
b. IV antibiotics and internal or external fixation
c. Early irrigation and debridement, IV antibiotics, and cast or splint placement
d. Early irrigation and debridement, IV antibiotics, and internal or external fixation
e. Early irrigation and debridement, IV antibiotics, compartment decompression, and internal or external fixation

446. A 6-year-old boy is brought into the emergency room by his mother for walking with a limp for several weeks. On examination, the patient has tenderness over his right thigh without evidence of external trauma. An x-ray of the pelvis shows a right femoral head that is small and denser than normal. Which of the following is the most likely diagnosis?
a. Slipped capital femoral epiphysis (SCFE)
b. Legg-Calve-Perthes (LCP) disease
c. Dysplasia of the hip
d. Talipes equinovarus
e. Blount disease

447. A 65-year-old man presents with acute onset of pain, swelling, and erythema of the left knee. He denies previous episodes or trauma to the knee. The differential diagnosis includes septic arthritis and gout. Which of the following is the best study to differentiate between gout and septic arthritis?

a. White blood cell count
b. X-ray of the knee
c. Magnetic resonance imaging (MRI) of the knee
d. Bone scan
e. Evaluation of synovial fluid aspirate

448. While playing with his children, a 44-year-old man falls and lands on his right shoulder. There is immediate pain and deformity. In an uncomplicated dislocation of the glenohumeral joint, the humeral head usually dislocates primarily in which of the following directions?

a. Anteriorly
b. Superiorly
c. Posteriorly
d. Laterally
e. Medially

449. A 29-year-old construction worker fell 15 ft from a roof and broke his right humerus, as depicted in the accompanying radiograph. Given his injury, which of the following nerves is most at risk?

a. Median nerve
b. Radial nerve
c. Posterior interosseous nerve
d. Ulnar nerve
e. Ascending circumflex brachial nerve

450. In a failed suicide gesture, a depressed student severs her radial nerve at the wrist. Which of the following is her expected disability?

a. Loss of ability to extend the wrist
b. Loss of ability to flex the wrist
c. Wasting of the intrinsic muscles of the hand
d. Sensory loss over the thenar pad and the thumb web
e. Palmar insensitivity

451. After being injured by a bull on his mother's farm, a young man is placed in a cast for a supracondylar fracture of his humerus. A few hours later he begins to experience intense pain, swelling, and weakness in the ipsilateral hand. Pulses are normal in bilateral upper extremities. Which of the following is the most appropriate initial management of this patient?

a. Observation
b. Repeat imaging of the humerus
c. Elevation of the extremity
d. Removal of the cast
e. Surgical decompression (fasciotomy)

452. A 39-year-old man presents with an isolated fracture of the tibia after being hit on the leg with a car. The patient is stable and a radiograph of the leg shows a tibial shaft fracture with severe dislocation. Which of the following is the most appropriate management of the fracture?

a. Closed reduction and application of a long leg cast
b. Intramedullary nailing
c. Surgical fixation with unreamed nailing
d. External fixation
e. Plate fixation

Questions 453 to 456

For each description, select the type of fracture or dislocation with which it is most likely to be associated. Each lettered option may be used once, more than once, or not at all.

a. Navicular (scaphoid) fracture
b. Monteggia deformity
c. Night stick fracture
d. Anterior shoulder dislocation
e. Fracture of the scapula

453. A patient presents with pain in the shoulder after a fall. On examination the shoulder is internally rotated.

454. A patient has tenderness over the forearm after being attacked by gang members with baseball bats.

455. A 30-year-old cyclist falls and injures her forearm. The radial head is dislocated and the proximal third of the ulna is fractured.

456. A patient has tenderness in the anatomical snuffbox.

Questions 457 to 460

For each description, select the type of bone disease with which it is most likely to be associated. Each lettered option may be used once, more than once, or not at all.

a. Osteogenesis imperfecta
b. Osteopetrosis
c. Osteitis fibrosa cystica
d. Osteomalacia
e. Osteitis deformans (synonym for Paget disease)

457. A patient with elevated parathyroid hormone levels presents with brown tumors in the long bones.

458. A patient with chronic renal failure presents with skeletal deformity and pain.

459. A genetically determined disorder in the structure or processing of type I collagen may require your patient to wear various orthoses to protect himself.

460. A patient presents with cortical thickening and cortical expansion of the bone with sclerotic areas.

Questions 461 to 463

For each description, select the type of lesion with which it is most likely to be associated. Each lettered option may be used once, more than once, or not at all.

a. Osteoid osteoma
b. Osteoblastoma
c. Osteosarcoma
d. Chondrosarcoma
e. Ewing sarcoma

461. An 11-year-old boy presents with pain in his right leg. A radiograph shows a circumscribed, densely sclerotic mass limited to the metaphysis of the lower femur.

462. A 9-year-old boy presents with severe pain in the left femur. The pain is relieved by aspirin. On plain film, a 0.5-cm lucent lesion, which is surrounded by marked reactive sclerosis, is seen.

463. A 12-year-old boy complains of pain in his left leg that is worse at night. He has been experiencing fevers and also has a 9-lb weight loss. X-ray demonstrates an aggressive lesion with a permeative pattern of bone lysis and periosteal reaction. There is an associated large soft tissue mass as well. Pathology demonstrates the tumor to be of the round cell type.

Orthopedics

Answers

444. The answer is b. (*Brunicardi, pp 1579-1580.*) Lachman test is a sensitive and reliable clinical test to evaluate for injury to the anterior cruciate ligament (ACL). The knee is held in slight extension and while holding the thigh steady with one hand the tibia is pulled anteriorly with the other hand. Anterior translation of the knee suggests a torn ACL. The posterior drawer test is used to evaluate for a posterior cruciate ligament injury and is essentially the reverse of the Lachman test with a slightly flexed knee. A "locked knee" occasionally occurs with a displaced meniscal tear and prevents full extension of the knee. Excessive valgus laxity (outward deviation of the leg) is associated with a medial cruciate ligament injury while excessive varus laxity can be seen with a lateral cruciate ligament injury.

445. The answer is e. (*Townsend, pp 547-551.*) Early irrigation and debridement are the mainstays in management of an open fracture. Debridement requires meticulous removal of all foreign material and resection of all nonviable tissue from the wound to reduce the bacterial count. IV antibiotics do not penetrate nonviable tissue. The wound is aggressively explored because the area of injury is always larger than expected from merely observing the wound. Irrigation with copious amounts of saline is performed with repeat debridements 48 to 72 hours later to assess for further necrosis. Given the significant amount of muscle damage in open fractures, fasciotomies are liberally performed during debridement. Skeletal stabilization is crucial for soft tissue healing in an open fracture. Compared to cast and splints, internal or external fixation allows greater access to wound care and is the preferred method of stabilization. Wound coverage is usually accomplished within 1 week of injury.

446. The answer is b. (*Brunicardi, pp 1604-1606.*) The patient's presentation and x-ray findings are most consistent with LCP. LCP can occur between the ages of 2 and 12, is 3 to 5 times more common in boys, and is bilateral in 10% to 20% of cases. The pathogenesis is thought to involve a period of ischemia in the proximal femoral epiphysis followed by revascularization.

Patients with LCP present with a limp and pain in the groin, thigh, or knee. Plain radiographs show a small and denser-than-normal femoral head on the affected side. Slipped capital femoral epiphysis is a disorder involving dissociation between the epiphysis and metaphysis of the proximal femur. SCFE usually occurs during the adolescent growth spurt and is bilateral in one-third of cases. Patients with SCFE also present with a limp and pain in the thigh or knee. The physical examination is most remarkable for limitation of internal rotation of the hip. Plain films of the pelvis in SCFE show displacement of the metaphysis of the proximal femur. Developmental dysplasia of the hip involves a spectrum of disorders with differing degrees of instability of the hip and underdevelopment of the acetabulum. Talipes equinovarus is "clubfoot." Blount disease involves infants born with physiologic genu varum (bow legs).

447. The answer is e. *(Brunicardi, p 1577.)* The patient's presentation is consistent with both septic arthritis and gout. The most definitive study to differentiate between the 2 diagnoses is synovial fluid aspiration. In gout, urate crystals are seen on analysis of the joint fluid. In septic arthritis, synovial fluid aspirate demonstrates bacteria and white blood cells with high neutrophils on differential count. White blood cell count can be elevated with both processes. X-ray and MRI would show tissue swelling around the joint consistent with both conditions. A bone scan would target the area of inflammation but not give any information as to the source of the inflammation.

448. The answer is a. *(Brunicardi, p 1581.)* The glenohumeral joint is bounded posteriorly by the teres minor and infraspinatus muscles and partially by the long head of the triceps. It is bounded laterally by the powerful deltoid muscle; superiorly, the acromion process precludes upward dislocation. However, anteriorly and inferiorly the pectoralis major and the long head of the biceps do not completely stabilize the glenohumeral joint; in this region the articular ligaments and joint capsule provide the major structural support. Thus, the joint is not strongly supported in its anteroinferior aspect and consequently anterior (or anteroinferior) dislocations are the most common glenohumeral dislocations. The humeral head is driven anteriorly, which tears the shoulder capsule, detaches the labrum from the glenoid, and produces a compression fracture of the humeral head. Most glenohumeral dislocations result from a posteriorly directed force on an arm that is partially abducted. Posterior dislocation is much rarer and should raise the possibility of a seizure as the precipitating cause. Clinical suspicion and physical examination are important in diagnosis of glenohumeral joint dislocations; diagnosis can be confirmed by radiologic plain films (anteroposterior, scapular lateral, and axillary views).

449. The answer is b. *(Brunicardi, pp 1574-1575.)* The radiograph demonstrates a transverse fracture of the distal half of the humeral shaft. The radial nerve runs in a groove on the posterior aspect of the humerus as it courses into the forearm compartment and is therefore at high risk of injury. If the nerve injury is apparent before any manipulation has been done, the fracture should be reduced; the nerve injury should be observed, since the nerve function will likely improve with time. If the nerve injury is present only after reduction, immediate surgical exploration is warranted because the nerve might be trapped in the fracture site. At this level of the arm, the ulnar and median nerves are well protected by muscle. The posterior interosseous nerve is a distal branch of the radial nerve and may be injured in fractures near the radial head, but it is in no danger from injuries at the level seen in this radiograph. There is no ascending circumflex brachial nerve.

450. The answer is d. *(Brunicardi, p 1615.)* An injury to the radial nerve at the wrist would cause primarily sensory abnormalities. The dorsum of the hand from the radial aspect of the fourth digit over the thumb, including the thenar pad and thumb web, becomes insensate after severance of the radial nerve at the wrist. Radial injuries more proximally would impair extension of the wrist and digits as well as forearm supination.

451. The answer is d. *(Brunicardi, p 1623.)* The patient has early compartment syndrome secondary to extrinsic compression from a cast that is circumferentially too tight. The cast needs to be immediately removed and the upper extremity needs to be thoroughly assessed. If the symptoms do not improve with removal of the splint then surgical decompression with fasciectomy is warranted. Compartment syndromes result from increasing pressures in the fascial compartments. Capillary blood flow is compromised first resulting in loss of oxygen delivery to tissues and increased extremity edema because of increased capillary permeability. Next, venous and lymphatic flow is compromised resulting in further edema. Arterial flow is the last to be compromised and therefore pulse changes are a late finding and normal pulses do not rule out a compartment syndrome. Extreme pain (out of proportion to the injury), pain on passive extension of the fingers or toes, pallor of the extremity, motor paralysis, and paresthesias are all components of the syndrome. The diagnosis can be confirmed by measuring intracompartmental pressures, but, whenever physical findings or symptoms are suspicious, the patient should be taken immediately to surgery. Observation, repeated imaging, and elevation would waste precious time and are not appropriate measures for a patient who is suspected of having a compartment syndrome.

452. The answer is b. (*Moore, pp 929-930.*) Surgical fixation with intramedullary nailing is the operation of choice for a stable patient with a severe tibial shaft fracture. Surgical fixation, as compared to closed treatment, provides better control of alignment, allows motion of the foot and ankle, and the possibility of earlier weight bearing. Multiple large clinic trials have demonstrated that unreamed nailing strategies have higher incidence of nonunion and malunion as opposed to fracture fixation with reamed cannulated nails. External fixation is most often used in the setting of high-energy trauma with significant soft tissue injury, vascular injuries needing repair, and in polytrauma patients as a "damage control" procedure. Plate fixation of tibial fractures is generally reserved for periarticular injuries too proximal or distal for intramedullary nailing. Closed treatment is the method of choice for tibial shaft fractures of minor severity and dislocation.

453 to 456. The answers are 453-d, 454-c, 455-b, 456-a. (*Brunicardi, pp 1574-1576, 1581, 1626-1627.*) Anterior shoulder dislocations can occur following minor or major trauma. Patients complain of local pain and present with an internally rotated shoulder. Closed reduction with a sling for comfort is usually sufficient therapy.

Dislocation of the radial head with a fracture of the proximal third of the ulna is known as Monteggia deformity. It is most often repaired with internal fixation of the ulna with closed reduction of the radial head. Late complications include heterotopic ossification and redislocation of the radial head.

Fractures of the navicular (scaphoid) bone of the wrist should be suspected in anyone, particularly a young person, who falls on an outstretched hand. Although x-rays are mandatory, it is important to realize that the fracture may not be seen on the initial x-ray and that a presumptive diagnosis can and should be made on clinical grounds alone. Typically, there will be tenderness to palpation at the anatomic suffbox. Immobilization at the time of injury in a thumb spica splint is required.

A night stick fracture refers to fractures of the ulnar shaft that result from a direct blow to the ulnar forearm by a club or night stick. These fractures are most commonly managed nonsurgically with a cast.

Fractures of the scapula can result from direct blows or falls onto the shoulder. Most scapula fractures are managed conservatively. Fractures with significant involvement of the glenoid require open reduction and internal fixation.

457 to 460. The answers are 457-c, 458-d, 459-a, 460-e. *(Brunicardi, pp 216, 1377-1378, 1596; Townsend, p 970.)* Osteitis fibrosa cystica is commonly associated with hyperparathyroidism. Increased bone turnover in this condition can be determined with an elevated serum alkaline phosphatase level. Brown or osteoclastic tumors and bone cysts may be present in the long bones. Treatment is parathyroidectomy.

Osteomalacia is characterized by lower bone turnover than osteitis fibrosa cystica. It is associated with skeletal deformity, fractures, and pain.

Osteogenesis imperfecta is a genetically determined disorder in the structure or processing of type I collagen. Patients present with osteopenia, low muscle mass, and hernias. There are 4 major subtypes with mild to lethal manifestations.

Osteitis deformans, or Paget disease, is characterized by large abnormal osteoclasts involved in increased bony resorption causing local lysis of bone. The rapid healing process that follows leads to the characteristic sclerosis, cortical thickening, and cortical expansion of the bone on radiographs.

Osteopetrosis is a rare skeletal deformity associated with increased density of the bones.

461 to 463. The answers are 461-d, 462-b, 463-f. *(Brunicardi, pp 1590-1595.)* Osteosarcoma, or osteogenic sarcoma, is the most common bone malignancy in children. It is most common in the distal femur, proximal tibia, and proximal humerus. On radiographs the tumor generally appears as a circumscribed, densely sclerotic mass. Treatment for periosteal osteogenic sarcomas is wide surgical excision with adjuvant radiation or chemotherapy.

An osteoid osteoma typically presents with severe pain that is characteristically relieved by aspirin. On radiograph, the lesion appears as a small lucency (usually < 1.5 cm) within the bone that is surrounded by reactive sclerosis. These lesions gradually regress over 5 to 10 years, but most are excised to relieve symptoms. Surgical extirpation is usually curative.

Ewing sarcoma is a round cell–type tumor. This is a highly malignant tumor that affects children (age range 5-15 years) and tends to occur in the diaphyses of long bones. The spine and pelvis can also be primary sites. There is a permeative pattern of bone lysis and periosteal reaction often associated with a large soft tissue mass. Fever and weight loss are common. The pain is often more pronounced at night. Treatment usually involves a combination of radiation and systemic chemotherapy.

Osteoblastoma is a rare bone-producing tumor that can present as a mass or local pain. The tumor is, by definition, > 1.5 cm and can occur anywhere. On radiograph the tumor appears as a purely lytic lesion. Treatment is simple excision.

Chondrosarcoma is a malignant neoplasm of cartilage most often seen in the pelvis, spine, proximal humerus, and the knee. It most frequently presents as pain and radiographs show an expansive destructive lesion of the bone with focal areas of calcification. Treatment consists of wide surgical excision.

Neurosurgery

Questions

464. A severely traumatized woman is seen in the emergency room (ER) with decreased mental status. Prior to intubation, she does not open her eyes, withdraws with all of her extremities, and makes incomprehensible sounds. What is her Glasgow coma scale score?

a. 3
b. 4
c. 5
d. 6
e. 7

465. A 25-year-old unhelmeted man involved in a motorcycle collision has multiple cerebral contusions on head computed tomographic (CT) scan. He is agitated but hemodynamically stable, with a heart rate of 80 beats per minute and a mean arterial pressure (MAP) of 90 mm Hg. An intracranial pressure monitor is placed, and the initial ICP reading is 30 mm Hg. Which of the following is the most appropriate in the management of his traumatic brain injury (TBI) over the next few days?

a. Hyperventilation to maintain a cerebral P_{CO_2} of 25 to 30 mm Hg
b. Administration of neosynephrine to increase his MAP and, consequently, his cerebral perfusion pressure (CPP)
c. Administration of mannitol (1 g/kg) to reduce his ICP
d. Placement of the patient in Trendelenburg position to increase cerebral perfusion
e. Avoidance of all sedating drugs in the first 24 to 48 hours in order to accurately assess his neurologic status

466. A 50-year-old woman complains of headaches and lateralizing weakness. A CT scan of the brain reveals an irregular mass in the right cerebral hemisphere. A biopsy documents that this is a glioblastoma. Which of the following is the best treatment strategy for potential cure?

a. Chemotherapy with temozolomide alone
b. Combination chemotherapy with carmustin, cisplatin, and temozolomide
c. External beam radiation alone
d. Surgical resection alone
e. Combined surgical resection, external beam radiation, and chemotherapy with temozolomide

467. A 60-year-old otherwise healthy woman presents to her physician with a 3-week history of severe headaches. A contrast CT scan reveals a small, circular, hypodense lesion with ringlike contrast enhancement. Which of the following is the most likely diagnosis?

a. Brain abscess
b. High-grade astrocytoma
c. Parenchymal hemorrhage
d. Metastatic lesion
e. Toxoplasmosis

468. A 16-year-old adolescent boy sustains head trauma in a motor vehicle collision. He has a GCS of 15 and an obvious depressed skull fracture with 1-cm displacement. During his hospital stay, he notices clear fluid draining from his nose. What is the best management strategy for this patient?

a. Immediate surgical elevation of the skull fracture
b. Delayed surgical elevation of the skull fracture
c. Immediate dural repair
d. Elevation of the head of the bed and placement of a lumbar drain
e. Antibiotic therapy for sinusitis

469. A 39-year-old man presents to his physician with the complaint of loss of peripheral vision. Which of the following findings are demonstrated by the subsequent magnetic resonance imaging (MRI) scan, shown here?

a. Cerebral atrophy
b. Pituitary adenoma
c. Optic glioma
d. Pontine hemorrhage
e. Multiple sclerosis plaque

470. An 18-year-old man is admitted to the ER following a motorcycle accident. He is alert and fully oriented, but witnesses to the accident report an interval of unresponsiveness following the injury. Skull films disclose a fracture of the left temporal bone. Following x-ray, the patient suddenly loses consciousness and dilation of the left pupil is noted. Which of the following is the most likely diagnosis?

a. A ruptured berry aneurysm
b. An acute subdural hematoma
c. An epidural hematoma
d. An intra-abdominal hemorrhage
e. A ruptured arteriovenous malformation

471. A 42-year-old woman presents to the ER with the worst headache of her life. A noncontrast CT scan of the head is negative for lesions or hemorrhage. She then undergoes a lumbar puncture, which appears bloody. All 4 tubes collected have red blood cell counts greater than 100,000/mL. Which of the following steps is the most appropriate management of this patient?

a. Repeat the head CT scan with intravenous contrast.
b. Perform an angiogram of the aorta and lumbar branches for immediate embolization of the injured vessel.
c. Perform a 4-vessel cerebral angiogram.
d. Administer a dose of mannitol.
e. Consult neurosurgery for immediate ventriculostomy.

472. A trauma patient with a closed-head injury is being monitored in the neurosurgical intensive care unit (ICU). His ICP measurement is seen to rise precipitously. An acute increase in ICP is characterized by which of the following clinical findings?

a. Respiratory irregularities
b. Decreased blood pressure
c. Tachycardia
d. Papilledema
e. Compression of the fifth cranial nerve

473. A 24-year-old patient with known neurofibromatosis type 2 undergoes an MRI for ringing in his ears. The MRI demonstrates lesions in bilateral auditory canals. Which of the following is the most likely diagnosis?

a. Gangioneuroma
b. Schwannoma
c. Ependymoma
d. Meningioma
e. Pituitary adenoma

474. An 18-year-old high school senior develops peripheral vision abnormalities. A CT scan of the brain reveals a cystic suprasellar mass with some calcification noted. Clinically, this is compatible with a craniopharyngioma. What is the best next step in treatment?

a. Growth hormone therapy
b. Cerebral angiography with tumor embolization
c. Transsphenoidal decompression of the optic nerve and optic chiasm
d. Surgical resection
e. Radiotherapy

475. Following significant head trauma, a 34-year-old woman undergoes a CT scan that demonstrates bilateral frontal lobe contusions of the brain. There is no midline shift. She has a GCS of 14. Which of the following is the best initial management of this patient?

a. Observation alone
b. Observation and administration of anticonvulsive medication for 1 week
c. Placement of an intracranial pressure monitor
d. Administration of 25 g of mannitol
e. Intubation and hyperventilation

476. A 45-year-old woman presents with left-sided weakness. A CT scan of the head demonstrates a well-circumscribed mass abutting the skull in the right hemisphere. Workup of the mass reveals a meningioma. Which of the following is the best next step in treatment?

a. Cerebral angiography with tumor embolization
b. Preoperative radiation therapy followed by surgical excision
c. Surgical excision
d. Chemotherapy with adriamycin
e. Chemoradiation

477. A middle-aged homeless man is brought to the ER by EMS for altered mental status, seizures, and vomiting. On physical examination he has no fever, neck stiffness, or evidence of head trauma. He does, however, have multiple dental caries and a focal neurologic deficit. Which of the following is the best next step in the patient's workup?

a. Lumbar puncture
b. Noncontrast head CT
c. Contrast-enhanced head CT
d. Placement of ICP monitor
e. Placement of ventriculoperitoneal shunt

Questions 478 and 479

For each description, select the type of vascular event with which it is most likely to be associated. Each lettered option may be used once, more than once, or not at all.

a. Subdural hematoma
b. Epidural hematoma
c. Carotid dissection
d. Brain contusion
e. Ruptured intracranial aneurysm

478. While watching a golf tournament, a 37-year-old man is struck on the side of the head by a golf ball. He is conscious and talkative after the injury, but several days later he is noted to be increasingly lethargic, somewhat confused, and unable to move his right side.

479. A 42-year-old woman complains of the sudden onset of a severe headache, stiff neck, and photophobia. She loses consciousness. She is later noted to have a dilated pupil.

Neurosurgery

Answers

464. The answer is e. *(Townsend, pp 484-487.)* The patient has a Glasgow coma scale (GCS) score of 7 prior to intubation (Eye opening = 1, Verbal = 2, Motor = 4). The Glasgow coma scale was developed to enable an initial assessment of the severity of head trauma. It is now also used to standardize serial neurologic examinations in the early post-injury period. It measures the level of consciousness using 3 parameters: verbal response (5 points), motor response (6 points), and eye opening (4 points); a "T" is used in lieu of a verbal score when the patient is intubated. The score is the sum of the highest number achieved in each category and ranges from 3 for a completely unresponsive patient to 15 for a fully oriented and alert patient. A score of 13 to 15 is considered a mild traumatic brain injury (TBI), 9 to 12 a moderate TBI, and 8 or less a severe TBI. The GCS score can be used to prognosticate outcome and likelihood of neurosurgical intervention.

Eye opening	No response	1
	To painful stimulus	2
	To verbal stimulus	3
	Spontaneous	4
Best verbal response	No response	1
	Incomprehensible sounds	2
	Inappropriate words	3
	Disoriented, inappropriate content	4
	Oriented and appropriate	5
Best motor response	No response	1
	Abnormal extension (decerebrate posturing)	2
	Abnormal flexion (decorticate posturing)	3
	Withdrawal	4
	Purposeful movements	5
	Obeys commands	6
Total		3-15

465. The answer is c. (*Townsend, pp 2090-2094.*) The cerebral perfusion pressure (CPP) is calculated as the difference between the MAP and the ICP; optimally the CPP should be maintained at greater than 70 mm Hg and the ICP at less than 20 mm Hg. Methods for reducing ICP include elevation of the head of the bed (reverse Trendelenburg), administration of mannitol or other diuretics to improve cerebral blood flow, use of short-acting sedatives to decrease patient agitation (the drugs should be intermittently held to perform neurological examinations), prevention of hypovolemia and treatment of hypotension, and prevention of hypoventilation and hypercapnia. Hypoventilation and hypercapnia cause vasodilation of the cerebral vessels, which increases the intracranial volume and pressure. Hyperventilation may still be used in cases of herniation or impending herniation to acutely lower ICP. However, prolonged hyperventilation is not recommended because of decreased perfusion (secondary to vasoconstriction) to an already ischemic brain. Furthermore, the brain resets to the new target P_{CO_2} within 48 to 72 hours, limiting the beneficial effects of hyperventilation and resulting in increased ICP when the P_{CO_2} is later normalized. Therefore, hypercarbia should be avoided, but hypocapnia below 30 mm Hg cannot be recommended except in extreme circumstances. Use of pressors to maintain a CPP above 70 mm Hg is controversial.

466. The answer is e. (*Townsend, p 2106.*) Glioblastoma multiforme is the most common form of primary intracranial neuroepithelial tumor. It is a heterogeneous glial cell tumor derived from the malignant degeneration of an astrocytoma or anaplastic astrocytoma. These tumors are most commonly found in the cerebral hemispheres during the fifth decade of life. CT and MRI scans typically reveal an irregular lesion with hypodense central necrosis, peripheral ring enhancement of the highly cellular tumor tissue, and surrounding edema and mass effect. Curative resections are rare. Standard therapy consists of surgical resection, external beam radiation, and chemotherapy. Temozolomide is an alkylating agent that is used to treat glioblastoma multiforme; carmustine and cisplatin have been the primary chemotherapeutic agents for treating malignant gliomas. Surgical resection alone is not curative. The course of the disease progresses rapidly after presentation, with median survival being 1 year; thus, treatment is often palliative and may involve any or a combination of the above-mentioned therapies.

467. The answer is d. (*Townsend, p 2110.*) The CT findings are consistent with any of the suggested lesions. However, the most likely diagnosis in an immunocompetent patient is metastatic disease, which has an incidence of approximately 150,000 to 250,000 cases per year as compared to primary intracranial tumors, which have an incidence of 35,000 per year. Roughly 15% to 30% of cancer patients develop intracranial metastases during the course of their disease. The cancers that most frequently metastasize to the brain parenchyma include those of the lung, breast, kidney, gastrointestinal (GI) tract, and melanomas. Leukemia shows a predilection for the leptomeninges. A large majority of these lesions become symptomatic owing to mass effect from white matter edema. Treatment is dependent on the number and size of the lesions and the physical condition of the patient, but may include a combination of surgery, radiosurgery, and whole-brain radiation therapy. Immunocompromised patients are at increased risk for toxoplasmosis and central nervous system lymphomas. Both immunocompetent and immunocompromised hosts can develop pyogenic brain abscesses, which typically occur in the setting of known infection (which can spread either locally or hematogenously).

468. The answer is c. *(Brunicardi, pp 1523-1524.)* This patient has a cerebrospinal fluid (CSF) leak from the nose or rhinorrhea associated with a depressed skull fracture. When a skull fracture occurs in the area of the paranasal sinuses, the mastoid air cells, or the middle ear, a tear in the meninges may result in CSF drainage from the ear or nose. The presence of rhinorrhea or otorrhea requires observation; although meningitis is a serious sequela, the role of prophylactic antibiotics is controversial. Otorrhea usually heals within a few days. Persistent cerebrospinal fluid from the nose or ear for more than 14 days requires surgical repair of the torn dura. Most skull fractures do not require surgical treatment unless they are depressed or compound. A general rule is that all depressed skull fractures—defined as fractures in which the cranial vault is displaced inward—should be surgically elevated, especially if they are depressed more than 1 cm, if a fragment is over the motor strip, or if small, sharp fragments are seen on x-ray (as they may tear the underlying dura). Compound fractures, defined as fractures in which the bone and the overlying skin are broken, must be cleansed and debrided and the wound must be closed.

469. The answer is b. *(Brunicardi, pp 1541-1542.)* This T1-weighted sagittal MRI scan reveals a dumbbell-shaped homogeneous mass involving the sella turcica and the suprasellar region. This lesion is most consistent with a pituitary adenoma, a benign tumor arising from the adenohypophysis.

Pituitary adenomas are the most common sellar lesion and constitute 10% to 15% of all intracranial neoplasms. Macroadenomas are greater than 1 cm in size and microadenomas less than 1 cm. Pituitary adenomas may be functional, resulting in endocrinopathies from excessive hormone secretion, such as prolactin (amenorrhea or galactorrhea), growth hormone (gigantism or acromegaly), or adrenocorticotrophic hormone (ACTH) (Cushing syndrome). The tumor pictured is a macroadenoma; these larger tumors may cause symptoms secondary to mass effect; for example, a bitemporal visual field defect can result from compression of the optic chiasm. This tumor's dumbbell shape results from impingement on the adenoma by the diaphragm of the sella turcica. The suprasellar extension seen here makes a frontal craniotomy rather than the more commonly utilized transsphenoidal approach more appropriate.

470. The answer is c. (*Brunicardi, p 1525.*) Epidural hematomas are typically caused by a tear of the middle meningeal artery, and they may be associated with linear skull fractures, usually in the temporal region. The lesion appears as a hyperdense biconvex mass between the skull and the brain on CT scan. Clinical presentation is highly variable, and outcome depends largely on promptness of diagnosis and surgical evacuation. The typical history is one of head trauma followed by a momentary alteration in consciousness and then a lucid interval lasting for up to a few hours. This is followed by a loss of consciousness, dilation of the pupil on the side of the epidural hematoma, and then hemiparesis of the contralateral side. If treated promptly, outcome is favorable in 85% to 90% of cases. Treatment consists of temporal craniectomy, evaluation of the hemorrhage, and control of the bleeding vessel.

471. The answer is c. (*Townsend, pp 2098-2102.*) The patient's history of the "worst headache of her life" and initial examination findings are highly suggestive of a subarachnoid hemorrhage. A CT scan without contrast will show a localized clot, diffusely distributed hemorrhage, intraventricular hemorrhage, or intraparenchymal hemorrhage 80% to 90% of the time. If the CT scan is negative, and the history and physical examination strongly support a subarachnoid hemorrhage, then a lumbar puncture is obtained. As opposed to traumatic lumbar taps, the red blood cell count does not diminish between the first and last tubes collected when a subarachnoid hemorrhage is present. Xanthochromia is the yellow appearance of cerebrospinal fluid caused by the degradation of heme to bilirubin in the red blood cells entering the CSF during the bleeding. Workup should then proceed to a 4-vessel cerebral angiogram to assess for a cerebral aneurysm. Given that only about 85% of cerebral aneurysms are identified on the initial study, a second angiogram should be performed within 7 to 10 days after the first study to completely rule out an aneurysm. Initial management consists of medical therapy to counteract vasospasm, blood pressure control, and anticonvulsant therapy. Although hydrocephalus can result from blockage of the arachnoidal channels, ventriculostomy is not the surgical management of choice. Surgical treatment should be initiated early and consists of craniotomy with clipping of the aneurysm.

472. The answer is a. *(Brunicardi, p 1521.)* The onset of irregular respirations, bradycardia, and, finally, increased blood pressure with acutely increasing ICP is termed the Cushing response or triad. Irregular respirations are due to hypoperfusion of the brainstem. The hypertension and bradycardia are due to decreased cerebral perfusion and the compensatory response. Cerebral perfusion pressure is the difference between the MAP and ICP. When the blood pressure is inadequate for cerebral perfusion, vasoconstriction and an increase in cardiac output occur to increased blood pressure and therefore CPP. The resultant hypertension stimulates the baroreceptors in the carotid bodies resulting in bradycardia. Focal mass lesions can result in herniation. Depending on the direction of the mass effect, the herniation can cause compression of different areas of the brain. Herniation of brain parenchyma through the tentorial incisura or foramen magnum causes brainstem compression. Herniation usually causes compression of the third cranial nerve and thus leads to a fixed and dilated pupil on that side. Papilledema is a finding with chronic increases in ICP.

473. The answer is b. *(Townsend, p 2108.)* Bilateral vestibular schwannomas are associated with neurofibromatosis type 2; patients with this disease also present with meningiomas and ependymomas. Benign schwannomas, or peripheral nerve sheath tumors that arise from perineural fibroblasts (Schwann cells) are treated with surgical excision. Malignant schwannomas, which are rare, are treated with radiation therapy if curative resection is not possible. Intracranial schwannomas most frequently originate in the vestibular branch of the eighth cranial nerve and represent 10% of all intracranial neoplasms. Symptoms include hearing loss, tinnitus, and vertigo. Neurofibromas are also Schwann cell tumors but are histologically distinguishable from schwannomas; patients with multiple neurofibromas typically have neurofibromatosis-1 or von Recklinghausen disease. Other peripheral nerve tumors include ganglioneuromas, neuroblastomas, chemodectomas, and pheochromocytomas.

474. The answer is d. (*Brunicardi, p 1542.*) Treatment of craniopharyngiomas consists of complete subfrontal or transsphenoidal excision if possible. If complete excision is not feasible, partial resection (rather than decompression of the optic chiasm alone) with adjuvant radiotherapy is recommended. Craniopharyngiomas are cystic tumors with areas of calcification and originate in the epithelial remnants of Rathke pouch. These usually benign tumors are found in the sellar and suprasellar region and lead to compression of the pituitary, optic tracts, and third ventricle. As a result, they show up on radiographic imaging as an area of sellar erosion with calcification within or above the sella. Craniopharyngiomas are most commonly found in children but may also present in adulthood. In children, they can cause growth retardation because of hypothalamic-pituitary dysfunction. Hormone replacement is not indicated in the absence of an enocrinopathy. There is no role for cerebral angiography with tumor embolization.

475. The answer is b. (*Brunicardi, p 1524-1525.*) Patients deemed to have a substantial contusion should receive anticonvulsive medication to prevent seizures in the early posttraumatic period. There is no role for placement of an intracranial pressure monitor as the patient has a mild traumatic brain injury and the clinical examination can be followed for signs of deterioration. Mannitol and intubation are not required in the setting of mild traumatic brain injury. Cerebral contusions are bruises of neural parenchyma that most commonly involve the convex surface of a gyrus. The most frequent sites of cerebral contusion are the orbital surfaces of the frontal lobes and the anterior portion of the temporal lobes. The etiology of the contusion is always traumatic. Injuries may be seen both at the site of impact (coup) and in parenchyma opposite the site (contrecoup).

476. The answer is c. (*Townsend, pp 2107-2108.*) The primary treatment of meningiomas is surgical excision with adjuvant radiation therapy if complete excision is not possible. Cerebral embolization has been used preoperatively to reduce blood loss and as a palliative option for patients who are poor surgical candidates, but is not a definitive therapeutic modality. Meningiomas are slow-growing, relatively benign tumors that arise from the arachnoid layer of the meninges. They occur predominantly in women, with a peak incidence at age of 45 years. They are treated primarily by surgical excision. Even after gross total resection, recurrence occurs in 11% to 15% of cases.

477. The answer is c. *(Townsend, p 2128.)* The patient's presentation is most consistent with a brain abscess, which is diagnosed by contrast-enhanced CT or MRI. In this condition, fever, elevated white blood cell count, and signs of meningeal irritation are often absent. Brain abscesses develop by either contiguous spread from adjacent structures or hematogenous spread from a distant site. Common sites of infection include paranasal sinus infection, dental caries, and ear infection. Contrast-enhanced CT and MRI reveal a ring-enhancing lesion usually at the gray-white interface with surrounding edema. Treatment involves accurate identification of the causative organism and appropriate antibiotic therapy, relief of mass effect with aspiration versus surgical excision, and treatment of the underlying cause. A lumbar puncture, ICP monitor, or ventriculoperitoneal shunt would not be helpful in the workup of a brain abscess. A noncontrast head CT is valuable in the workup of an intracranial hemorrhage. It does not provide the images needed to diagnose a brain abscess.

478 and 479. The answers are 478-a, 479-e. *(Townsend, pp 2098-2102, 2112-2116.)* Subdural hematomas usually arise from tears in the veins bridging from the cerebral cortex to the dura or venous sinuses, often after only minor head injuries. They can become apparent several days after the initial injury. On CT scan, a subdural hematoma appears to be crescent-shaped.

Reproduced, with permission, from Feliciano DV, Mattox KL, Moore EE. Trauma. 6th ed. New York: McGraw-Hill, 2008. Fig. 20-1.

Reproduced, with permission, from Feliciano DV, Mattox KL, Moore EE. Trauma. 6th ed. New York: McGraw-Hill, 2008. Fig. 20-2A.

Treatment is drainage of the hematoma through a burr hole; a formal craniotomy may be required if the fluid reaccumulates. Significant brain contusions from blunt trauma are usually associated with at least transient loss of consciousness; similarly, epidural hematomas result in a period of unconsciousness, although a lucid interval may follow, during which neurologic findings are minimal. Epidural hematomas usually arise as a result of an injury to the middle meningeal artery. They appear "lenticular" or biconvex or lens-shaped on CT scan.

Reproduced, with permission, from Doherty GM. Current Diagnosis & Treatment: Surgery. 13th ed. New York: McGraw-Hill, 2010. Fig. 36-22.

Subarachnoid hemorrhage (SAH) in the absence of antecedent trauma most commonly arises from a ruptured intracranial aneurysm, which typically is found at the bifurcation of the major branches of the circle of Willis. Other, less frequent causes of SAH include hypertensive hemorrhage, trauma, and bleeding from an arteriovenous malformation. Patients typically present with the sudden onset of an excruciating headache. Complaints of a stiff neck and photophobia are common. Loss of consciousness may be transient or may evolve into frank coma. Cranial nerve palsies are seen as a consequence both of increased ICP because of hemorrhage and pressure of the aneurysm on adjacent cranial nerves. CT scans classically demonstrate blood in the spaces normally filled with cerebrospinal fluid at the base of the brain and around the brainstem.

CT scans followed by cerebral arteriography help to confirm the diagnosis as well as to identify the location of the aneurysm. Treatment consists of surgical ligation of the aneurysm by placing a clip across its neck. Early surgical intervention (within 72 hours of SAH) may prevent aneurysmal rebleeding and allow aggressive management of posthemorrhage vasospasm. Nimodipine, which is a calcium channel blocker, has been shown to reduce ischemic complications from SAH presumably by ameliorating vasospasm.

Otolaryngology

Questions

480. A 14-year-old boy is brought to medical attention because of nasal fullness and bleeding. Inspection reveals enlarged cervical lymph nodes as well. Biopsy of a lymph node confirms nasopharyngeal carcinoma. What is the best management strategy for this patient?

a. Chemoradiation
b. External beam radiation therapy
c. Intracavitary radiation therapy
d. Surgical resection
e. Surgical resection followed by adjuvant chemoradiation

481. A young motorcycle driver is thrown against a concrete bridge abutment and sustains severe trauma about the face, with marked periorbital edema and ecchymosis as well as epistaxis. He is obtunded with rapid, shallow breathing. Which of the following is the next appropriate step in his workup and management?

a. Evaluation of the cervical spine.
b. Blind nasopharyngeal intubation with cervical in-line stabilization.
c. Oropharyngeal intubation with cervical in-line stabilization.
d. Emergency tracheostomy.
e. Emergency cricothyroidotomy.

482. A 48-year-old man with a strong history of cigarette use and heavy alcohol intake presents with an intraoral mass. Biopsy shows squamous cell cancer. Chest x-ray shows hyperinflated lungs but is otherwise normal. Which of the following is indicated as part of his staging workup?

a. Measurement of serum alkaline phosphatase and calcium levels.
b. Bronchoscopy.
c. Esophagoscopy.
d. Echocardiography.
e. No further workup is necessary.

483. Your patient presents with a complaint of a mass on her right cheek, which has been slowly enlarging. Biopsy shows a pleomorphic adenoma. Which is the next step in her management?

a. Superficial parotidectomy with preservation of the facial nerve
b. Superficial parotidectomy with resection of the facial nerve
c. Total parotidectomy with preservation of the facial nerve
d. Total parotidectomy with resection of the facial nerve
e. Enucleation of the adenoma

484. A 5-year-old child presents with a small mass near the anterior border of the sternocleidomastoid muscle. The mass is associated with localized erythema and induration, and the child is febrile. Which of the following is the definitive treatment of this problem?

a. Antibiotic therapy
b. Incision and drainage
c. Incision and drainage followed by complete excision after resolution of the inflammation and infection
d. Partial excision followed by clinical observation
e. Immediate excision followed by postoperative antibiotic therapy for 1 week

485. A 21-year-old woman asks you to evaluate a small painless lump in the midline of her neck that moves with swallowing. You make the clinical diagnosis of thyroglossal duct cyst. Which of the following is the most appropriate management of this patient?

a. Excision of the cyst
b. Excision of the cyst and the central portion of the hyoid bone
c. Excision of the cyst, the central portion of the hyoid bone, and the tract to the base of the tongue
d. Excision of the cyst, the central portion of the hyoid bone, and the tract to the base of the tongue, with sampling of central cervical lymph nodes
e. Excision of the cyst, the central portion of the hyoid bone, and the tract to the base of the tongue, with biopsy of the thyroid gland

486. A 60-year-old smoker is seen because of a 3-cm midline ulcerating mass that is visualized when he sticks out his tongue. Biopsy establishes that this is squamous cell carcinoma. Which of the following is the most appropriate treatment of his cancer?

a. Radiation therapy alone
b. Partial glossectomy
c. Partial glossectomy and cervical lymph node sampling
d. Partial glossectomy and bilateral neck dissections
e. Partial glossectomy followed by chemoradiation

487. A 38-year-old woman who underwent total thyroidectomy for multi-nodular goiter 6 months ago presents with persistent hoarseness. Which of the following nerves was most likely injured during her operation?

a. Superior laryngeal nerve
b. Bilateral recurrent laryngeal nerves
c. Unilateral recurrent laryngeal nerve
d. Hypoglossal nerve
e. Marginal mandibular branch of the facial nerve

488. A 4-year-old boy is brought into the emergency room by his parents for difficulty in breathing and swallowing. On physical examination the child is febrile, tachycardic, and tachypneic. He is anxious, drooling, and becomes increasingly exhausted while struggling to breathe. A lateral cervical spine radiograph is shown here. Which of the following is the most appropriate management of this patient?

Reproduced, with permission, from Knoop KJ, Stack LB, Storrow AB, et al. Atlas of Emergency Medicine. 3rd ed. New York: McGraw-Hill, 2009. Fig. 5-46. Photo contributor: Kevin J. Knoop, MD, MS.

a. Examine the larynx at bedside
b. IV antibiotics and admission to the floor
c. Immediate endotracheal intubation in the emergency room
d. Immediate endotracheal intubation in the operating room
e. Immediate tracheostomy in the operating room

489. A 58-year-old man is found to have a small mass in the right neck on a yearly physical examination. The patient reports that the mass has been slowly growing for the last few months and is not associated with pain or drainage. He has an otherwise negative review of systems. On examination there is a hard, mobile 2-cm mass along the mid-portion of the right sternocleidomastoid muscle. Which of the following is the most appropriate initial step in the workup of the neck mass?

a. No further workup is needed. Reevaluate the mass after a course of antibiotics for 2 weeks.
b. Fine-needle aspiration (FNA).
c. Core needle biopsy.
d. Incisional biopsy.
e. Excisional biopsy.

490. A 62-year-old man presents with a 3-month history of an enlarged lymph node in the left neck. He is a long-time smoker of cigarettes and denies fevers, night sweats, fatigue, or cough. On physical examination there is a 1.5-cm hard, fixed mass below the angle of the mandible in the left neck. Which of the following is the most likely cause of an enlarged lymph node in the neck?

a. Thyroglossal duct cyst
b. Dermoid tumor
c. Carotid body tumor
d. Branchial cleft cyst
e. Metastatic squamous cell carcinoma

Otolaryngology

Answers

480. The answer is a. (*Brunicardi, p 502.*) Chemoradiation is standard therapy for nasopharyngeal carcinoma. Intracavitary radiation may be used in addition to external beam radiation therapy, but is not definitive treatment in and of itself. Surgical resection is not typically used to treat nasopharyngeal carcinoma, but can be considered for local recurrences. Risk factors for nasopharyngeal carcinoma include environment, ethnicity, and tobacco. There is an unusually high incidence of nasopharyngeal cancer in southern China, Africa, Alaska, and in Greenland Eskimos. A strong association exists with Epstein-Barr virus (EBV) infections, such that EBV titers may be used to follow a patient's response to treatment. The incidence of nasopharyngeal carcinoma has a bimodal distribution in the teen years and between ages 45 and 55. Most patients present with a neck mass, and up to 20% of patients may already have bilateral cervical nodal involvement at that time. Less than 5% of patients have distant metastases on presentation. Diagnosis of nasopharyngeal cancer, which tends to arise in relatively young people, should be made by biopsy of the primary tumor.

481. The answer is c. (*Mulholland, pp 354-356.*) In patients with severe facial or mandibular trauma, airway difficulties may develop secondary to the effects of massive hemorrhage, tissue swelling, or associated laryngeal trauma. Periorbital ecchymosis (ie, raccoon eyes) can be indicative of a concomitant basilar skull fracture. Oropharyngeal intubation with cervical in-line stabilization should be attempted first in this patient given his facial injuries, respiratory distress, and decreased mental status. Blind nasopharyngeal intubation should not be attempted because of the risk of placement of the tube into the brain due to disruption of the cribriform plate. If oral or nasotracheal intubation cannot be performed easily, cricothyroidotomy or emergency tracheostomy should be performed. Evaluation of the cervical spine is a top priority and should be performed in any patient with head trauma after stabilization of the ABCs (airway, breathing, and circulation) and prior to further facial studies. Although most facial fractures can be diagnosed easily with a standard radiographic facial series, computed tomography (CT) is more accurate and allows assessment of areas (eg, intracerebral contents) that cannot be evaluated by conventional techniques. CT is the preferred method of evaluation for patients with severe maxillofacial trauma. Maxillary fractures are categorized by the LeFort classification, and, unlike other facial fractures, are frequently associated with severe nasal and nasopharyngeal hemorrhage. This may be treated with head elevation and ice compresses. Nasal packing also affords good control of hemorrhage, and in extreme cases ligation or embolization of the internal maxillary artery may be necessary. Definitive reduction and fixation of fractures may be delayed while other injuries and medical problems are addressed. In addition to control of hemorrhage, initial management of facial fractures may include temporary stabilization and wound closure.

482. The answer is c. *(Townsend, pp 815-816.)* Because of the chance of a synchronous cancer in the aerodigestive tract, bronchoscopy and esophagoscopy are recommended, although the former may be omitted in the face of a normal chest radiologic study. Serum alkaline phosphatase and calcium levels are tumor markers that may be helpful but are not standard. Imaging modalities such as CT, MRI, positron emission tomography (PET), or ultrasound may be useful in preoperative planning. Echocardiography is not part of the staging workup but may be indicated to gauge operative risk in the setting of cardiac risk factors. Squamous cell cancers of the head and neck appear to arise as a response to tobacco in general (including chewing tobacco), rather than just to cigarette smoking, especially when used in combination with alcohol ingestion. Chemotherapy for squamous cell pharyngeal cancer has been used very successfully in childhood and adolescence, although its role in adult pharyngeal cancer is uncertain. Treatment of nasopharyngeal squamous cell carcinoma is by radiation, followed by radical neck dissection if lymph node metastases have not been controlled. Oropharyngeal cancers have responded equally well to surgery and radiation, and both treatments are routinely employed. In the hypopharynx, surgery is the optimal treatment, often supplemented by postoperative radiation therapy. Surgery for hypopharyngeal cancers includes radical neck dissection because lymph node metastases occur frequently and are not well controlled by radiation alone.

483. The answer is a. *(Brunicardi, pp 507-508.)* The treatment for pleomorphic adenomas (mixed tumors) of the parotid gland is superficial parotidectomy with preservation of the facial nerve. Unless adequately excised, they tend to recur locally in a high percentage of cases. Enucleation is not recommended given that tumor spillage at the time of resection can increase the chance of recurrence. Pleomorphic adenomas can occur in either the major (submandibular, parotid, and sublingual) or minor salivary glands. These round tumors have a rubbery consistency and are slow-growing; all are potentially malignant. The sites most commonly affected by pleomorphic adenomas of the salivary glands are the lips, tongue, and palate.

484. The answer is c. (*Mulholland, pp 1844-1846.*) The child has a branchial cleft remnant (branchial cleft cysts, sinuses, and fistulas). These more commonly arise from the first and second branchial pouches, while those from the third and fourth branchial pouches are rarer. This child has an infected cyst due to accumulation of secretions. The treatment is incision and drainage and then complete excision when the infection has resolved. Acute inflammation and infection predisposes patients to recurrence from incomplete excision and nerve injury.

The internal opening of the first branchial remnant is the external auditory canal; for the second, it is the posterolateral pharynx below the tonsillar fossa. The facial nerve may be injured during dissection of the first fistula. The second branchial tract passes between the carotid bifurcation and adjacent to the hypoglossal nerve. The third and fourth branchial remnants have an internal opening in the piriform sinus.

485. The answer is b. (*Mulholland, pp 1847-1849.*) Surgical resection is the standard therapy for thyroglossal duct cysts. The Sistrunk procedure, which involves local resection of the cyst and the central portion of the hyoid bone along with the tract all the way to the base of the tongue, is the operation of choice. Simple excision of the cyst results in an unacceptably high recurrence rate. Thyroglossal duct cysts result from retention of an epithelial tract between the thyroid and its embryologic origin in the foramen cecum at the base of the tongue. This tract usually penetrates the hyoid bone. There is no sex predilection, and although these cysts are more frequently detected in children, they may not become symptomatic until adulthood. The most common presentation is a painless swelling in the midline of the neck that moves with protrusion of the tongue or swallowing. They should not be confused with midline ectopic thyroid tissue. The cysts are prone to infection and progressive enlargement. Although rare

(< 1%), epidermoid or papillary carcinomas do occur within thyroglossal duct cysts. Arbitrary sampling of cervical lymph nodes is not indicated during surgical resection.

486. The answer is d. (*Mulholland, pp 622-623.*) Treatment is surgical—wide local excision of the tumor and neck dissection as needed. For patients with a localized tumor less than 2 cm, elective neck dissections are not indicated. Otherwise, unilateral or bilateral (for midline lesions) elective nodal dissections are performed for prognostic purposes. Cancers of the tongue commonly present on the lateral or ventral surface of the tongue. Metastases to the submandibular or cervical nodes are common. Local invasion may result in tongue deviation due to involvement of the hypoglossal nerve or decreased sensation due to involvement of the lingual nerve.

487. The answer is c. (*Townsend, pp 840-841.*) Recurrent laryngeal nerve damage can occur as a result of previous surgery such as thyroidectomy, malignancy, or chronic diseases such as collagen vascular disease. Unilateral recurrent laryngeal nerve injury can result in hoarseness, voice changes, weak cough, or difficulty swallowing. Bilateral recurrent laryngeal nerve injury is more serious and can result in complete airway obstruction and may require tracheostomy. Treatment of persistent hoarseness, suggesting injury versus paralysis to the recurrent laryngeal nerve, is with medialization of the vocal cord. Superior laryngeal nerve injury, which is also common after thyroid surgery, is manifested by voice weakness and difficulties with pitch, particularly high notes. Injury to the hypoglossal nerve causes deviation of the tongue toward the side of the injury. The marginal mandibular branch of the facial nerve innervates the muscles to the lower lip.

488. The answer is d. (*Mulholland, p 1843.*) The patient's history, physical examination, and radiographic findings are classic for acute epiglottitis. The "thumb sign" is a characteristic radiographic finding on lateral neck x-ray that is a result of a thickened epiglottis which resembles the distal thumb. An airway should be emergently secured in the operating room; the surgeon should be prepared to perform a tracheostomy if endotracheal intubation is unsuccessful. Attempts to visualize the patient's larynx, such as at the bedside or in the emergency room, may result in sudden airway occlusion with aspiration and respiratory arrest. Therefore, examination of the patient's airway must be undertaken only in the operating room with personnel prepared to perform endotracheal intubation.

Acute epiglottitis most commonly occurs in children 2 to 4 years of age, and is caused by *Haemophilus influenzae* in more than 90% of the cases. It presents as a rapidly progressive illness with symptoms of stridor, airway obstruction, drooling, and difficulty swallowing and signs of systemic toxicity (leukocytosis, fever, and/or tachycardia). If the child's condition permits, lateral neck x-rays can be obtained which show edema of the epiglottis and ballooning of the hypopharynx (the thumb sign). In advanced cases, the child is anxious and will sit erect and lean forward.

489. The answer is b. (*Townsend, p 837.*) Neck masses in adults represent malignancy until proven otherwise. One of the initial steps in the workup of neck masses is fine-needle aspiration. FNA has an overall accuracy of 95% for benign neck masses and 87% for malignant masses. It is the least invasive method to biopsy tissue but is more than adequate for identifying benign versus malignant tissue. CT scanning assists in evaluating the masses and potential primary sites, but cannot delineate between benign versus malignant masses.

490. The answer is e. (*Townsend, pp 837-838.*) Most commonly, lymphadenopathy in an adult is indicative of metastatic squamous cell cancer (SCC). Metastatic SCC originates most frequently from the nasopharynx, oropharynx, or hypopharynx. In addition to lymphadenopathy, persistent lateral neck masses in adults may represent neuromas, neurofibromas, carotid body tumors, branchial cleft cysts, lipomas, sebaceous cysts, parathyroid cysts, or a primary soft tissue tumor. Midline neck masses may represent thyroglossal duct cysts, dermoid tumors, thyroid masses, lipomas, or sebaceous cysts.

Pediatric Surgery

Questions

491. A neonate is examined in the nursery and found to have no anal orifice; only a small perineal fistulous opening is visualized. A complete workup is negative for any cardiac, esophageal, genitourinary, or musculoskeletal anomalies. Which of the following is the best next step in the management of this patient?

a. Diverting colostomy only
b. Posterior sagittal anorectoplasty only
c. Posterior sagittal anorectoplasty with diverting colostomy
d. Perineal operation only
e. Perineal operation with diverting colostomy

492. A 2-month-old boy is examined because he has been straining while passing stool and has a distended abdomen. He is very low on the growth chart for age. The primary care physician suspects that the boy has Hirschsprung disease. Which of the following findings on workup is diagnostic?

a. Absence of ganglion cells on full-thickness rectal biopsy 2 cm above the dentate line
b. Absence of ganglion cells on full-thickness rectal biopsy 1 cm above the dentate line
c. Absence of ganglion cells on suction rectal biopsy 1 cm above the dentate line
d. Identification of a transition zone between the sigmoid colon and the distal rectum on barium enema
e. Inhibition of the resting anal inhibitory reflex on anorectal manometry

493. A newborn has a midline defect in the anterior abdominal wall. The parents ask what, if anything, should be done. Spontaneous closure of which of the following congenital abnormalities of the abdominal wall generally occurs by the age of 4?

a. Umbilical hernia
b. Patent urachus
c. Patent omphalomesenteric duct
d. Omphalocele
e. Gastroschisis

494. A neonate is found to have an imperforate anus. As the pediatric surgeon you recommend studies to search for other anomalies. Which of the following is an associated abnormality?

a. Congenital pulmonary airway malformation
b. Hydrocephalus
c. Duodenal atresia
d. Congenital heart disease
e. Corneal opacities

495. A 36-hour-old infant presents with bilious vomiting and an increasingly distended abdomen. At exploration, the segment pictured here is found as the point of obstruction. What is the best next step in management?

a. Gentle, persistent traction on the specimen
b. Enteroenterostomy
c. Small bowel resection with exteriorization of the ends
d. Small bowel resection with anastomosis
e. Lysis of Ladd band

496. A 1-year-old child has repeated episodes of vomiting and abdominal distention. An x-ray shows obstruction at the second portion of the duodenum. Laparotomy is performed and an annular pancreas is discovered. For a symptomatic partial duodenal obstruction secondary to an annular pancreas, which of the following is the operative treatment of choice?

a. A Whipple procedure
b. Gastrojejunostomy
c. Vagotomy and gastrojejunostomy
d. Partial resection of the annular pancreas
e. Duodenoduodenostomy

497. Approximately 2 weeks after a viral respiratory illness, an 18-month-old child complains of abdominal pain and passes some bloody mucus per rectum. A long, thin mass is palpable in the right upper quadrant of the abdomen. No peritoneal signs are present. Intussusception is suspected. Which of the following is the most appropriate next step?

a. Diagnostic air enema with subsequent observation and serial abdominal examinations
b. Hydrostatic reduction with air enema
c. Diagnostic laparoscopy with laparoscopic reduction
d. Exploratory laparotomy with bowel resection
e. Decompressive colonoscopy with placement of a rectal tube

498. An 18-year-old woman presents with abdominal pain, fever, and leukocytosis. With the presumptive diagnosis of appendicitis, a right lower quadrant (McBurney) incision is made and a lesion 60 cm proximal to the ileocecal valve is identified (see photo). Which of the following is the most likely diagnosis?

a. Intestinal duplication
b. Mesenteric cyst
c. Meckel diverticulum
d. Ileoileal intussusception
e. "Christmas tree" type of ileal atresia

499. A newborn infant born from a mother with polyhydramnios presents with excessive salivation along with coughing and choking with the first oral feeding. An x-ray of the abdomen shows gas in stomach and a nasogastric tube coiled in the esophagus. Which of the following is the most likely diagnosis?

a. Esophageal atresia
b. Tracheoesophageal fistula
c. Esophageal atresia and tracheoesophageal fistula (TEF)
d. Omphalocele
e. Gastroschisis

500. An infant is born with a defect in the anterior abdominal cavity. Upon examination there are abdominal contents (small bowel and liver) protruding directly through the umbilical ring. Which of the following should be considered in the management of this condition?

a. No further workup is indicated prior to closure of the abdominal wall defect.
b. A Silastic silo should be placed with immediate reduction of the viscera into the abdominal cavity.
c. Broad-spectrum intravenous antibiotics should be administered prophylactically.
d. Topical antimicrobial solutions should be administered prophylactically.
e. Enteral feeds for nutritional support should be initiated early prior to operative management.

501. A 2-week-old infant presents with sudden onset of bilious emesis. Plain films of the abdomen show evidence of an intestinal obstruction. An upper gastrointestinal (UGI) contrast series reveals a midgut volvulus with the site of obstruction at the third portion of the duodenum. Which of the following is the most likely diagnosis?

a. Necrotizing enterocolitis (NEC)
b. Intussusception
c. Hirschsprung disease
d. Anomalies of intestinal rotation and fixation
e. Hypertrophic pyloric stenosis

502. A 29-week-old previously healthy male infant presents with fevers, abdominal distention, feeding intolerance, and bloody stools at 3 weeks of age. The patient undergoes x-ray and ultrasound examination for possible necrotizing enterocolitis. Which of the following findings on imaging is an indication for surgical management?

a. Pneumoperitoneum
b. Ascites
c. Portal venous gas
d. Ileus
e. Pneumatosis intestinalis

503. A newborn presents with signs and symptoms of distal intestinal obstruction. Abdominal x-rays reveal dilated loops of small bowel, absence of air-fluid levels, and a mass of meconium within the right side of the abdomen mixed with gas to give a ground-glass appearance. Which of the following should be performed as the initial management of the patient?

a. Administration of oral polyethylene glycol
b. Bowel rest with nasogastric tube decompression and broad-spectrum intravenous antibiotics
c. Contrast enema
d. Surgical evacuation of the luminal meconium
e. Resection of the dilated terminal ileum

504. A 4-week-old male infant presents with projectile, nonbilious emesis. Ultrasound of the abdomen reveals a pyloric muscle thickness of 8 mm (normal 3-4 mm). Which of the following is the best initial management of this patient?

a. Urgent pyloromyotomy
b. Urgent pyloroplasty
c. Urgent gastroduodenostomy
d. Fluid hydration and correction of electrolyte abnormalities prior to operative management
e. Administration of sodium bicarbonate to correct aciduria prior to operative management

505. A 1-month-old female infant presents with persistent jaundice. A serum direct bilirubin is 4.0 mg/dL and an ultrasound of the abdomen shows a shrunken gallbladder and inability to visualize the extrahepatic bile ducts. Which of the following is the most appropriate initial management of this patient?

a. NPO and total parenteral nutrition
b. Oral choleretic bile salts
c. Methylprednisolone
d. IV antibiotics
e. Exploratory laparotomy

506. A full-term male newborn experiences respiratory distress immediately after birth. A prenatal sonogram was read as normal. An emergency radiograph is shown here. The patient is intubated and placed on 100% O_2. Arterial blood gases reveal pH 7.24, P_{O_2} 60 kPa, and P_{CO_2} 52 kPa. The baby has sternal retractions and a scaphoid abdomen. Which of the following should be performed in the management of this patient?

a. Administration of intravenous steroids
b. Placement of bilateral tube thoracostomies
c. Immediate thoracotomy with lung resection
d. Immediate laparotomy with repair of the diaphragm
e. Mechanical ventilation with low tidal volumes

507. A 2-year-old asymptomatic child is noted to have a systolic murmur, hypertension, and diminished femoral pulses. Which of the following should be performed as part of the preoperative workup and management of this child's disorder?

a. Administration of indomethacin if there is a patent ductus arteriosus
b. Ligation of a patent ductus arteriosus
c. Echocardiography
d. Aortogram with bilateral lower extremity runoffs
e. Cardiac catheterization

508. A 35-week-term infant presents with cyanosis shortly after birth. His arterial oxygen saturation is only 30%. Which of the following is the most likely diagnosis?

a. Patent ductus arteriosus
b. Coarctation of the aorta
c. Atrial septal defect
d. Ventricular septal defect
e. Transposition of the great vessels

Questions 509 and 510

For each patient, select the most likely congenital cardiac anomaly. Each lettered option may be used once, more than once, or not at all.

a. Tetralogy of Fallot
b. Ventricular septal defect
c. Tricuspid atresia
d. Transposition of the great vessels
e. Patent ductus arteriosus

509. A noncyanotic 2-day-old child has a systolic murmur along the left sternal border; examination is otherwise normal. Chest x-ray and electrocardiogram are normal.

510. A 3-year-old child has congenital cyanosis.

Pediatric Surgery

Answers

491. The answer is d. (*Brunicardi, pp 1437-1438; Townsend, pp 2065-2067.*) The neonate has low imperforate anus, the treatment of which is a perineal operation only. Imperforate anus is a type of anorectal malformation that affects males and females with approximately the same frequency, occurring in 1 in 5000 live births. It is due to failure of descent of the urorectal septum. Anorectal malformations can be associated with other anomalies such as esophageal atresia or a tethered spinal cord which explains why a complete workup for associated lesions is important. The management of imperforate anus is dependent on whether the lesion is high or low, which is defined by the location of the end of the rectum relative to the level of the levator ani complex. The rectal fistula may end in the prostatic urethra or vagina in the high cases, while the low cases terminate in a perineal fistula. In females, high imperforate anus often occurs with a persistent cloaca (where the rectum, vagina, and urethra share a single perineal orifice). The neonate in the scenario has a low imperforate anus. For the low cases, only a perineal operation may be required, and these children will be expected to be continent. A 2-stage procedure—diverting colostomy followed by a subsequent pull-through procedure such as a posterior sagittal anoplasty—will be required for the high imperforate anus, and the likelihood of continence is smaller. If there is doubt about the level or location of the termination of the rectum, it is better to perform a temporary colostomy than to risk future incontinence.

492. The answer is a. (*Brunicardi, pp 1435-1437; Townsend, pp 2064-2065.*) Hirschsprung disease, which is the congenital absence of ganglion cells in the rectum or rectosigmoid colon, is definitively diagnosed by full-thickness rectal biopsy at least 2 cm above the dentate line. In neonates, suction rectal biopsy can be performed at the bedside. In older children, full-thickness rectal biopsy should be obtained. The biopsy should be taken at least 2 cm above the dentate line since the finding of aganglionosis at the level of the internal sphincter may be normal. Findings on barium enema—a distal narrow segment of bowel with markedly distended colon proximally (possibly with a transition zone) or lack of elimination of contrast after 24 hours—are suggestive of Hirschsprung disease. Symptoms may go unrecognized in the newborn period, with consequent development of malnutrition or enterocolitis. Initial treatment is colostomy decompression. Definitive repair is best delayed until nutritional status is adequate and the chronically distended bowel has returned to normal size. Unlike the situation with imperforate anus, which is associated with a high incidence of genitourinary tract anomalies and risk of long-term fecal incontinence, in Hirschsprung disease repair leads to satisfactory bowel function in most affected patients.

493. The answer is a. (*Brunicardi, pp 1441-1443.*) In most children, umbilical hernias close spontaneously by the age of 4 and need not be repaired unless incarcerated or symptomatic. Omphalocele and gastroschisis result in evisceration of bowel and require emergency surgical treatment to effect immediate or staged reduction and abdominal wall closure. Patent urachal or omphalomesenteric ducts result from incomplete closure of embryonic connections from the bladder and ileum, respectively, to the abdominal wall. They are appropriately treated by excision of the tracts and closure of the bladder or ileum.

494. The answer is d. (*Townsend, pp 2055-2056.*) Congenital anorectal anomalies are frequently associated with other congenital anomalies, including heart disease, esophageal atresia (EA), abnormalities of the lumbosacral spine, double urinary collecting systems, hydronephrosis, and communication between the rectum and the urinary tract, vagina, or perineum. Patients may present with a number of anomalies collectively known as the VACTERL syndrome: **V**ertebral anomalies, **A**nal atresia, **C**ardiac defect (eg, ventricular septal defect [VSD]), **T**racheo**E**sophageal fistula, **R**enal anomalies, and **L**imb defects (eg, radial dysplasia). They occur in approximately 1 in 5000 live births. A variety of surgical procedures have been devised to treat the problem, depending on the type of anomaly (whether the rectum ends above or below the level of the levator ani complex). However, even when anatomic integrity is established, the prognosis for effective toilet training is poor. In 50% of cases, continence is never achieved. Congenital pulmonary airway malformation, hydrocephalus, duodenal atresia, and corneal opacities have no significant association with congenital anorectal anomalies.

495. The answer is d. (*Brunicardi, pp 1427-1428; Townsend, pp 2059-2060.*) This is an example of an ileal atresia, which is treated with small bowel resection and primary anastomosis in this case. Whether the atresia is jejunal or ileal does not affect treatment, and there is no predilection for one site over the other. The basis of jejunoileal atresia is probably a mesenteric vascular accident during intrauterine growth. Resection and anastomosis should be performed if possible. If there is evidence of bowel ischemia or necrosis due to volvulus, the bowel should be exteriorized (ie, ileostomy and mucus fistula). Enteroenterostomy is the treatment for duodenal atresia (ie, Duodenoduodenostomy). Lysis of Ladd bands, incidental appendectomy, and detorsion of the bowel and repositioning of the small bowel on the right and colon on the left side of the abdomen are the treatment for malrotation. Gentle, persistent traction is not indicated for any of these disorders.

496. The answer is e. (*Mulholland, pp 1992-1993.*) A bypass procedure is the operation of choice for obstruction secondary to an annular pancreas. A Whipple procedure (pancreaticoduodenectomy) is too radical a therapy for this benign condition, and a partial resection of the annular pancreas often is complicated by fistula and does not treat the underlying problem of duodenal obstruction. Duodenoduodenostomy is much more physiologic than gastrojejunostomy and does not require a vagotomy to prevent marginal ulceration; it is therefore the procedure of choice.

497. The answer is b. (*Brunicardi, pp 1433-1434; Townsend, pp 2063-2064.*) Air (or barium) contrast enema is both diagnostic and therapeutic in patients with ileocolic intussusception without evidence of peritonitis. Intussusception is the result of invagination of a segment of bowel into distal bowel lumen. The most common type is ileocolic, which typically appears as a coiled spring on barium enema. Ileoileal and colocolic intussusceptions occur less commonly and are not easily diagnosed on enema. If bloody mucus (often described as "currant jelly stool"), peritonitis, or systemic toxicity has not developed, nonoperative management is preferred. Hydrostatic reduction by air enema is the appropriate initial treatment (although barium enema has also been traditionally used). Most patients are successfully managed this way and do not require surgical intervention. Immediate treatment should be instituted to avert the danger of bowel infarction. If signs of peritonitis or bowel ischemia are present, then surgical exploration, either open or laparoscopic, is indicated. Bowel resection may be required if reduction is not possible or there is evidence of ischemia/necrosis. Recurrence is surprisingly uncommon after either surgical or nonsurgical treatment. Decompressive colonoscopy with placement of a rectal tube is not indicated at any time in the management of intussusception.

498. The answer is c. *(Brunicardi, pp 1427-1438.)* This is an inflamed Meckel diverticulum. This common lesion is often clinically indistinguishable from acute appendicitis. It is the remnant of the vitelline duct. Meckel diverticula are usually located 60 cm proximal to the ileocecal valve, are antimesenteric, and may contain either gastric and pancreatic or only pancreatic tissue. Complications from a Meckel diverticulum include hemorrhage and obstruction, which are more common than inflammation. A technetium 99m (^{99m}Tc) pertechnetate scan ("Meckel scan") can be useful in the workup of a child with an occult source of lower gastrointestinal hemorrhage. Since complications are relatively rare, most surgeons do not recommend removing asymptomatic diverticula when they are incidentally discovered during abdominal procedures. Those diverticula with a narrow neck, palpable heterotopic tissue, or nodularity are prone to obstruction and should be excised. In addition, patients explored for abdominal pain of unknown etiology should also undergo diverticulectomy, as should those operated on for appendicitis who are to be left with a scar of the right lower quadrant.

Intestinal duplications are rare, mucosa-lined cysts that can occur anywhere along the gastrointestinal tract, but occur more frequently in the ileum. Mesenteric cysts are similar to intestinal duplications but do not contain mucosa or muscular wall. Intusussceptions occur when one piece of bowel telescopes into more proximal bowel. The "Christmas tree" anomaly describes a type of ileal atresia whereby the bowel distal to the atresia is vascularized in a retrograde fashion from the right colic or ileocolic artery.

499. The answer is c. *(Brunicardi, pp 1420-1424.)* The diagnosis of esophageal atresia (EA) should be entertained in an infant who presents with excessive salivation along with coughing and choking during the first oral feeding. A maternal history of polyhydramnios is often present. The inability to pass a nasogastric tube into the stomach is seen with EA. If gas is present in the gastrointestinal tract, then an associated tracheoesophageal fistula (TEF) is confirmed. In an infant with EA and TEF, the air is introduced into the stomach via the fistula between the distal esophagus and the trachea with each inspired breath. Reflux of gastric contents into the trachea through the TEF may result in cough, tachypnea, apnea, or cyanosis. After evaluating for VACTERL abnormalities (described in question 494), surgical repair of the EA and TEF is performed.

500. The answer is c. *(Brunicardi, pp 1442-1443; Townsend, pp 2067-2069.)* The infant has an omphalocele, which is treated initially with broad-spectrum prophylactic intravenous antibiotics, prevention of hypothermia, cardiopulmonary resuscitation, and gastric decompression. During normal development of the embryo, the midgut herniates outward through the umbilical ring and continues to grow. It returns back into the abdominal cavity by the eleventh week of gestation and undergoes normal rotation and fixation. If the intestines fail to return, the infant is born with abdominal contents protruding through the umbilical ring, termed an omphalocele. A sac composed of the peritoneum on the inside and amnion on the outside covers the bowel protecting it from the surrounding amniotic fluid. Sometimes the sac is torn in utero and the bowel is exposed to the amniotic fluid. This abdominal wall defect is called a gastroschisis and the defect is always seen on the right side of the umbilical ring with an intact umbilical cord. The risk for associated anomalies with gastroschisis is low. In contrast, more than half of infants with an omphalocele have other major or minor malformations, and karyotype abnormalities are present in roughly 30% of infants (including trisomies 13, 18, and 21). Thus, operative intervention for omphaloceles should be delayed until the patient has had a full evaluation for other abnormalities. In giant omphaloceles a Silastic silo allows for gradual reduction of the viscera into the abdominal cavity over several days. Acute attempts at reduction and tight dressings should be avoided so as to prevent rupture of the sac, interruption of venous return, or development of abdominal compartment syndrome. Topical solutions may be used in patients who cannot undergo operative therapy (but are not routinely used for prophylaxis), including topical antimicrobials such as silver sulfadiazine. In patients with gastroschisis, the intestine is often thickened, edematous, matted together, and foreshortened leading to impaired motility, digestion, and absorption. Both conditions are repaired surgically.

501. The answer is d. *(Townsend, pp 2060-2061.)* The patient's presentation and radiologic findings are most consistent with anomalies of intestinal rotation and fixation (aka malrotation). Rotational anomalies may present as a volvulus, duodenal obstruction, or intermittent or chronic abdominal pain. When the midgut returns to the abdominal cavity by the eleventh week of gestation, it rotates around the axis of the superior mesenteric artery for 270° in a counterclockwise direction placing the final position of the ligament of Treitz in the left upper quadrant and the cecum in the right lower quadrant of the abdomen. Interruption or reversal of any of these coordinated movements leads to the range of anomalies seen. The most frequently encountered anomaly is complete nonrotation of the midgut, in which the proximal jejunum and ascending colon are fused together as one pedicle. The midgut volvulus occurs on this pedicle leading to ischemic necrosis of the entire midgut. Necrotizing enterocolitis (NEC), Hirschsprung disease, hypertrophic pyloric stenosis, and intussusception are not associated with a midgut volvulus.

502. The answer is a. (*Brunicardi, pp 1429-1433; Townsend, pp 2061-2062.*) The patient's presentation and radiologic findings are classic for necrotizing enterocolitis (NEC). All of the listed radiologic findings can be seen in neonates with NEC, but the main indication for surgical management is intestinal perforation as evidenced by free air or pneumoperitoneum. NEC is the most common gastrointestinal emergency in the neonatal period. Prematurity is the single most important risk factor. Other significant risk factors include ischemia, bacteria, cytokines, and enteral feeding. About 80% of cases occur within the first month of life. The radiologic hallmark of NEC is pneumatosis intestinalis (air within the walls of the bowel). The distal ileum and ascending colon are usually affected, but the entire gastrointestinal tract may be involved (NEC totalis). Initial management consists of bowel rest with nasogastric tube decompression, fluid resuscitation, and broad-spectrum antibiotics. Medical management is successful in half of cases and surgery is reserved for patients with overall clinical deterioration, abdominal wall cellulitis, falling white blood cell count or platelet count, palpable abdominal mass, persistent fixed loop on abdominal films, or intestinal perforation. NEC is the single most common cause of short gut syndrome in children. Intestinal strictures may develop after either medical or surgical management of NEC in roughly 10% of infants.

503. The answer is c. (*Brunicardi, p 1429; Townsend, pp 2062-2063.*) The patient has a simple meconium ileus; the initial management is a contrast enema. In meconium ileus, the terminal ileum is dilated and filled with thick, tarlike, inspissated meconium. Meconium ileus in the newborn represents the earliest clinical manifestation of cystic fibrosis. The initial treatment of a simple meconium ileus is a water-soluble contrast enema. This is successful in relieving the obstruction in up to 75% of cases with a bowel perforation rate of less than 3%. Operative management is required when the contrast enema fails to relieve the obstruction. The surgical treatment of choice is to perform an enterotomy through the dilated distal ileum and then to irrigate the proximal and distal bowel with either warm saline or 4% N-acetylcysteine (Mucomyst). Meconium can then be milked into the distal colon or carefully removed through the enterotomy, which is closed in 2 layers at the end of the case.

504. The answer is d. *(Townsend, pp 2058-2059.)* The patient's symptoms and findings on ultrasound are consistent with hypertrophic pyloric stenosis. The treatment is pyloromyotomy (a partial-thickness cut at the pylorus through muscle but not mucosa) after fluid resuscitation and correction of electrolyte and acid–base abnormalities. Loss of gastric hydrochloric acid with vomiting results in a hypokalemic, hypochloremic, metabolic alkalosis. Before surgery, it is important to hydrate the infant and slowly correct the metabolic alkalosis with normal saline. Because the compensatory mechanism for metabolic alkalosis is hypoventilation/respiratory acidosis, correction is necessary to prevent postoperative apnea. Dehydration initially results in loss of bicarbonate in the urine to maintain a normal pH. However, because the renal mechanism for restoring volume status is aldosterone-mediated, hydrogen and potassium ions are excreted in the urine when sodium is reabsorbed leading to "paradoxical aciduria" (in the setting of alkalosis). Administration of bicarbonate is therefore not indicated.

505. The answer is e. *(Townsend, pp 2077-2078.)* This infant has findings consistent with biliary atresia and the treatment is laparotomy with Kasai hepatoportoenterostomy. An infant with persistent jaundice after the first few weeks of life needs to be evaluated with laboratory studies and an abdominal ultrasound. Biliary atresia is characterized by progressive obliteration of the extrahepatic and intrahepatic bile ducts. Delay in the diagnosis of biliary atresia leads to irreversible hepatic fibrosis. Success with surgical correction is much improved if undertaken before 60 days of life. If an abdominal ultrasound or liver-needle biopsy is consistent with biliary atresia, exploratory laparotomy is performed expeditiously. The initial goal at surgery is to confirm the diagnosis with demonstration of fibrotic biliary remnants and absent proximal and distal bile duct patency. Surgical correction of biliary atresia is with the Kasai hepatoportoenterostomy.

506. The answer is e. *(Brunicardi, pp 1416-1418; Townsend, pp 2072-2074.)* This radiograph of a child with a scaphoid abdomen and respiratory disease is characteristic of a congenital diaphragmatic hernia (CDH). These patients require cardiopulmonary stabilization prior to any operative repair. Severe hypoxia and respiratory distress at birth are a result of primary pulmonary hypertension due to hypoplasia rather than from compression of the lung from abdominal contents. Low tidal volumes and permissive hypercapnia are strategies of mechanical ventilation to prevent barotrauma. While pneumothoraces can occur (typically on the side opposite the CDH), bilateral tube thoracostomies are not indicated as initial management strategies. There is no role for intravenous steroids. Medical therapies for pulmonary hypertension such as inhaled nitric oxide have been used. In CDH infants with refractory hypoxia, extracorporeal membrane oxygenation (ECMO) has been used to stabilize the patient prior to repair. Closure of the diaphragmatic defect, which occurs posterolaterally (Bochdalek hernia), can be performed from the abdomen or the chest.

507. The answer is c. (*Mulholland, pp 1439-1440.*) This child has coarctation of the aorta, which is a congenital anomaly that usually causes narrowing of the aorta just distal to the left subclavian artery in the area of the ligamentum arteriosum. Coarctation is diagnosed by echocardiography; cardiac catheterization is rarely needed. CT angiography or MRI may be helpful, but aortogram with bilateral lower extremity runoffs is not necessary. Claudication is not a common feature of this disorder. Preoperative management includes administration of prostaglandins to reopen the ductus arteriosus which improves flow distal to the coarctation and to the lower body. Without surgery, complications in adults arise with eventual death from cardiac failure, rupture of aortic aneurysms or of a cerebral artery, and bacterial endocarditis. Coarctation is often associated with VSDs and aortic stenosis. Patients who are operated on earlier in life have a better chance of becoming normotensive.

508. The answer is e. (*Mulholland, pp 1425-1448.*) With the exception of coarctation, in which no shunt (or cyanosis) exists, the anomalies listed cause a shunting of blood between the systemic and lower-pressure pulmonary circulation. Transposition of the great vessels is a right-to-left shunt that leads to cyanosis. Except where there is persistent congenital pulmonary hypertension, patent ductus arteriosus and atrial septal defects cause a shunting of oxygenated blood from the aorta and left atrium, respectively, back into the pulmonary artery and right atrium. These anomalies cause recirculation of oxygenated blood within the cardiopulmonary circuit but not cyanosis. When a VSD is combined with pulmonary artery atresia (tetralogy of Fallot), the resulting undercirculation in the pulmonary system joins transposition as a cause of cyanosis. Other, less common congenital lesions in which the pulmonary arterial blood flow is relatively decreased include tricuspid atresia, Ebstein anomaly, and hypoplastic right ventricle.

509 and 510.   The answers are 509-b, 510-a. *(Mulholland, pp 1425-1448.)* VSD accounts for 20% to 30% of all congenital cardiac anomalies. It may lead to cardiac failure and pulmonary hypertension if the defect is larger than 1 cm, or it may be asymptomatic if the defect is small. Surgery is not indicated for the asymptomatic patient with a small defect since a substantial number of these anomalies close spontaneously during the first few years of life. Operation is indicated in infants with congestive heart failure or rising pulmonary vascular resistance (owing to the left-to-right shunt). Additionally, operation is indicated if the VSD has not closed by age of 5. Tetralogy of Fallot, transposition, and tricuspid atresia are cyanotic lesions. Congenital cyanosis that persists beyond the age of 2 years is associated, in the vast majority of cases, with tetralogy of Fallot. Patent ductus arteriosus is associated with the characteristic continuous machinery murmur.

Bibliography

Brunicardi FC, Andersen DK, Billiar TR, et al, eds. *Schwartz's Principles of Surgery.* 9th ed. New York, NY: McGraw-Hill; 2010.

Doherty GM. *Current Surgical Diagnosis & Treatment.* 13th ed. New York, NY: McGraw-Hill; 2010.

Moore EE, Mattox KL, DV Feliciano, et al, eds. *Trauma.* 6th ed. New York, NY: McGraw-Hill; 2007.

Mulholland MW, Lillemoe KD, Doherty GM, et al, eds. *Greenfield's Surgery Scientific Principles & Practice.* 5th ed. Philadelphia, PA: Lippincott, Williams & Wilkins; 2011.

Townsend CM Jr, Beauchamp RD, Evers BM, et al, eds. *Sabiston Textbook of Surgery.* 18th ed. Philadelphia, PA: Saunders; 2007.

Index